Menopause

Antonio Cano
Editor

Menopause

A Comprehensive Approach

Second Edition

Springer

Editor
Antonio Cano
Full Professor of Obstetrics and Gynecology
Salus Vitae Women's Health Clinical Center
Valencia, Spain

ISBN 978-3-031-83978-8   ISBN 978-3-031-83979-5 (eBook)
https://doi.org/10.1007/978-3-031-83979-5

© The Editor(s) (if applicable) and The Author(s), under exclusive license to Springer Nature Switzerland AG 2017, 2025

This work is subject to copyright. All rights are solely and exclusively licensed by the Publisher, whether the whole or part of the material is concerned, specifically the rights of translation, reprinting, reuse of illustrations, recitation, broadcasting, reproduction on microfilms or in any other physical way, and transmission or information storage and retrieval, electronic adaptation, computer software, or by similar or dissimilar methodology now known or hereafter developed.
The use of general descriptive names, registered names, trademarks, service marks, etc. in this publication does not imply, even in the absence of a specific statement, that such names are exempt from the relevant protective laws and regulations and therefore free for general use.
The publisher, the authors and the editors are safe to assume that the advice and information in this book are believed to be true and accurate at the date of publication. Neither the publisher nor the authors or the editors give a warranty, expressed or implied, with respect to the material contained herein or for any errors or omissions that may have been made. The publisher remains neutral with regard to jurisdictional claims in published maps and institutional affiliations.

This Springer imprint is published by the registered company Springer Nature Switzerland AG
The registered company address is: Gewerbestrasse 11, 6330 Cham, Switzerland

If disposing of this product, please recycle the paper.

Preface

The years since the last edition of this book have witnessed more profound changes in phenomena that, for the most part, were already announced or had barely begun. One important circumstance is that science has focused its attention on the ageing process. Ageing in good health and with an acceptable quality of life has become a widely shared goal for most disciplines of medicine, both clinical and experimental. This issue is of particular importance for women, who have a longer life expectancy than men. Today, there are more women, already around 700 million, experiencing menopausal transition and early postmenopause worldwide. In addition, women are more and better educated. The worldwide spread of the Internet and the availability of devices within easy reach, such as smartphones, favor access to and interest in health issues. Where is menopause care situated and what is its importance in this scenario? Menopause is confirmed, even more, as a milestone in the postreproductive stage. This universally experienced event has changed its meaning, so that it is no longer the gateway to old age. Poor quality of life is becoming less and less acceptable for women, and healthy ageing is understood from a holistic perspective, where social and psychological variables are closely integrated with biological changes. Demands extend to the control of vasomotor symptoms, but also to the quality of sleep, sexual life, or appropriate changes in the workplace.

The comprehensive philosophy of this book incorporates the latest achievements in the areas mentioned. Rigorous scientific evidence has remained a major driver in each chapter. Among the important changes, the alarm about menopausal hormone therapy has largely been defused, mainly because the data associated with safety are now more consistent. Additional evidence has confirmed that hormones protect against osteoporosis and, under appropriate conditions, also against cardiovascular disease. More evidence has accumulated on combinations with lower risk, while the achievement of reduced mortality continues to be confirmed. New discoveries of the neuroendocrinological mechanisms of vasomotor symptoms, and corresponding new therapies, have been a major advance, and concepts such as frailty remain strong indicators of the ageing process. Lifestyle continues to accumulate more favorable evidence because in a world with advances in precision medicine, selective agents against most noncommunicable diseases remain insufficient or nonexistent. This is the case for the worrying diseases of the central nervous system, such as dementia or Parkinson's, but also for cardiovascular diseases, malignant neoplasms, or osteoporosis.

This is the new ground that supports the main paths along which this second edition has been developed.

I cannot but thank the authors, who have once again given their best in each chapter, and Springer, for its continued support.

Valencia, Spain   Antonio Cano

Contents

Part I Biological Background

1. **Menopause, a Stage in the Life of Women** 3
   Gita D. Mishra and Hsin-Fang Chung

2. **Menopause: The Concepts and the Biological Background** 11
   Antonio Cano, Aitana Monllor-Tormos, Amparo Carrasco-Catena, and Rocío Belda-Montesinos

3. **Premature Ovarian Insufficiency** 27
   Agnieszka Podfigurna, Adam Czyzyk, Monika Grymowicz, Anna Szeliga, Roman Smolarczyk, and Blazej Meczekalski

Part II Impact of Estrogen Depletion on Symptoms and Quality of Life

4. **Clinical Symptoms and Quality of Life: Vasomotor Symptoms and Mood** 75
   Placido Llaneza and Cristina Llaneza-Suarez

5. **Clinical Symptoms and Quality of Life: Insomnia and Muscle/Joint Aches** 89
   Juan Enrique Blümel, María Soledad Vallejo, and Eugenio Arteaga

6. **Genitourinary Syndrome of Menopause. Vaginal Health and Microbiota** 105
   María Jesús Cancelo Hidalgo and Llaura Barrera Coello

7. **Sexual Health**... 129
   Nicolás Mendoza Ladrón de Guevara, Ana Rosa Jurado, and Loreto Mendoza Huertas

Part III The Impact of Estrogen Depletion on Disease Susceptibility

8. **Postmenopausal Osteoporosis** 147
   Amparo Carrasco-Catena, Aitana Monllor-Tormos, Nicolás Mendoza Ladrón de Guevara, Miguel Ángel García-Pérez, and Antonio Cano

| 9 | The Metabolic Syndrome During Female Midlife and Beyond | 169 |

Peter Chedraui and Faustino R. Pérez-López

| 10 | The Impact of Estrogen Decline on Other Noncommunicable Diseases | 187 |

Esperanza Navarro-Pardo, Tomi S. Mikkola, Tommaso Simoncini, Marta Millán, María Dolores Juliá, and Antonio Cano

Part IV Management of Menopause

| 11 | Hormone Therapy (I): Estrogens, Progestogens, and Androgens | 211 |

Francisco Quereda

| 12 | Hormone Therapy (II): Tibolone and the TSEC Concept | 231 |

Santiago Palacios and Mariella Lilue

| 13 | The Effect of Menopause Hormone Therapy on Climacteric Symptoms | 249 |

Camil Castelo-Branco, Laura Ribera, and Claudio Hernández-Angeles

| 14 | The Impact of Hormone Therapy on Other Noncommunicable Diseases: Central Nervous System, Cardiovascular Tree, Osteoarthritis, and Cancer | 263 |

Esperanza Navarro-Pardo, Tomi S. Mikkola, Tommaso Simoncini, Marta Millán, María Dolores Juliá, and Antonio Cano

| 15 | Nonhormonal Management of the Menopause | 289 |

Jenifer Sassarini and Mary Ann Lumsden

| 16 | Complementary and Alternative Therapies for Vasomotor Symptoms During Climacteric and Beyond | 303 |

Camil Castelo-Branco, Laura Ribera, and María Fernanda Garrido Oyarzún

| 17 | Lifestyle: Physical Activity | 317 |

Nicolás Mendoza Ladrón de Guevara, Carlos de Teresa Galván, and Débora Godoy Izquierdo

| 18 | Nutritional Management of Menopausal Women | 329 |

Annamaria Colao and Roberta Scairati

Part V Menopause in the Context of Healthy Ageing

| 19 | Frailty and Comorbidities: Frailty in Women | 351 |

Esperanza Navarro-Pardo, Patricia Villacampa-Fernández, Ruth E. Hubbard, Emily Gordon, and Antonio Cano

20	**Muscle Strength, Dynapenia, and Sarcopenia During Female Midlife and Beyond**	365
	Faustino R. Pérez-López, Pascual García-Alfaro, and Ignacio Rodríguez	
21	**Empowerment of Women and Lifestyle: The Help of Digital Technologies**	375
	Amparo Carrasco-Catena, Gema Ibáñez-Sánchez, Vicente Traver, and Antonio Cano	

About the Editor

Antonio Cano graduated in Medicine and Surgery from the University of Valencia, Spain. He received his PhD from the University of Bologna and completed a postdoctoral stay at the Imperial Cancer Research Fund in London, UK. His academic career includes a position as Assistant Professor at two Spanish universities, Murcia and Valencia, where he has become Professor of Obstetrics and Gynecology.

His activities in scientific societies include the European Menopause and Andropause Society (EMAS), of which he has been President, and the International Menopause Society (IMS), of which he is a member of both the Educational Committee and the Board of Directors. He is also Secretary General of the International Society of Gynecological Endocrinology (ISGE).

He serves on the editorial boards of several women's health journals, including *Climacteric* (associate editor), *Maturitas* (senior editorial advisor), *European Journal of Obstetrics, Gynecology and Reproductive Biology* (gynecology editor), and is a member of the editorial boards of *Gynecological Endocrinology* and *Gynecologic Reproductive Endocrinology and Metabolism*.

His area of research has been the action of steroids on reproductive tissues, later extended to the hormonal regulation of vasculature and bone cells, with relevance to cardiovascular disease in women and osteoporosis. He has incorporated frailty as an innovative research topic related to menopause and with relevance to healthy ageing in women.

Contributors

Eugenio Arteaga Departamento de Endocrinología, Facultad de Medicina, Pontificia Universidad Católica de Chile, Santiago, Chile

Rocío Belda-Montesinos Service of Obstetrics and Gynecology, University General Hospital, Valencia, Spain

Juan Enrique Blümel Medicina Interna Sur. Facultad de Medicina, Universidad de Chile, Santiago, Chile

Antonio Cano Full Professor of Obstetrics and Gynecology, Salus Vitae Women's Health Clinical Center, Valencia, Spain

Amparo Carrasco-Catena Clinical Area Women's Health, Hospital Universitario y Politécnico La Fe, Valencia, Spain

Camil Castelo-Branco Clinic Institute of Gynecology, Obstetrics and Neonatology, Hospital Clinic-Institut d'Investigacions Biomèdiques August Pi i Sunyer, University of Barcelona, Barcelona, Spain

Peter Chedraui Escuela de Postgrado en Salud, Universidad Espíritu Santo, Samborondón, Ecuador

Hsin-Fang Chung Australian Women and Girls' Health Research Centre, School of Public Health, The University of Queensland, Herston, Australia

Llaura Barrera Coello Obstetrics and Gynecology Department of University Hospital of Guadalajara, University of Alcalá, Madrid, Spain

Annamaria Colao Department of Clinical Medicine and Surgery, Unit of Endocrinology, Diabetology, Andrology and Nutrition; "Federico II" University of Naples, Naples, Italy

Adam Czyzyk TFP Fertility, Zielona Gora, Poland

Pascual García-Alfaro Department of Obstetrics and Gynecology, Hospital Universitario Dexeus, Barcelona, Spain

Miguel Ángel García-Pérez Faculty of Biological Sciences, Department of Cellular Biology, Functional Biology and Physical Anthropology, University of Valencia, Valencia, Spain

Débora Godoy Izquierdo Instituto Universitario de Investigación de Estudios de las Mujeres y de Género, Department of Personality, Psychological Assessment and Treatment, University of Granada, Granada, Spain

Emily Gordon Geriatric Medicine, Princess Alexandra Hospital, School of Medicine and Centre for Research in Geriatric Medicine, The University of Queensland, Woolloongabba, Australia

Monika Grymowicz Department of Gynecological Endocrinology, Medical University of Warsaw, Warsaw, Poland

Nicolás Mendoza Ladrón de Guevara Department of Obstetrics and Gynaecology, University of Granada, Granada, Spain

Claudio Hernández-Angeles Hospital Ginecoobstetricia Número 4 "Luis Castelazo Ayala", Instituto Mexicano del Seguro Social, Torreón, Mexico

María Jesús Cancelo Hidalgo Obstetrics and Gynecology Department of University Hospital of Guadalajara, University of Alcalá, Madrid, Spain

Ruth E. Hubbard PA Southside Clinical Unit, Centre for Research in Geriatric Medicine, Translational Research Institute, The University of Queensland, Brisbane, Australia

Loreto Mendoza Huertas Department of Obstetrics and Gynecology, University of Granada, Granada, Spain

Gema Ibáñez-Sánchez University Institute of Information and Communication Technologies (ITACA), Valencia, Spain

María Dolores Juliá Department of Pediatrics, Obstetrics and Gynecology, University of Valencia, Valencia, Spain

Section of Gynecology and Reproduction, University and Polytechnic Hospital La Fe, Valencia, Spain

Ana Rosa Jurado Department of Obstetrics and Gynecology, University of Granada, Granada, Spain

Instituto Europeo de Sexologia, Marbella, Málaga, Spain

Mariella Lilue Palacios Clinic of Women's Health, Madrid, Spain

Placido Llaneza Gynecological Endocrinology and Human Reproduction Unit, Hospital Central de Asturias, Universidad de Oviedo, Oviedo, Spain

Cristina Llaneza-Suarez Severo Ochoa Health Center, SESPA, Universidad de Oviedo, Oviedo, Spain

Mary Ann Lumsden University of Glasgow, Glasgow, UK

Blazej Meczekalski Department of Gynecological Endocrinology, Poznan University of Medical Sciences, Poznan, Poland

Tomi S. Mikkola Department of Obstetrics and Gynecology, Helsinki University Central Hospital, Helsinki, Finland

Marta Millán Hospital Universitario Marqués Valdecilla, University of Cantabria, Santander, Spain

Gita D. Mishra Australian Women and Girls' Health Research Centre, School of Public Health, The University of Queensland, Herston, Australia

Aitana Monllor-Tormos Service of Obstetrics and Gynecology, Hospital Clinic Universitari, Valencia, Spain

Women's Health Research Group, INCLIVA – Hospital Clínico Universitario, Valencia, Spain

Esperanza Navarro-Pardo Department of Developmental and Educational Psychology, University of Valencia, Valencia, Spain

María Fernanda Garrido Oyarzún Clínica Universidad de los Andes, Santiago de Chile, Chile

Santiago Palacios Palacios Clinic of Women's Health, Madrid, Spain

Faustino R. Pérez-López Department of Obstetrics and Gynecology, Universidad de Zaragoza Facultad de Medicina, Zaragoza, Spain

Agnieszka Podfigurna Department of Gynecological Endocrinology, Poznan University of Medical Sciences, Poznan, Poland

Francisco Quereda Hospital Universitario de San Juan de Alicante, Miguel Hernández University, Alicante, Spain

Laura Ribera Clinic Institute of Gynecology, Obstetrics and Neonatology, Hospital Clinic-Institut d'Investigacions Biomèdiques August Pi i Sunyer, University of Barcelona, Barcelona, Spain

Ignacio Rodríguez Department of Obstetrics and Gynecology, Hospital Universitario Dexeus, Barcelona, Spain

Jenifer Sassarini Glasgow Royal Infirmary, University of Glasgow, Glasgow, UK

Roberta Scairati Department of Clinical Medicine and Surgery, Unit of Endocrinology, Diabetology, Andrology and Nutrition; "Federico II" University of Naples, Naples, Italy

Tommaso Simoncini Division of Obstetrics and Gynecology, Department of Clinical and Experimental Medicine, University of Pisa, Pisa, Italy

Roman Smolarczyk Department of Gynecological Endocrinology, Medical University of Warsaw, Warsaw, Poland

Anna Szeliga Department of Gynecological Endocrinology, Poznan University of Medical Sciences, Poznan, Poland

Carlos de Teresa Galván Centro Andaluz de Medicina del Deporte, Granada, Granada, Spain

Vicente Traver University Institute of Information and Communication Technologies (ITACA), Valencia, Spain

Joint Unit for Healthcare Processes Reengineering (eRPSS)—Health Research Institute University and Polytechnic Hospital La Fe, Valencia, Spain

María Soledad Vallejo Obstetricia y Ginecología, Hospital Clínico, Universidad de Chile, Santiago, Chile

Patricia Villacampa-Fernández Department of Developmental and Educational Psychology, University of Valencia, Valencia, Spain

Part I
Biological Background

Menopause, a Stage in the Life of Women

Gita D. Mishra and Hsin-Fang Chung

Abstract

The timing of menopause is an indicator of underlying health and can act as a sentinel for future health status. The average age at natural menopause is 50–51 years in high-income countries. Premature ovarian insufficiency (menopause before the age of 40 years) and early menopause (between 40 and 44 years) have been linked with a range of chronic diseases, including cardiovascular disease and premature mortality. In this chapter, we use a life course approach to understand how early life experiences and exposures influence the timing of natural menopause and subsequent health outcomes. We also highlight common symptoms experienced during the menopausal transition.

1.1 Introduction

Menopause is the end of menstruation following the cessation of ovulation [1]. It may be spontaneous (natural menopause) or iatrogenic (including bilateral oophorectomy and chemotherapy or pelvic radiation treatment for cancer) [1]. Natural menopause is determined after a woman has experienced 12 consecutive months of amenorrhea without any other obvious pathologic or physiologic causes [2]. In contrast, the removal of both ovaries (bilateral oophorectomy) in premenopausal women, which results in an abrupt reduction in sex hormones, will cause surgical menopause [2]. Women who have a premenopausal hysterectomy or unilateral oophorectomy do not go straight into menopause, but they may reach menopause 1–2 years earlier than those who do not have these procedures [3, 4].

G. D. Mishra (✉) · H.-F. Chung
Australian Women and Girls' Health Research Centre, School of Public Health,
The University of Queensland, Herston, Australia
e-mail: g.mishra@uq.edu.au; h.chung1@uq.edu.au

Humans, gorillas, killer whales, and short-finned pilot whales are the only species known to experience menopause [5, 6]. While discussion on the reasons for the existence of menopause is still under debate, from an evolutionary perspective, there are three main explanatory hypotheses. The *grandmother hypothesis*, which speculates that older (nonreproductive) mothers help their childbearing daughters and thus increase her reproductive fitness. The *mother hypothesis* assumes that older women stop reproducing because it is too risky for them to give birth and to increase the chance of survival of their offspring [6]. A more recent proposition, the *reproductive conflict hypothesis* (also known as the *mother-in-law conflict hypothesis*) suggests that the cost of intergenerational reproductive conflict between older females and younger females of the same social unit impacts the reproductive fitness calculations [7]. A Finnish study, using birth, death, and marriage records kept by the Lutheran church from 1702 and 1908, found that when both mothers-in-law and daughters-in-law gave birth around the same time, their offspring had a 66% lower chance of survival, with offspring of the older mothers having even lower chance of survival (50%) [8].

1.2 Age at Natural Menopause

Menopause is a natural stage of aging that usually occurs between the ages of 45 and 55 years. The International Collaboration for a Life Course Approach to Reproductive Health and Chronic Disease Events (InterLACE) consortium pooled individual-level data from half a million women in high-income countries and reported that the average age at natural menopause was 50.5 years (95% confidence intervals: 50.2–50.8 years). However, there were substantial variations across studies and racial/ethnic groups, with the youngest mean age at menopause for South Asian women (48.8 years) [9]. A previous meta-analysis of 46 studies across 24 countries also showed that age at natural menopause varied by geographical region, with the lowest being among Latin American, Middle Eastern, African, and Asian countries and the highest in Europe and Australia [10].

A woman's age at natural menopause is not only a marker of reproductive ageing but is also an indicator of underlying health and can even act as a sentinel for her future health status [11]. Cessation of menstruation before the age of 40 years is defined as premature ovarian insufficiency (POI), and menopause that occurs between 40 and 44 years is termed early menopause [12]. In high-income countries, around 1 in 10 women have POI (2%) or early menopause (7.6%) [13]. Global estimates from 31 studies reported a higher prevalence of POI (3.7%) and early menopause (12.2%), potentially reflecting a lower mean age at natural menopause in low- and middle-income countries [14]. Meta-analyses and pooled analyses from InterLACE showed that POI and early menopause were associated with an increased risk of coronary heart disease, stroke, type 2 diabetes, fracture, chronic obstructive pulmonary disease, lung cancer, and premature mortality [15–20]. However, later menopause was associated with an increased risk of breast and endometrial cancer [21, 22]. This does not necessarily imply any causal relationships but could result from common risk factors, including genetic, lifestyle factors, and exposures in early life. For example, this may be the case for cardiovascular disease (CVD), where recent findings suggest that preexisting risk factors, such as cigarette smoking and raised total serum cholesterol and blood pressure, are associated with both earlier menopause and CVD [23, 24].

1.3 Risk Factors for Early Age at Natural Menopause

1.3.1 Genetic Factors

Factors across the life course have been shown to be associated with the timing of menopause, which appears to reflect a complex interplay of factors, from genetic, cumulative socioeconomic, and lifestyle factors to female reproductive factors. Family studies have revealed that genetic factors influence roughly half of the variation in age at natural menopause, with estimated heritability of 42% in the United Kingdom, 44% in the Netherlands, and 52% in the United States [25–27]. Supporting evidence from observational studies suggests that family history of early menopause or POI is a strong predictor (six-fold increased odds) of having menopause before age 45 years [28, 29]. Genome-wide association studies have also identified specific genetic variants associated with the timing of menopause that provide insight into biological mechanisms for ovarian aging [30].

1.3.2 Early Life Factors

Epidemiological evidence indicates an important role for factors in early life, including childhood nutrition and childhood socioeconomic status. For instance, women who experienced prenatal and childhood famine (particularly severe famine between ages 2 and 6 years) [31, 32], low body weight at age 2 years [33, 34], or not having been breastfed [33, 34] had earlier age at menopause. Low socioeconomic position and adverse life events in childhood have been found to have a greater impact on age at natural menopause than the experience of such circumstances in adulthood [34–37]. More specifically, early emotional stress may impact reproductive aging, with evidence that women who experienced parental divorce early in life (before 5 years) and paternal absence (between ages 6 and 11 years) tended to have earlier age at menopause [35, 37]. Early experience of abuse may also affect ovarian function and reproductive aging via dysregulation of stress responses [38, 39]. Women with a history of childhood sexual abuse and intimate partner violence had earlier age at menopause [37, 40], and the association was substantially mediated through cigarette smoking [40].

1.3.3 Lifestyle Factors

Of the various lifestyle and environmental factors in adulthood known to affect the timing of menopause, only cigarette smoking and underweight are consistently related to early menopause [10, 24, 41], whereas being overweight or obese is associated with later age at menopause [41, 42]. Dose-response relationships were observed that higher intensity, longer duration, higher cumulative dose, earlier age at start smoking, and short time since quitting were all associated with a higher risk of POI and early menopause, but the risk was considerably lower for former smokers [24]. Smokers who had quit smoking for more than 10 years (preferably before 30 years) had a similar risk of POI and early menopause as never smokers [24]. Underweight women had over twice the risk of early menopause, and the risk remained after adjusting for smoking status [42].

1.3.4 Reproductive Factors

Several reproductive factors have been shown to be associated with POI and early menopause. InterLACE data showed that having early menarche (≤ 11 vs 13 years) increased the risk of POI by 80%, and the risk was doubled for nulliparous women compared with those having two or more children [13]. Early menarche and nulliparity also increased the risk of early menopause but to a much lesser extent [13]. The combination of early menarche and nulliparity resulted in a five-fold increased risk of POI and two-fold increased risk of early menopause compared with women having later menarche and two or more children [13]. The sparse evidence from low- and middle-income countries (e.g., India and China) also suggested that early age at menarche and nulliparity were associated with POI and early menopause [43, 44]. Furthermore, a history of infertility and recurrent pregnancy loss (especially three or more miscarriages and two or more stillbirths) were associated with an increased risk of POI and early menopause, compared with those without these fertility issues [45]. The associations seemed to differ by race, with stronger associations for Asian women with such fertility issues [45]. The Nurses' Health Study II demonstrated that women with short cycle length (≤ 25 vs 26–31 days), very regular cycles (vs irregular cycles or no periods), premenstrual disorders, and endometriosis had a higher risk of early natural menopause (<45 years) [46–48].

1.4 Timing and Duration of Perimenopause

While a significant body of research has been conducted on identifying the factors associated with the timing of menopause, limited evidence exists on the timing and duration of perimenopause. The length of perimenopause has been shown to have an adverse effect on quality of life. Using data from the 1946 British birth cohort, it was found that women who experienced prolonged perimenopause had a higher decline in two aspects of quality of life: perceived physical health (including energy level) and psychosomatic status (such as nervous emotional state, ability to concentrate) [49]. This is consistent with an earlier study from the United States that found longer perimenopause was associated with a higher rate of medical consultations [50].

1.5 Symptoms During the Menopausal Transition

Vasomotor symptoms (including hot flushes and night sweats), virginal dryness, and sleep disturbance are the common physiological symptoms attributable to menopause [51, 52]. Each woman experiences menopausal symptoms differently. Many feel minor discomfort for a short period of time, while others have more severe symptoms over several years. InterLACE data showed that over 40% of women (median age 50 years, interquartile range 49–51 years) never experienced vasomotor symptoms, while 15% experienced severe vasomotor symptoms [53]. Similar figures were found for sleeping difficulty (39% reported never and 14% severe). The study demonstrated that women with severe vasomotor symptoms were more likely to have incident depressed mood over 3 years of follow-up compared with those without vasomotor symptoms, but sleeping difficulty largely explained the observed association [53]. Some groups of women are more likely to experience vasomotor symptoms during the menopausal transition, including those who are overweight or obese, smokers, less educated, and those with anxiety and depressed mood or feel stressed [54, 55].

Recently, epidemiological studies have attempted to provide a more detailed picture of the various distinct trajectories of symptoms experienced through the menopausal transition and into postmenopause. For instance, findings from two studies have both shown that women whose vasomotor symptoms peaked strongly either before or after age at natural menopause tended to decline relatively quickly in postmenopause [56, 57]. Such trajectories for the severity of these symptoms were not evident when based on chronological age, but only when their timing was examined with respect to the age at natural menopause. In the future, this information may help guide women in the management of their symptoms in selection of appropriate treatment options.

In addition to these common symptoms, menopausal transition is accompanied by accelerated gains in fat mass and simultaneous losses in lean mass [58]. These changes in body composition continue until 2 years after menopause [58]. A recent US study found that the rate of increase in total fat and lean mass is 0.32 kg per year in premenopause and 0.4 kg per year during the menopausal transition [58]. Factors associated with weight gain in midlife include a lack of exercise, unhealthy diet, lower levels of education, insufficient sleep, parity, and a family history of obesity [59].

1.6 Future Research

Overall, risk factors from prenatal stage through to adult life influence the age at menopause, with consequent implications for health risks in later life. Our understanding from epidemiological studies of the effects of menopausal transition on women and the factors that influence its duration and timing remains unclear and incomplete, especially on those from low- and middle-income countries. Expanding life course research in these countries will demonstrate whether social trends, such as growing income inequality during childhood and adulthood and upward mobility, similarly relate to women's age at menopause as is the case in rich nations. One way forward lies in expanding studies such as InterLACE that combine individual-level data from numerous international studies of women's health [60, 61]. This would provide a more comprehensive and detailed picture of the menopausal transition, its timing and long-term health implications, for women not just in high-income countries but from across regions and from diverse populations.

Conflict of Interest None declared.

Funding Gita D Mishra is supported by Australian National Health and Medical Research Council Leadership Fellowship (APP2009577). The InterLACE Consortium is funded by Australian National Health and Medical Research Council project grant (APP1027196) and Centres of Research Excellence grant (APP1153420).

References

1. Davis SR, et al. Menopause. Nat Rev Dis Primers. 2015;1:15004.
2. Mishra GD, et al. Optimising health after early menopause. Lancet. 2024;403(10430):958–68.
3. Rosendahl M, Simonsen MK, Kjer JJ. The influence of unilateral oophorectomy on the age of menopause. Climacteric. 2017;20(6):540–4.
4. Moorman PG, et al. Effect of hysterectomy with ovarian preservation on ovarian function. Obstet Gynecol. 2011;118(6):1271–9.
5. Atsalis S, Margulis SW. Perimenopause and menopause: documenting life changes in aging female gorillas. Interdiscip Top Gerontol. 2008;36:119–46.
6. Thomas P. The post-reproductive lifespan: evolutionary perspectives. BioSci Master Rev. 2013;5(1):1–9.
7. Croft DP, et al. Reproductive conflict and the evolution of menopause in killer whales. Curr Biol. 2017;27(2):298–304.
8. Lahdenpera M, et al. Severe intergenerational reproductive conflict and the evolution of menopause. Ecol Lett. 2012;15(11):1283–90.
9. InterLace Study Team. Variations in reproductive events across life: a pooled analysis of data from 505 147 women across 10 countries. Hum Reprod. 2019;34(5):881–93.
10. Schoenaker DA, et al. Socioeconomic position, lifestyle factors and age at natural menopause: a systematic review and meta-analyses of studies across six continents. Int J Epidemiol. 2014;43(5):1542–62.
11. Mishra GD, Cooper R, Kuh D. A life course approach to reproductive health: theory and methods. Maturitas. 2010;65(2):92–7.
12. European Society for Human Reproduction and Embryology (ESHRE) Guideline Group on POI, et al. ESHRE guideline: management of women with premature ovarian insufficiency. Hum Reprod. 2016;31(5):926–37.
13. Mishra GD, et al. Early menarche, nulliparity and the risk for premature and early natural menopause. Hum Reprod. 2017;32:679.
14. Golezar S, et al. The global prevalence of primary ovarian insufficiency and early menopause: a meta-analysis. Climacteric. 2019;22(4):403–11.
15. Muka T, et al. Association of age at onset of menopause and time since onset of menopause with cardiovascular outcomes, intermediate vascular traits, and all-cause mortality: a systematic review and meta-analysis. JAMA Cardiol. 2016;1(7):767–76.

16. Chung HF, et al. Ethnic differences in the association between age at natural menopause and risk of type 2 diabetes among postmenopausal women: a pooled analysis of individual data from 13 cohort studies. Diabetes Care. 2023;46(11):2024–34.
17. Zhu D, et al. Age at natural menopause and risk of incident cardiovascular disease: a pooled analysis of individual patient data. Lancet Public Health. 2019;4(11):e553–64.
18. Liang C, et al. Female reproductive histories and the risk of chronic obstructive pulmonary disease. Thorax. 2024;79:508.
19. Anagnostis P, et al. Association between age at menopause and fracture risk: a systematic review and meta-analysis. Endocrine. 2019;63(2):213–24.
20. Chung HF, Gete DG, Mishra GD. Age at menopause and risk of lung cancer: a systematic review and meta-analysis. Maturitas. 2021;153:1–10.
21. Wu Y, et al. Age at menopause and risk of developing endometrial cancer: a meta-analysis. Biomed Res Int. 2019;2019:8584130.
22. Collaborative Group on Hormonal Factors in Breast, C. Menarche, menopause, and breast cancer risk: individual participant meta-analysis, including 118 964 women with breast cancer from 117 epidemiological studies. Lancet Oncol. 2012;13(11):1141–51.
23. Kok HS, et al. Heart disease risk determines menopausal age rather than the reverse. J Am Coll Cardiol. 2006;47(10):1976–83.
24. Zhu D, et al. Relationships between intensity, duration, cumulative dose, and timing of smoking with age at menopause: a pooled analysis of individual data from 17 observational studies. PLoS Med. 2018;15(11):e1002704.
25. Morris DH, et al. Familial concordance for age at natural menopause: results from the breakthrough generations study. Menopause. 2011;18(9):956–61.
26. Murabito JM, et al. Heritability of age at natural menopause in the Framingham heart study. J Clin Endocrinol Metab. 2005;90(6):3427–30.
27. van Asselt KM, et al. Heritability of menopausal age in mothers and daughters. Fertil Steril. 2004;82(5):1348–51.
28. Cramer DW, Xu H, Harlow BL. Family history as a predictor of early menopause. Fertil Steril. 1995;64(4):740–5.
29. Torgerson DJ, Thomas RE, Reid DM. Mothers and daughters menopausal ages: is there a link? Eur J Obstet Gynecol Reprod Biol. 1997;74(1):63–6.
30. Ruth KS, et al. Genetic insights into biological mechanisms governing human ovarian ageing. Nature. 2021;596(7872):393–7.
31. Yarde F, et al. Prenatal famine, birthweight, reproductive performance and age at menopause: the Dutch hunger winter families study. Hum Reprod. 2013;28(12):3328–36.
32. Elias SG, et al. Caloric restriction reduces age at menopause: the effect of the 1944-1945 Dutch famine. Menopause. 2018;25(11):1232–7.
33. Mishra G, Hardy R, Kuh D. Are the effects of risk factors for timing of menopause modified by age? Results from a British birth cohort study. Menopause. 2007;14(4):717–24.
34. Hardy R, Kuh D. Does early growth influence timing of the menopause? Evidence from a British birth cohort. Hum Reprod. 2002;17(9):2474–9.
35. Hardy R, Kuh D. Social and environmental conditions across the life course and age at menopause in a British birth cohort study. BJOG. 2005;112(3):346–54.
36. Lawlor DA, Ebrahim S, Smith GD. The association of socio-economic position across the life course and age at menopause: the British Women's heart and health study. BJOG. 2003;110(12):1078–87.
37. Magnus MC, et al. Childhood psychosocial adversity and female reproductive timing: a cohort study of the ALSPAC mothers. J Epidemiol Community Health. 2018;72(1):34–40.
38. Allsworth JE, et al. Ovarian function in late reproductive years in relation to lifetime experiences of abuse. Epidemiology. 2001;12(6):676–81.
39. Allsworth JE, et al. Longitudinal study of the inception of perimenopause in relation to lifetime history of sexual or physical violence. J Epidemiol Community Health. 2004;58(11):938–43.
40. Mishra GD, et al. The role of smoking in the relationship between intimate partner violence and age at natural menopause: a mediation analysis. Womens Midlife Health. 2018;4:1.

41. Tao X, et al. Body mass index and age at natural menopause: a meta-analysis. Menopause. 2015;22(4):469–74.
42. Zhu D, et al. Body mass index and age at natural menopause: an international pooled analysis of 11 prospective studies. Eur J Epidemiol. 2018;33(8):699–710.
43. Wang M, et al. Factors related to age at natural menopause in China: results from the China Kadoorie Biobank. Menopause. 2021;28(10):1130–42.
44. Dasgupta D, Pal B, Ray S. Factors that discriminate age at menopause: a study of Bengali Hindu women of West Bengal. Am J Hum Biol. 2015;27(5):710–5.
45. Liang C, et al. Is there a link between infertility, miscarriage, stillbirth, and premature or early menopause? Results from pooled analyses of 9 cohort studies. Am J Obstet Gynecol. 2023;229(1):47 e1–9.
46. Whitcomb BW, et al. Menstrual cycle characteristics in adolescence and early adulthood are associated with risk of early natural menopause. J Clin Endocrinol Metab. 2018;103(10):3909–18.
47. Yang Y, et al. Premenstrual disorders, timing of menopause, and severity of vasomotor symptoms. JAMA Netw Open. 2023;6(9):e2334545.
48. Thombre Kulkarni M, et al. Association between laparoscopically confirmed endometriosis and risk of early natural menopause. JAMA Netw Open. 2022;5(1):e2144391.
49. Mishra G, Kuh D. Perceived change in quality of life during the menopause. Soc Sci Med. 2006;62(1):93–102.
50. McKinlay SM, Brambilla DJ, Posner JG. The normal menopause transition. Maturitas. 2008;61(1–2):4–16.
51. Al-Safi ZA, Santoro N. Menopausal hormone therapy and menopausal symptoms. Fertil Steril. 2014;101(4):905–15.
52. NIH. NIH state-of-the-science conference statement on management of menopause-related symptoms. NIH Consens State Sci Statements. 2005;22(1):1–38.
53. Chung HF, et al. The role of sleep difficulties in the vasomotor menopausal symptoms and depressed mood relationships: an international pooled analysis of eight studies in the InterLACE consortium. Psychol Med. 2018;48(15):2550–61.
54. Thurston RC, Joffe H. Vasomotor symptoms and menopause: findings from the study of Women's health across the nation. Obstet Gynecol Clin N Am. 2011;38(3):489–501.
55. Anderson DJ, et al. Obesity, smoking, and risk of vasomotor menopausal symptoms: a pooled analysis of eight cohort studies. Am J Obstet Gynecol. 2020;222(5):478 e1–478 e17.
56. Mishra GD, Kuh D. Health symptoms during midlife in relation to menopausal transition: British prospective cohort study. BMJ. 2012;344:e402.
57. Mishra GD, Dobson AJ. Using longitudinal profiles to characterize women's symptoms through midlife: results from a large prospective study. Menopause. 2012;19(5):549–55.
58. Greendale GA, et al. Changes in body composition and weight during the menopause transition. JCI Insight. 2019;4(5):e124865.
59. Davis SR, et al. Understanding weight gain at menopause. Climacteric. 2012;15(5):419–29.
60. Mishra GD, et al. InterLACE: a new international collaboration for a life course approach to women's reproductive health and chronic disease events. Maturitas. 2013;74(3):235–40.
61. Mishra GD, et al. The InterLACE study: design, data harmonization and characteristics across 20 studies on women's health. Maturitas. 2016;92:176–85.

Menopause: The Concepts and the Biological Background

Antonio Cano, Aitana Monllor-Tormos, Amparo Carrasco-Catena, and Rocío Belda-Montesinos

Abstract

The biological basis of menopause stems from the exhaustion of follicular endowment in the ovary and clinically manifests as loss of menses and of fertility. Menopause is preceded by a series of clinical stages, as depicted in the Staging of Reproductive Aging Workshop (STRAW). The updated version STRAW+10 includes the different reproductive stages, together with the clinically impactful menopausal transition and end of reproductive life represented by the postmenopausal phase. Epidemiological studies show that age at menopause, generally considered to be around 50 years, shows significant variations across different world regions. High socioeconomic conditions may delay menopause, but other variables are at work. The hormonal background of each stage has been well described. The clinical implications are mainly represented by cycle irregularities and menopausal symptoms. Predicting age at menopause remains uncertain at the individual level.

A. Cano (✉)
Full Professor of Obstetrics and Gynecology, Salus Vitae Women's Health Clinical Center, Valencia, Spain
e-mail: Antonio.cano@uv.es

A. Monllor-Tormos
Service of Obstetrics and Gynecology, Hospital Clinic Universitari, Valencia, Spain
e-mail: monllor_ait@gva.es

A. Carrasco-Catena
Clinical Area Women's Health, Hospital Universitario y Politécnico La Fe, Valencia, Spain
e-mail: carrasco_ampcat@gva.es

R. Belda-Montesinos
Service of Obstetrics and Gynecology, University General Hospital, Valencia, Spain
e-mail: belda_roc@gva.es

© The Author(s), under exclusive license to Springer Nature Switzerland AG 2025
A. Cano (ed.), *Menopause*, https://doi.org/10.1007/978-3-031-83979-5_2

2.1 Menopause and the Menopause Transition

Natural menopause is the permanent cessation of menstruation caused by exhaustion of the ovarian follicles. Unlike the testicles, ovaries undergo spontaneous functional disappearance at a relatively early age. Lack of follicular replication after fetal life at approximately 20 weeks of gestation [1] leaves a predetermined follicular endowment with a limited duration. The specific pattern of follicular attrition, with successive waves of growing follicles at regular time intervals, progressively reduces the resident population in the ovary until complete depletion. Hormonal support for the menstrual cycle in the last years of ovarian life may be insufficient, causing heterogeneity in the cycle pattern. Some women maintain acceptable regularity until the last menstrual period (LMP), while others suffer from irregular cycles with fluctuating ovulation and anovulation. There may be periods of amenorrhea lasting several months and bleeding disturbances, which may be accompanied by a list of symptoms resulting in frequent medical consultations and expenses.

The clinical implications of this changing pattern in the years leading up to the menopause form the basis of another important concept, the menopausal transition. In 1994, the World Health Organization proposed a conceptual difference between menopause and perimenopause. Menopause was defined only when 1 year has elapsed since LMP in the absence of any other obvious physiological or pathological causes [2], a definition which means that menopause can only be known retrospectively. Perimenopause is the interval in which some women have irregular menstrual cycles before menopause. This period overlaps with the menopausal transition but also includes the extra year required for confirmation of menopause. This WHO distinction has been incorporated by most of the world's scientific societies [3].

The term "climacteric" has been used as a more holistic concept, integrating the entire period of change and including psychological and other domains. Such a broad approach exceeds the framework of parameters commonly used in the clinical setting [4].

2.1.1 The Staging of Reproductive Aging Workshop (STRAW)

The need to standardize the follicular and ovarian hormonal changes of reproductive aging prompted a group of experts from different scientific societies to set up the Staging of Reproductive Aging Workshop (STRAW) initiative in 2001 [5]. The objective of STRAW was to obtain a consensus on the different stages detectable throughout a woman's reproductive life.

The STRAW initiative evaluated both menstrual characteristics and their corresponding hormonal, biological background. Menopausal symptoms were also included when present. A refined version, the STRAW+10, was published in 2012 to incorporate data from several additional studies (Fig. 2.1) [6]. Evidence supporting staging of clinical and biological events in women's later reproductive years comes from data obtained in four large epidemiological studies: the Study of Women Across the Nation (SWAN)

2 Menopause: The Concepts and the Biological Background

	MENARCHE						FMP (0)			
Stage	-5	-4	-3b	-3a	-2	-1	+1a	+1b	+1c	+2
Terminology	REPRODUCTIVE				MENOPAUSAL TRANSITION		POSTMENOPAUSE			
	Early	Peak	Late		Early	Late	Early			Late
						Perimenopause				
Duration	Variable				Variable	1-3 years	2 years (1+1)		3-6 years	Remaining lifespan
PRINCIPAL CRITERIA										
Menstrual Cycle	Variable to regular	Regular	Regular	Subtle changes in Flow/Length	Variable Length Persistent ≥7-day difference in length of consecutive cycles	Interval of amenorrhea of ≥60 days				
SUPPORTIVE CRITERIA										
Endocrine FSH			Low	Variable*	↑Variable*	↑ >25 IU/L**	↑ Variable	Stabilizes		
AMH			Low	Low	Low	Low	Low	Very Low		
Inhibin B				Low	Low	Low	Low	Very Low		
Antral Follicle Count			Low	Low	Low	Low	Very low	Very Low		
DESCRIPTIVE CHARACTERISTICS										
Symptoms						Vasomotor symptoms Likely	Vasomotor symptoms Most Likely			Increasing symptoms of urogenital atrophy

* Blood draw on cycle days 2-5 ↑=elevated
**Approximate expected level based on assays using current international pituitary standard

Figure is a modification of work found in Harlow et al. (3)

Fig. 2.1 The Stages of Reproductive Aging Workshop (STRAW) outline the seven principal stages of the reproductive life of women, including the perimenopause and postmenopausal phases. Each stage is typified by the menstrual cycle pattern, principal accompanying symptoms, and supporting information in the form of biochemical or imaging features. Reproduced with the permission of the American Society for Reproductive Medicine from Ref. [6]. Permission conveyed through Copyright Clearance Center, Inc.

[7], the Melbourne Women's Midlife Health Project [8], the Seattle Midlife Women's Health Project [9], and the TREMIN Research Program on Women's Health, currently the world's longest ongoing study of menstrual pattern [10].

STRAW divided the female reproductive period into three main phases: reproductive, menopausal transition, and postmenopause. Each phase was then subdivided into stages, making a total of 10. Each STRAW stage is supported by three types of criteria: primary, supportive, and descriptive. The primary criterion is the menstrual pattern at all stages, while supporting criteria include hormone levels and follicular parameters. The latter are quantitatively defined as the number of antral follicles identified by antral follicle count (AFC) by ultrasonography. The system also adds descriptive characteristics of associated clinical symptoms when present.

2.1.2 The Menopausal Transition in STRAW

The menopausal transition is the STRAW+10 phase that bridges the reproductive and postmenopausal phases. Prior to the menopausal transition, the late reproductive phase already shows very subtle changes affecting the menstrual pattern and hormonal background. These changes are so slight that they often go unnoticed clinically.

The menopausal transition includes two stages, early (stage −2) and late (stage −1) in STRAW+10 (Fig. 2.1). The distinguishing feature of the menopausal transition is that it is usually symptomatic. Cycle irregularities and menopausal symptoms including mood swings and vasomotor alterations such as hot flashes and night sweats form the most frequent symptomatic pattern.

For obvious reasons, it is more complicated to apply either the WHO definition or the STRAW classification to women with natural menopause who have undergone hysterectomy or to those using hormonal treatments, either the pill or progestin-bearing intrauterine devices (IUDs).

2.1.2.1 The Menstrual Cycle During the Menopausal Transition

The appearance of irregular menstrual cycles heralds the onset of the menopausal transition. More specifically, stage −2 STRAW defines menstrual cycles of persistent variable duration ≥7 days apart in consecutive cycles, whereas stage −1 already requires intervals of amenorrhea ≥60 days.

Much of what is known about menstrual patterns during the menopausal transition comes from the huge prospectively collected database initiated in the 1930s by Alan Treloar [11]. Variability in cycle length, including short and long cycles, was already reported by 10%–15% of women 6 years before menopause. An additional 30% of women reported variability between 2 and 3 years before menopause. Interestingly, a residual 4.5% of women will still have one or more menses after a year of amenorrhea at age 52 years. This observation should be kept in mind when evaluating women with postmenopausal bleeding as although malignancy should be ruled out, fortunately the cause is often remaining follicle activity.

Cycle irregularity in women going through the menopausal transition may be accompanied by episodes of heavy bleeding. There is already a progressive increase in blood loss volume with age in regular cycles [12]. Published after the Treloar study, an interesting Australian study recruiting 250 women between 45 and 55 years of age who were followed prospectively for 4 years [13] provided data integrating both cycle irregularities and changes in flow. Comparing the last 3 months with the previous 12 months, 30% of women reported no changes, 10% experienced changes in bleeding frequency but not amount, 22% changes in amount but not frequency, 26% in both frequency and amount, and 12% reported three or more months of amenorrhea.

2.2 Epidemiological Data

The age at menopause has remained relatively stable throughout history and across different regions worldwide; 50 years has been considered a good approximation. However, there are some differences whose mechanisms are not yet clear, and research interest in this field is justifiable given the studies suggesting that age at menopause may be a marker of general health. A later menopause seems to predispose to cancer of the reproductive tissues (endometrium, ovary) and breast but confers an advantage against osteoporosis and cardiovascular disease. The balance appears positive and later menopause is associated with longer survival [14], whereas the opposite occurs for both survival and cardiovascular risk in women with premature menopause or early-onset menopause [15–19].

A systematic review [20] has found that natural menopause generally occurs slightly later in developed countries. The highest mean age is found in Australia (51.3 years) and Europe (50.5 years), followed by the United States (49.1 years). Age at menopause is lower in Asia (48.8 years) and Africa (48.4 years), and the lowest ages are observed in the Middle East (47.4 years) and Latin America (47.2 years). Some studies have proposed that the difference may be influenced by an increase in the age at menopause in developed countries [21], suggesting that environmental, nutritional, or other factors could have an effect [22]. Several biological, genetic, and/or other influences may also be at play, as indicated by the considerable variation from woman to woman, which can range from 45 to 55 years of age. Nonetheless, the majority of the population cluster around the median age, with a variation of less than 3 years [23].

The age at which the menopausal transition begins is also subject to variation. Data from the Massachusetts Women's Health Study (MWHS) showed a median age at onset of perimenopause of 47.5 years and that its duration was almost 4 years in that population [24]. In addition, longer duration of perimenopause was associated with increased symptom reporting and a higher number of medical consultations.

2.3 Variables Affecting Menopause Age

Prediction of age at menopause is still not possible at the individual level despite significant advances [25]. However, research has suggested some key potential factors.

2.3.1 Genetics

Heritability of age at menopause has been detected in twin registries and family history studies. Community-based epidemiological studies, such as the multigenerational Framingham Heart Study, confirmed this association and genetic factors were found to explain at least 50% of interindividual variability in menopausal age [26]. The genetic basis of menopause has been identified primarily via studies of premature ovarian failure, and more detailed information can be found in the corresponding chapter of this book. When considering natural menopause, the task becomes more difficult. A systematic review reports that robot linkage analyses and genome-wide association studies (GWAS) have found regions containing promising candidate genes. Association studies, however, have yielded poor results. A GWAS analysis of nearly 70,000 women identified 44 common susceptibility loci for age at natural menopause [27], but they accounted for only 2.5–4.1% of the observed variation [28]. From another perspective, polygenic risk scores constructed using single nucleotide polymorphisms identified from GWAS have confirmed an association with age at menopause in women included in the SWAN cohort [29]. Building on the GWAS data, the use of more advanced technology such as whole transcriptome association has identified additional candidate genes in samples from 69,360 women of European ancestry [30].

2.3.2 Lifestyle

Environmental and socioeconomic factors appear to influence the timing of menopause, as suggested by the later age of menopause in wealthy countries. Lifestyle underlies at least some of these factors.

Current smoking is a persistently detected variable [31–36]. Tobacco use appears to be toxic to the follicular pool, possibly via polycyclic aromatic hydrocarbons in cigarette smoke [37]. According to a systematic review, smoking is responsible for a 1-year reduction in the age at natural menopause [20] and for approximately 5% of the risk of early menopause [38]. Smoking also appears to shorten perimenopause [24]. The limited data on former smokers do not seem to support an association with age at menopause [20], and when an association is detected, it is weaker [39].

The notion that diet affects age at menopause is derived from both indirect and direct evidence. Weight gain and significant weight swings have shown some impact on delayed age at menopause in older [39] and more recent studies [20, 40–43]. The suggestion that this finding may be owing to the influence of diet has been reinforced by data showing that food deprivation, even in childhood, has an association with earlier menopause [44].

Physical activity at an intensive level has been associated with anovulation and amenorrhea, but the relationship with changes in age at menopause is unclear. Data from the SWAN cohort suggest that having less physical activity is associated with later age at menopause [45].

Little is known about the effects of other environmental or occupational factors, but being employed was also associated with later age at natural menopause in SWAN [45]. This factor may reflect the effect of stress associated with unemployment or lower socioeconomic status, given that exposure to stress, even in early life, has been associated with earlier menopause [46].

2.3.3 Other Factors

Data from different cohorts have shown that both early menarche ($\leq$11 years) and nulliparity (vs. giving birth to two or more children) increase the risk of premature (LMP <40 years) and early menopause (LMP 40–44 years) [47]. In fact, women with early menarche and nulliparity had a more than five-fold increased risk of premature menopause and two-fold increased risk of early menopause [48].

Attempts have been made to predict age at menopause based on other factors, such as maternal age at menopause. However, individual predictions in the clinical setting remain elusive at present [25, 49].

2.4 The Biological Basis of Menopause

The natural history of ovarian function is influenced by the rate of attrition of the follicles residing in the ovary. The almost complete depletion of the follicular population in the late menopausal transition leads to a significant reduction in the production of estrogen, resulting in insufficient endometrium proliferation for subsequent shedding and concomitant bleeding. Menopause is confirmed when this follicular insufficiency continues for at least 1 year, despite possible bursts of more active follicular waves.

Ovarian depletion occurs because follicles are not replaced in a clearly detectable way after fetal life. The existence of a certain follicular regenerative capacity has been described in rodents [50, 51], in very specific experimental conditions in humans [52], and was more recently demonstrated with pluripotent cells [53], so cannot be definitively ruled out. Nonetheless, even if occurring in humans under physiological conditions, its effect is obviously minimal.

Follicular loss is exponential from the intrauterine phase onward, with dramatic changes in the population of follicles ranging from a maximum of 6–7 million to only 300,000 at puberty. Following this considerable drop, the follicle population continues to decline at a good pace and only about 450 oocytes will reach ovulation.

2.4.1 Regulators of Folliculogenesis and Menopause

Unlike previous theories limiting folliculogenesis to the 2 weeks before ovulation in each menstrual cycle, the landmark contributions of Gougeon clearly showed that follicle cohorts begin to grow about 3 months before ovulation [54]. A high number of follicles make up the initial cohort, but they progressively become apoptotic and only one will reach the ovulation stage.

2.4.1.1 Constitution of the Follicular Cohort: Initial Steps

The clock marking the endocrinological lifespan of the ovary is governed by certain mechanisms which determine folliculogenesis initiation, crucial among which is recruitment of specific primordial follicles (the follicular structure of resting follicles in the ovary) that will be activated and join the growing cohort. A complex set of local factors act on the population of primordial follicles to determine which will begin to grow and which will remain dormant [55]. Anti-Müllerian hormone (AMH) plays a key role by regulating the size of the follicular cohort and helping maintain an adequate ovarian reserve. This function of AMH was demonstrated in classic rodent experiments in which silencing of the AMH gene was followed by early depletion of follicles in the ovary [56].

Our understanding of how other agents contribute through autocrine and paracrine mechanisms is still in its infancy. These agents include Kit ligand, also called stem cell factor (SCF), along with a variety of others that have demonstrated the ability to stimulate the growth of preantral follicles, such as the tyrosine kinase receptor, the serine kinase receptor, or the wingless receptor, while the Hippo pathway limits follicular growth. All of them act in a concatenated way although the details of their specific role have not been sufficiently described [57].

2.4.1.2 Progression of the Cohort and Follicle Maturation

Once initiated, the growth of the follicular cohort is governed mostly by the follicular stimulating hormone (FSH) at a certain stage of follicular development. Together with luteinizing hormone (LH), FSH is produced in the pituitary gonadotroph, which is why they are commonly called gonadotropins. Gonadotropins regulate granulosa and theca cells, which extend along the follicle wall and around the oocyte, to stimulate ovarian steroidogenesis. Hormonal production includes estrogens, but also androgens and progesterone [58].

Folliculogenesis includes two phases of follicle growth, tonic and exponential. The latter begins approximately 3 weeks prior to ovulation and is characterized by a high sensitivity to gonadotropins [54]. Nonetheless, the tonic phase is also sensitive to these hormones since FSH receptors are already detected in the granulosa cells of secondary follicles at the beginning of the tonic phase of growth. The precise contribution of FSH in these early phases of folliculogenesis is still unclear.

2.4.2 Changes in the Late Reproductive Stage in STRAW+10

The progressive reduction in size of follicular waves over time is accompanied by a parallel decrease in circulating levels of AMH. Another hormonal feature in this late STRAW+10 reproductive stage involves inhibins A and B, two dimeric proteins also secreted by granulosa cells in the ovary. Both inhibin isoforms are composed of two subunits, α and β, with the difference that the β isoform has two forms and can be βA and βB for inhibin A and B, respectively (Fig. 2.2). Inhibin isoforms differ in their expression during the menstrual cycle [59]. Decreased inhibin B production has been considered the main cause of monotropic increase in FSH, which is a selective increase in circulating FSH detected at the beginning of the menstrual cycle before the menopausal transition [60, 61] (Fig. 2.3). Inhibin A has been also suggested to play a role by reducing circulating levels prior to menopause, with a similar timing to inhibin B [62].

Reduced corpus luteum activity is another variable that has been suggested by some researchers. Some level of deficiency in the corpus luteum in the previous cycle, attributable to a possible deterioration in follicular quality, contributes to further increasing FSH at the beginning of the cycle [63, 64].

Increased FSH has been considered responsible for the trend toward shorter, but still regular, cycles experienced by women in the late reproductive stage of STRAW+10. Higher FSH levels accelerate the growth of these last surviving

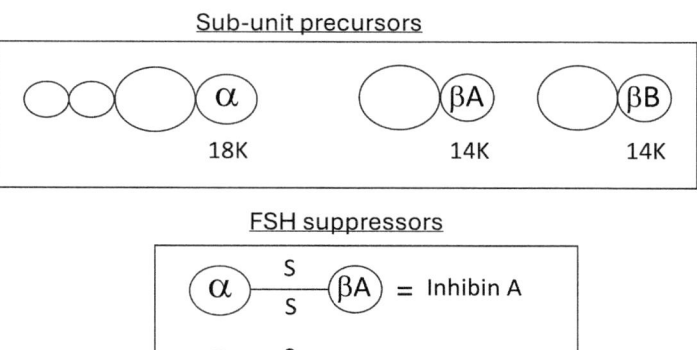

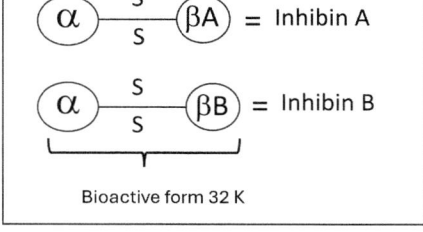

Fig. 2.2 Molecular structures of inhibin (**A**) and inhibin (**B**). Both isoforms are heterodimers deriving from precursors, peptides of bigger size that generate the corresponding subunits after proteolytic cleavage. The specificity of each isoform is dependent on the β subunit since the α subunit is common. The two "S"s in the inter-subunit linker represent a single disulfide bond

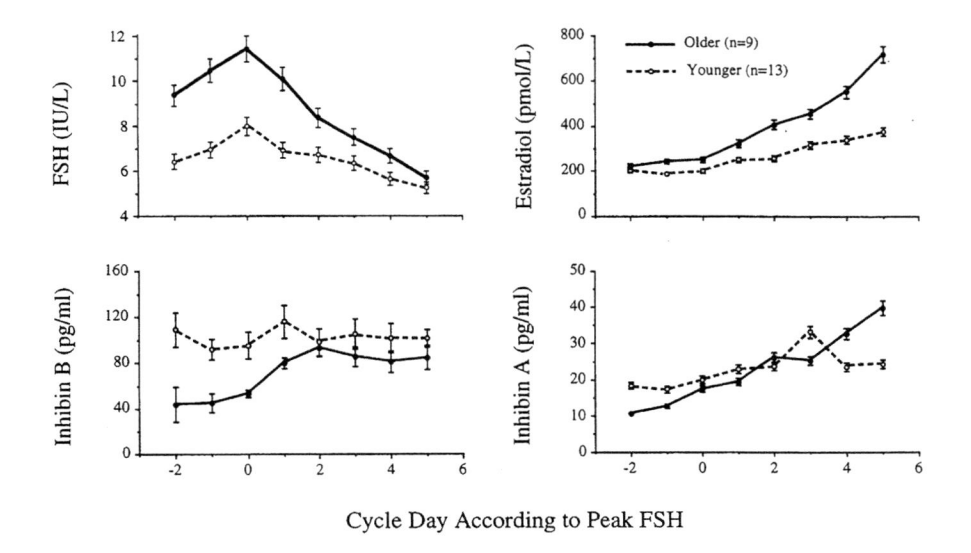

Fig. 2.3 The panel shows the pattern of FSH, inhibin (**B**), estradiol, and inhibin (**A**) as obtained from two groups of ovulatory women, who were divided into older (age 40–45) and younger (age 20–25). The "monotropic" increase of FSH in older women is a reflection of the corresponding decrease in inhibin B. Estradiol production is higher in older women during the follicular phase of the cycle. With permission of Elsevier from Ref. [65]. Permission obtained through Copyright Clearance Center, Inc.

follicles, just before the process of selection and dominance of the ovulatory follicle. Furthermore, higher FSH levels likely favor greater estrogen production, a paradoxical feature of the late reproductive stages found in a proportion of women [65]. Consistent with this observation, P450aro (aromatase) expression is increased in granulosa cells aspirated from follicles of older women [66].

It therefore seems that as well as reducing in number, cellular components of follicles, granulosa cells, and oocytes undergo changes in their functional performance. Despite so, the cycle remains regular and only the production of inhibins and some deterioration of luteal function seem to be affected. Fertility, on the contrary, is affected a few years earlier. Oocytes therefore seem to be more sensitive to age than the hormonal machinery of the theca-granulosa complex.

The reasons for the functional deterioration of follicles in the last reproductive years are not clear. Among the proposed mechanisms, previous studies suggested oxidative stress [67]. According to this hypothesis, the accumulation of reactive oxygen species (ROS) occurs continuously in mitochondria as a consequence of leakage of high-energy electrons in the mitochondrial electron transport chain. More recent updates confirm transcriptomic changes affecting both granulosa cells and oocytes. There is sufficient molecular evidence to confirm that ROS overproduction would condition a series of effects such as mitochondrial DNA inactivation and/or mutation, as well as accumulation of abnormal proteins and changes in the lipid component of cell membranes [68]. The cellular components of the follicles from the last cycles are strong candidates for accumulating functional abnormalities due to longer exposure to this process in the ovary.

2.4.3 The Menopausal Transition

A hallmark of the menopausal transition is the onset of irregular cycles. A difference of ≥ 7 days in the length of consecutive menstrual cycles marks the early stage (stage -2 STRAW+10) of the menopausal transition, of undefined duration [6]. There is an increasing trend toward anovulatory cycles, which can reach 10–15% [64]. The Daily Hormonal Study was a sub-cohort of the SWAN which made a parallel study of hormones and menstrual cycle patterns in 511 women. An absence of luteal activity, which can be interpreted as anovulatory cycles, increased progressively until reaching around 15–18% between -4 and -3 years of menopause [64]. The relatively high prevalence of appreciable estrogen levels in conjunction with anovulation favors abnormal bleeding episodes.

Menopausal symptoms, such as vasomotor symptoms (VMS) or irritability, appear as a consequence of hypoestrogenic intervals, although they are more common in the next stage, -1. A feeling of bloating can also occur as the result of hyperestrogenic episodes.

Women are considered to enter the late stage (stage -1 STRAW+10) when there is amenorrhea lasting ≥ 60 days. The duration of this stage has been established at 1–3 years. The endocrine pattern is accentuated, so FSH levels are on average higher and estrogen levels lower, although there are still some fluctuations. Concomitant increases in LH also occur, although normally closer to menopause. This change in gonadotropin secretion results from an increase in GnRH, which changes both the pulsatile pattern and the mass of peptide released as a result of decreased estradiol feedback, adding to the reduced levels of inhibin B. Local changes in brain peptides, kisspeptin, and others mediate the change [58]. The anovulation rate reaches around 80% in the year before the LMP and often manifests as amenorrheic anovulation due to lower estrogen levels.

The symptoms of menopause (such as VMS, irritability, and poor sleep quality) appear more frequently due to these increased hypoestrogenic periods, and the symptoms associated with hyperestrogenism, if present, slowly disappear.

There has been some debate as to whether the concomitant aging process of the central nervous system also plays a role. Experiences with rodents have clearly shown that positive feedback to estradiol via hypothalamic-pituitary blockade deteriorates at midlife [69]. The basis of the dysfunction is reduced availability of hypothalamic neuropeptides and a loss of coordination necessary to produce adequate bursts of GnRH. Similar dysfunctions have been reported since decades ago in women who suffer perimenopausal anovulatory cycles with severe bleeding disorders [70].

In contrast, negative feedback remains unchanged for longer, as demonstrated by the reduction in circulating gonadotropin levels when estrogen or a combination of estrogen and progesterone is administered [71].

2.4.4 Postmenopause

The postmenopausal state is divided into two periods in the STRAW+10: early and late postmenopause. Although the hormonal changes capable of causing endometrial proliferation to a stage leading to a hemorrhagic episode cannot be provided, the ovary still harbors a residual follicular population with some hormonal activity. However, this is progressively reduced because of the continuous loss of follicles. The decline in estradiol levels stabilizes approximately a couple of years after menopause [72]. Gonadotropins remain stable but also decrease by approximately 30% around age 75. According to one study, this change is due to a 22% reduction in GnRH pulse rate and 30% reduction in pituitary sensitivity to GnRH in older women [58].

The postmenopausal ovary maintains some steroidogenic activity of the spindle cells of the ovarian stroma. These cell populations meet the conditions to remain hormonally active, due to persistence of a certain vascular structure [73] and a good population of LH receptors. Indeed, studies on ovarian vein blood from postmenopausal women have shown that the postmenopausal ovary contributes significantly to the circulating reserve of testosterone and that the contribution can persist up to 10 years after menopause [74]. This androgen production may have an impact on some psychological states or libido, as suggested by the clinical effects observed with testosterone replacement in surgical and natural menopausal women [75, 76].

Testosterone production from the ovary can act as a substrate for aromatase, the enzyme that converts androgens to estrogens. Aromatase is expressed in multiple tissues, including fat and brain, where the enzyme may act as an alternative source of estrogen. Thanks to aromatase expression, local production of estrogens provides the biological basis for the concept of intracrinology [77, 78]. This type of self-sufficiency is achieved without affecting other tissues, by taking steroids from the ovary or adrenal glands as a substrate. For example, circulating dehydroepiandrosterone (DHEA) can fuel steroid-forming enzymes to meet the physiological needs of different target tissues. A good example of tissue with a high level of local estrogen is the breast, which can amplify this function in the event of malignant transformation [79].

2.5 Conclusion

The ovary is a gland with two main hormone-producing compartments, the follicular apparatus and the stroma. Follicles enclose oocytes surrounded by different layers of theca and granulosa cells, which are responsible for most of the production of steroid hormones. Three species of steroid hormones are produced: estrogens, progesterone, and androgens. The stromal compartment produces androgens and survives follicular decline for an undetermined number of years. The decrease in follicular support conditions different endocrinological profiles, which provide the basis for the clinical forms of the menopausal transition. These forms incorporate variable patterns, including irregular bleeding and a combination of symptoms that reflect hormonal deprivation, such as VMS or mood swings, or hormonal excess, such as breast tenderness. The reduction of the resident follicular population below a certain threshold marks the end of uterine bleeding, which by consensus is considered definitive after 1 year of amenorrhea.

The incidence of endometrial proliferative or hyperplastic changes often accompanies the anovulatory substrate and may be the underlying reason for abnormal bleeding. The possibility of a pathological background in the form of benign (leiomyoma, adenomyosis, etc.) or malignant conditions should prompt appropriate evaluation of these women, particularly in the postmenopause period. Even at that stage, nonetheless, some cases can be explained by bursts of estrogen resulting from sporadic follicular growth.

References

1. Strauss JF III, Williams CJ. The ovarian life cycle. In: Strauss III JF, Barbieri RL, editors. Yen & Jaffe's reproductive endocrinology. Philadelphia: Elsevier Saunders; 2014. p. 157–91.
2. WHO. Scientific group on research on the menopause in the 1990s, WHO technical report series. Geneva: WHO; 1996. http://apps.who.int/iris/bitstream/10665/41841/1/WHO_TRS_866.pdf. Accessed Dec 7, 2023.
3. Menopause: diagnosis and management (NICE Guideline 23), https://www.nice.org.uk/guidance/ng23. Accessed Nov 3, 2023.

4. Blümel JE, Lavín P, Vallejo MS, Sarrá S. Menopause or climacteric, just a semantic discussion or has it clinical implications? Climacteric. 2014;17:235–41. https://doi.org/10.3109/1369713 7.2013.838948.
5. Soules MR, Sherman S, Parrott E, Rebar R, Santoro N, Utian W, et al. Executive summary: stages of reproductive aging workshop (STRAW). Fertil Steril. 2001;76:874–8.
6. Harlow S, Gass M, Hall JE, Lobo R, Maki P, Rebar RW, et al. Executive summary of the stages of reproductive aging workshop + 10: addressing the unfinished agenda of staging reproductive aging. Fertil Steril. 2012;97:843–51.
7. Gold EB, Sternfeld B, Kelsey JL, Brown C, Mouton C, Reame N, et al. Relation of demographic and lifestyle factors to symptoms in a multi-racial/ethnic population of women 40-55 years of age. Am J Epidemiol. 2000;152:463–73. https://doi.org/10.1093/aje/152.5.463.
8. https://researchdata.edu.au/melbourne-womens-midlife-health-project/97876. Accessed 3 Nov 2023.
9. Woods NF, Mitchell ES. The Seattle midlife women's health study: a longitudinal prospective study of women during the menopausal transition and early postmenopause. Womens Midlife Health. 2016;2:6. https://doi.org/10.1186/s40695-016-0019-x.
10. Mansfield PK, Carey M, Anderson A, Barsom SH, Koch PB. Staging the menopausal transition: data from the TREMIN research program on women's health. Womens Health Issues. 2004;14:220–6. https://doi.org/10.1016/j.whi.2004.08.002.
11. Treloar AE, Boynton RE, Behn BG, Brown BW. Variation of the human menstrual cycle through reproductive life. Int J Fertil. 1967;12(1 Pt 2):77–126.
12. Hallberg L, Högdahl AM, Nilsson L, Rybo G. Menstrual blood loss--a population study. Variation at different ages and attempts to define normality. Acta Obstet Gynecol Scand. 1966;45:320–51.
13. Dudley EC, Hopper JL, Taffe J, Guthrie JR, Burger HG, Dennerstein L. Using longitudinal data to define the perimenopause by menstrual cycle characteristics. Climacteric. 1998 Mar;1(1):18–25. https://doi.org/10.3109/13697139809080677.
14. Shadyab AH, Macera CA, Shaffer RA, Jain S, Gallo LC, Gass ML, et al. Ages at menarche and menopause and reproductive lifespan as predictors of exceptional longevity in women: the women's health initiative. Menopause. 2017;24:35–44.
15. Muka T, Oliver-Williams C, Kunutsor S, Laven JS, Fauser BC, Chowdhury R, et al. Association of age at onset of menopause and time since onset of menopause with cardiovascular outcomes, intermediate vascular traits, and all-cause mortality: a systematic review and meta-analysis. JAMA Cardiol. 2016;1:767–76.
16. Honigberg MC, Zekavat SM, Aragam K, Finneran P, Klarin D, Bhatt DL, et al. Association of premature natural and surgical menopause with incident cardiovascular disease. JAMA. 2019;322:2411–21. https://doi.org/10.1001/jama.2019.19191.
17. Okoth K, Chandan JS, Marshall T, Thangaratinam S, Thomas GN, Nirantharakumar K, et al. Association between the reproductive health of young women and cardiovascular disease in later life: umbrella review. BMJ. 2020;371:m3502. https://doi.org/10.1136/bmj.m3502.
18. Xu Z, Chung HF, Dobson AJ, Wilson LF, Hickey M, Mishra GD. Menopause, hysterectomy, menopausal hormone therapy and cause-specific mortality: cohort study of UK Biobank participants. Hum Reprod. 2022;37:2175–85. https://doi.org/10.1093/humrep/deac137.
19. Schuermans A, Nakao T, Uddin MM, Hornsby W, Ganesh S, Shadyab AH, et al. Age at menopause, leukocyte telomere length, and coronary artery disease in postmenopausal women. Circ Res. 2023;133:376–86. https://doi.org/10.1161/CIRCRESAHA.123.322984.
20. Schoenaker DA, Jackson CA, Rowlands JV, Mishra GD. Socioeconomic position, lifestyle factors and age at natural menopause: a systematic review and meta-analyses of studies across six continents. Int J Epidemiol. 2014;43:1542–62.
21. Dratva J, Gómez Real F, Schindler C, Ackermann-Liebrich U, Gerbase MW, Probst-Hensch NM, et al. Is age at menopause increasing across Europe? Results on age at menopause and determinants from two population-based studies. Menopause. 2009;16:385–94.

22. Elias SG, van Noord PAH, Peeters PHM, Tonkelaar ID, Grobbee DE. Caloric restriction reduces age at menopause: the effect of the 1944–1945 Dutch famine. Menopause. 2018;25:1232–7. https://doi.org/10.1097/GME.0000000000001224.
23. te Velde ER, Pearson PL. The variability of female reproductive ageing. Hum Reprod Update. 2002;8:141–54. https://doi.org/10.1093/humupd/8.2.141.
24. McKinlay SM, Brambilla DJ, Posner JG. The normal menopause transition. Maturitas. 2008;61:4–16.
25. Nelson SM, Davis SR, Kalantaridou S, Lumsden MA, Panay N, Anderson RA. Anti-Müllerian hormone for the diagnosis and prediction of menopause: a systematic review. Hum Reprod Update. 2023;29:327–46. https://doi.org/10.1093/humupd/dmac045.
26. Murabito JM, Yang Q, Fox C, Wilson PW, Cupples LA. Heritability of age at natural menopause in the Framingham heart study. J Clin Endocrinol Metab. 2005;90:3427–30.
27. Day FR, Ruth KS, Thompson DJ, Lunetta KL, Pervjakova N, Chasman DI, et al. Large-scale genomic analyses link reproductive aging to hypothalamic signaling, breast cancer susceptibility and BRCA1-mediated DNA repair. Nat Genet. 2015;47:1294–303. https://doi.org/10.1038/ng.3412.
28. Laven JS, Visser JA, Uitterlinden AG, Vermeij WP, Hoeijmakers JH. Menopause: genome stability as new paradigm. Maturitas. 2016;92:15–23.
29. Zhao W, Smith JA, Bielak LF, Ruiz-Narvaez EA, Yu M, Hood MM, et al. Associations between polygenic risk score for age at menarche and menopause, reproductive timing, and serum hormone levels in multiple race/ethnic groups. Menopause. 2021;28:819–28. https://doi.org/10.1097/GME.0000000000001775.
30. Shi J, Wu L, Li B, Lu Y, Guo X, Cai Q. Transcriptome-wide association study identifies susceptibility loci and genes for age at natural menopause. Reprod Sci. 2019;26:496–502. https://doi.org/10.1177/1933719118776788.
31. Oboni JB, Marques-Vidal P, Bastardot F, Vollenweider P, Waeber G. Impact of smoking on fertility and age of menopause: a population-based assessment. BMJ Open. 2016;6:e012015.
32. Henderson K, Bernstein L, Henderson B, Kolonel L, Pike MC. Predictors of the timing of natural menopause in the multiethnic cohort study. Am J Epidemiol. 2008;167:1287–94.
33. Morris DH, Jones ME, Schoemaker MJ, McFadden E, Ashworth A, Swerdlow AJ. Body mass index, exercise, and other lifestyle factors in relation to age at natural menopause: analyses from the breakthrough generations study. Am J Epidemiol. 2012;175:998–1005.
34. Hyland A, Piazza K, Hovey KM, Tindle HA, Manson JE, Messina C, et al. Associations between lifetime tobacco exposure with infertility and age at natural menopause: the women's health initiative observational study. Tob Control. 2016;25:706–14. https://doi.org/10.1136/tobaccocontrol-2015-052510.
35. Mishra GD. Body mass index and age at natural menopause: an international pooled analysis of 11 prospective studies. Eur J Epidemiol. 2018;33:699–710. https://doi.org/10.1007/s10654-018-0367-y.
36. Wang M, Kartsonaki C, Guo Y, Lv J, Gan W, Chen ZM, et al. Factors related to age at natural menopause in China: results from the China Kadoorie Biobank. Menopause. 2021;28:1130–42. https://doi.org/10.1097/GME.0000000000001829.
37. Mattison DR, Thorgeirsson SS. Smoking and industrial pollution, and their effects on menopause and ovarian cancer. Lancet. 1978;1:187–9.
38. Pelosi E, Simonsick E, Forabosco A, Garcia-Ortiz JE, Schlessinger D. Dynamics of the ovarian reserve and impact of genetic and epidemiological factors on age of menopause. Biol Reprod. 2015;92:130.
39. Willett W, Stampfer MJ, Bain C, Lipnick R, Speizer FE, Rosner B, et al. Cigarette smoking, relative weight, and menopause. Am J Epidemiol. 1983;117:651–8.
40. Aydin ZD. Determinants of age at natural menopause in the Isparta menopause and health study: premenopausal body mass index gain rate and episodic weight loss. Menopause. 2010;17:494–505.
41. Zhu D, Chung HF, Pandeya N, Dobson AJ, Kuh D, Crawford SL, et al. Association between body mass index, waist circumference, and age at natural menopause: a population-based

cohort study in Chinese women. Women Health. 2021;61:902–13. https://doi.org/10.1080/03630242.2021.1992066.
42. Szegda KL, Whitcomb BW, Purdue-Smithe AC, Boutot ME, Manson JE, Hankinson SE, et al. Adult adiposity and risk of early menopause. Hum Reprod. 2017;32:2522–31. https://doi.org/10.1093/humrep/dex304.
43. Li Y, Zhao D, Wang M, Sun JY, Liu J, Qi Y, et al. Association between body mass index, waist circumference, and age at natural menopause: a population-based cohort study in Chinese women. Women Health. 2021;61:902–13. https://doi.org/10.1080/03630242.2021.1992066.
44. Hardy R, Kuh D. Does early growth influence timing of the menopause? Evidence from a British birth cohort. Hum Reprod. 2002;17:2474–9.
45. Gold EB, Crawford SL, Avis NE, Crandall CJ, Matthews KA, Waetjen LE, et al. Factors related to age at natural menopause: longitudinal analyses from SWAN. Am J Epidemiol. 2013;178:70–83.
46. Mishra GD, Cooper R, Tom SE, Kuh D. Early life circumstances and their impact on menarche and menopause. Womens Health (Lond). 2009;5:175–90.
47. Mishra GD, Chung HF, Cano A, Chedraui P, Goulis DG, Lopes P, et al. EMAS position statement: predictors of premature and early natural menopause. Maturitas. 2019;123:82–8. https://doi.org/10.1016/j.maturitas.2019.03.008.
48. Mishra GD, Pandeya N, Dobson AJ, Chung HF, Anderson D, Kuh D, et al. Early menarche, nulliparity and the risk for premature and early natural menopause. Hum Reprod. 2017;32:679–86. https://doi.org/10.1093/humrep/dew350.
49. Depmann M, Broer SL, van der Schouw YT, Tehrani FR, Eijkemans MJ, Mol BW, et al. Can we predict age at natural menopause using ovarian reserve tests or mother's age at menopause? A systematic literature review. Menopause. 2016;23:224–32.
50. Johnson J, Canning J, Kaneko T, Pru JK, Tilly JL. Germline stem cells and follicular renewal in the postnatal mammalian ovary. Nature. 2004;428:145–50. https://doi.org/10.1038/nature02316.
51. Johnson J, Bagley J, Skaznik-Wikiel M, Lee HJ, Adams GB, Niikura Y, et al. Oocyte generation in adult mammalian ovaries by putative germ cells in bone marrow and peripheral blood. Cell. 2005;122:303–15. https://doi.org/10.1016/j.cell.2005.06.031.
52. White YA, Woods DC, Takai Y, Ishihara O, Seki H, Tilly JL. Oocyte formation by mitotically active germ cells purified from ovaries of reproductive-age women. Nat Med. 2012;18:413–21.
53. Yoshino T, Suzuki T, Nagamatsu G, Yabukami H, Ikegaya M, Kishima M, et al. Generation of ovarian follicles from mouse pluripotent stem cells. Science. 2021;373:eabe0237. https://doi.org/10.1126/science.abe0237.
54. Gougeon A. Dynamics of follicular growth in the human: a model from preliminary results. Hum Reprod. 1986;1:81–7.
55. McGee EA, Raj RS. Regulators of ovarian preantral follicle development. Semin Reprod Med. 2015;33:179–84.
56. Durlinger AL, Kramer P, Karels B, de Jong FH, Uilenbroek JT, Grootegoed JA, et al. Control of primordial follicle recruitment by anti-Müllerian hormone in the mouse ovary. Endocrinology. 1999;140:5789–96.
57. Hsueh AJ, Kawamura K, Cheng Y, Fauser BC. Intraovarian control of early folliculogenesis. Endocr Rev. 2015;36:1–24. https://doi.org/10.1210/er.2014-1020.
58. Hall JE. Endocrinology of the menopause. Endocrinol Metab Clin N Am. 2015;44:485–96.
59. Groome NP, Illingworth PJ, O'Brien M, Pai R, Rodger FE, Mather JP, et al. Measurement of dimeric inhibin B throughout the human menstrual cycle. J Clin Endocrinol Metab. 1996;81:1401–5.
60. Klein NA, Illingworth PJ, Groome NP, McNeilly AS, Battaglia DE, Soules MR. Decreased inhibin B secretion is associated with the monotropic FSH rise in older, ovulatory women: a study of serum and follicular fluid levels of dimeric inhibin A and B in spontaneous menstrual cycles. J Clin Endocrinol Metab. 1996;81:2742–5.

61. Klein NA, Battaglia DE, Clifton DK, Bremner WJ, Soules MR. The gonadotropin secretion pattern in normal women of advanced reproductive age in relation to the monotropic FSH rise. J Soc Gynecol Investig. 1996;3:27–32.
62. Overlie I, Mørkrid L, Andersson AM, Skakkebaek NE, Moen MH, Holte A. Inhibin A and B as markers of menopause: a five-year prospective longitudinal study of hormonal changes during the menopausal transition. Acta Obstet Gynecol Scand. 2005;84:281–5. https://doi.org/10.1111/j.0001-6349.2005.00490.x.
63. Santoro N, Crawford SL, Lasley WL, Luborsky JL, Matthews KA, McConnell D, et al. Factors related to declining luteal function in women during the menopausal transition. J Clin Endocrinol Metab. 2008;93:1711–21. https://doi.org/10.1210/jc.2007-2165.
64. Santoro N, Roeca C, Peters BA, Neal-Perry G. The menopause transition: signs, symptoms, and management options. J Clin Endocrinol Metab. 2021;106:1–15. https://doi.org/10.1210/clinem/dgaa764.
65. Soules MR, Battaglia DE, Klein NA. Inhibin and reproductive aging in women. Maturitas. 1998;30:193–204.
66. Shaw ND, Srouji SS, Welt CK, Cox KH, Fox JH, Adams JA, et al. Compensatory increase in ovarian aromatase in older regularly cycling women. J Clin Endocrinol Metab. 2015;100:3539–47.
67. Tarín JJ. Potential effects of age-associated oxidative stress on mammalian oocytes/embryos. Mol Hum Reprod. 1996;2:717–24. https://doi.org/10.1093/molehr/2.10.717.
68. Wang S, Zheng Y, Li J, Yu Y, Zhang W, Song M, et al. Single-cell transcriptomic atlas of primate ovarian aging. Cell. 2020;180:585–600.e19. https://doi.org/10.1016/j.cell.2020.01.009.
69. Downs JL, Wise PM. The role of the brain in female reproductive aging. Mol Cell Endocrinol. 2009;299:32–8.
70. Cano A, Gimeno F, Fuente T, Parrilla JJ, Abad L. The positive feedback of estradiol on gonadotropin secretion in women with perimenopausal dysfunctional uterine bleeding. Eur J Obstet Gynecol Reprod Biol. 1986;22:353–8.
71. Gill S, Lavoie HB, Bo-Abbas Y, Hall JE. Negative feedback effects of gonadal steroids are preserved with aging in postmenopausal women. J Clin Endocrinol Metab. 2002;87:2297–302.
72. Randolph JF Jr, Zheng H, Sowers MR, Crandall C, Crawford S, Gold EB, et al. Change in follicle-stimulating hormone and estradiol across the menopausal transition: effect of age at the final menstrual period. J Clin Endocrinol Metab. 2011;96:746–54.
73. Nicosia SV. The aging ovary. Med Clin North Am. 1987 Jan;71(1):1–9.
74. Fogle RH, Stanczyk FZ, Zhang X, Paulson RJ. Ovarian androgen production in postmenopausal women. J Clin Endocrinol Metab. 2007;92:3040–3.
75. Shifren JL, Braunstein GD, Simon JA, Casson PR, Buster JE, Redmond GP, et al. Transdermal testosterone treatment in women with impaired sexual function after oophorectomy. N Engl J Med. 2000;343:682–8.
76. Shifren JL, Davis SR, Moreau M, Waldbaum A, Bouchard C, DeRogatis L, et al. Testosterone patch for the treatment of hypoactive sexual desire disorder in naturally menopausal women: results from the INTIMATE NM1 study. Menopause. 2006;13:770–9.
77. Labrie F. All sex steroids are made intracellularly in peripheral tissues by the mechanisms of intracrinology after menopause. J Steroid Biochem Mol Biol. 2015;145:133–8.
78. Labrie F, Bélanger A, Pelletier G, Martel C, Archer DF, Utian WH. Science of intracrinology in postmenopausal women. Menopause. 2017;24:702–12. https://doi.org/10.1097/GME.0000000000000808.
79. McNamara KM, Sasano H. The intracrinology of breast cancer. J Steroid Biochem Mol Biol. 2015;145:172–8.

Premature Ovarian Insufficiency

Agnieszka Podfigurna, Adam Czyzyk, Monika Grymowicz, Anna Szeliga, Roman Smolarczyk, and Blazej Meczekalski

Abstract

Premature ovarian insufficiency can be defined as cessation of ovarian function in women younger than 40 years old and is linked to the development of hypergonadotropic hypogonadism.

Generally, the incidence of POI is estimated as 1% of women. Specifically, it can be stated that it occurs in 1% of women younger than 40 years old and in 0.4% in women aged less than 35 years old. The detailed epidemiological data regarding POI is very limited. Pathogenesis of POI is very complex and still not fully understood. Genetic causes are regarded as leading pathomechanism of POI. Other causes are referred to autoimmune, metabolic, and infectious background. Due to oncological treatment of adolescents and young women, iatrogenic actions constitute essential part of POI causes. Idiopathic cause of POI still requires elucidation.

In patients with spontaneous POI, amenorrhea or oligomenorrhea may be accompanied by vasomotor symptoms (hot flashes and night sweats), dyspareunia related to vaginal dryness, lack of libido, sleep disturbance, and arthralgia. Symptoms of estrogen deficiency develop in many, but not all, patients. In women experiencing menopause induced by surgery or cancer treatment, the symptoms of estrogen deficiency are often more severe and longer lasting. The strongest evidence of autoimmune mechanisms involvement in pathology of POI comes from the high incidence of coexistence of POI with other autoimmune disorders. It is estimated that around 10–55% of patients with POI have associated autoimmune diseases.

The effect of POI-associated estrogen deficiency on bone is the most clearly established adverse consequences of POI condition although hypoestrogenism can be asymptomatic in aspect of bones for many years in most women until fracture occurs. Low bone mineral density (BMD), usually assessed by dual energy X-ray absorptiometry (DEXA), is a risk factor of fracture and widely used as a surrogate in assessing fracture risk and treatment effects. The main reason of shortened life expectancy in POI patients is cardiovascular disease. To date, it has been shown that POI women present several risk factors for the development of cardiovascular disease: endothelial dysfunction, autonomic dysfunction, metabolic disturbances, and increased inflammatory factors.

Therefore, early initiated estrogen-progestin replacement therapy is recommended in POI women to treat menopausal symptoms, maintain bone health and prevent osteoporosis, and control the future risk of cardiovascular disease The treatment should be continued at least until the average age of natural menopause.

3.1 Introduction

3.1.1 Definition and Clinical Diagnostic Criteria

Premature ovarian insufficiency (POI) can be defined as cessation of ovarian function in women younger than 40 years old and is linked to the development of hypergonadotropic hypogonadism. The hypogonadism clinically presents as amenorrhea, which sometimes is preceded by oligomenorrhea and decreased circulating estradiol levels. Different clinical definitions of POI have been proposed. Recently, European Society of Human Reproduction and Embryology (ESHRE) appointed Special Interest Group Reproductive Endocrinology to develop a contemporary guideline for POI diagnosis and management. According to this guideline, for diagnosing POI, finding menstrual abnormalities and biochemical confirmation is required as follows:

- Oligo−/amenorrhea for at least 4 months.
- An elevated FSH level >25 IU/l on two occasions >4 weeks apart [1].

This definition is in line with other proposals. For example, European Menopause and Andropause Society stated that diagnosis can be made in women younger than 40 with primary or secondary amenorrhea (of at least 4 months duration), increased follicle-stimulating hormone (FSH) serum concentration above 40 IU/L, an estradiol (E2) level below 50 pmol/L, and infertility [2].

Many other terms have been proposed for POI. In professional literature, aside from POI, it is most frequently called primary ovarian insufficiency, premature ovarian failure, and premature menopause [3]. Our current understanding of this condition makes it possible to consider it as an early menopause. There are several important differences between POI and menopause. First, menopause is a physiological process, whereas POI is a pathology. In menopause, the cessation of gonadal function is complete, while some POI patients sporadically produce estrogen and ovulate. For the same reason, professional societies recommend to omit the "premature ovarian failure" term, which also suggests permanent lack of gonadal function [1, 2]. The last but very significant difference between menopause and POI is long-term consequences. The POI is related to number of specific issues related to physical health, reproductive function, and psychological problems, which are not present in women undergoing menopause (see Sect. 3.5). Some authors suggest the term early menopause for describing menopause occurring between 40th and 44th year of life.

3.2 Pathogenesis of POI

Pathogenesis of POI is very complex and still not fully understood. Genetic causes are regarded as leading pathomechanism of POI. Other causes are referred to autoimmune, metabolic, and infectious background. Due to oncological treatment of adolescents and young women, iatrogenic actions constitute essential part of POI causes. Idiopathic cause of POI still requires elucidation.

3.2.1 Genetic Causes

It is reported that up to 40% of POI can be attributed to genetic causes. POI genetic background is referred to polygenic nature. Chromosomal abnormality accounts for approximately 10–12% of POI patients. The majority is referred to X chromosome abnormality [4]. Therefore, karyotype examination should be performed in all POI patients without iatrogenic background.

Classification of POI genetic background can be arranged in different ways. Here, we present classification based on non-syndromic POI and syndromic POI causes [5].

Genetic background of POI still requires further elucidation. New technologies in molecular biology such as genome-wide association study (GWAS) and next-generation sequencing (NGS) are regarded as promising tool for the POI genetic research.

Classification of POI Genetic Background
I. Non-syndromic POF.
  1. Ligands of TGF-beta family.
     – BMP-15.
     – GDF-9.
     – INHA.

2. FMR1.
3. G-protein-coupled receptors.
   – Gonadotropin receptors.
   – GPR3.
4. NR5A1 (SF-1).
5. Other transcription factors.
   – FOXO3a.
   – NOBOX.
   – FIGLA.
II. Syndromic POF.
   1. Turner syndrome.
   2. CDGs syndrome and galactosemia.
   3. Pseudohypoparathyroidism type 1a (PHP1A).
   4. Autoimmune polyglandular syndrome type 1.
   5. Progressive external ophthalmoplegia.
   6. Ovarioleukodystrophy.
   7. Ataxia telangiectasia.
   8. Demirhan syndrome.
   9. Blepharophimosis, ptosis, epicanthus inversus syndrome (BPES).

3.2.1.1 Non Syndromic POF

Ligands of TGF-Beta Family

BMP-15
BMP-15 encodes for an oocyte-specific member of TGF-β superfamily factor of growth factors [6]. This protein plays an essential role for stimulation follicle development and follicle maturation. For the first time in 2004, Di Pasquale et al. reported heterozygous missense mutation p.Tyr235Cys which resulted in functionally compromised mutant BMP15 protein and POI [7]. Possible mechanism is referred to impairment of granulosa cells signaling and augmentation of follicle atresia.

GDF-9
GDF-9 is a member of transforming growth factor beta (TGF-β) superfamily, and like other TGF-β proteins, it is translated as a preproprotein [8]. GDF-9 protein is responsible for proper steroidogenesis and granulosa cells function.

Numerous studies confirmed role of GDF-9 variants in POI pathogenesis [9]. However, Takebayashi et al. [10] did not find any GDF-9 mutations in women with polycystic ovary syndrome and POI.

Inhibin A (INHA)
Inhibin a-subunit (INHA) is responsible for regulating the pituitary secretion of FSH, acting in negative feedback control of FSH. It is essential in the recruitment and development of follicles during folliculogenesis. A decrease in serum INHA concentration occurs when ovarian follicular pool begins to reduce [11].

Mutations in the INHα gene, which may cause a decrease in the amount of bioactive inhibin, result in an increased FSH concentration, leading to a premature depletion of follicle, typical feature of POI ovaries [12, 13]. It is possible that some GDF-9 variants may occur in POI women some ethnicities more than in others [14].

FMR1
FMR1 gene is located in Xq27.3 outside the Xq POI critical region [15]. This gene codes for a protein called fragile X mental retardation protein, or FMRP. The FMR1 gene is expressed in oocytes and encodes an RNA-binding protein involved in translation [16]. The accumulation of FMRP may impair the expression of genes required for oocyte development.

FMR1-related POI, defined as cessation of menses before age 40 years, has been observed in carriers of premutation alleles. POI occurs in approximately 20% of females who have an FMR1 premutation. Premutation carriers have been identified in 0.8–7.5% of women with sporadic form of primary insufficiency [17]. According to ESHRE Statement, fragile X permutation testing is indicated in POI women [1].

G-Protein-Coupled Receptors
– Gonadotropin receptors.
– GPR3.

G-protein-coupled receptor 3 is a protein encoded by the GPR3 gene in humans which is involved in signal transduction [18]. GPR3 plays an important role as a link between oocytes and the surrounding somatic tissue and is expressed in mammalian oocytes where it maintains meiotic arrest and is thought [19]. The results of two studies suggested that mutations in GPR3 are not a common cause of POI in Chinese women [20, 21].

SF-1 (NR5A1)
Steroidogenic factor 1 (SF-1) also known as NR5A1 is described as nuclear receptor and regulator of multiple genes involved in adrenal and gonadal development, steroidogenesis, and the reproductive axis [22]. Several variants of SF-1 gene were identified and were characterized as associated with POI pathogenesis [23].

Other Transcription Factors

FOXO3a
FOXO3a gene belongs to the forehead gene family [24]. Watkins et al. [25] found potentially causal mutations in FOXO3A (2/90; 2.2%) and FOXO1A (1/90; 1.1%) were identified in POF patients. Functional studies should be used to clarify the role of different FOXO3a variants in POI pathogenesis.

NOBOX
NOBOX is an oocyte-specific homeobox gene that plays a critical role in early folliculogenesis. Studies performed by Qin revealed the role of NOBOX mutations in

POI pathogenesis [26, 27]. Bouilly et al. [28]found that NOBOX mutations can be responsible for 5–6% of POI in Caucasian and African population.

FIGLA

FIGLA gene is localized on chromosome 2 (2p12) [8]. FIGLA is expressed in the human fetal ovary and plays essential role in primordial follicle formation [29].

Different variants (p.140 delN); p.Arg83Cys) of FIG alpha were found respectively in Chinese and Indian population with POI [30, 31].

3.2.1.2 Syndromic POF

Turner Syndrome

Turner syndrome is characterized as chromosomal abnormality associated with a complete or partial absence of one X chromosome in a phenotypic female [32]. Germ cells atresia and the extent of ovarian failure vary based on the mosaicism level. The prevalence of Turner syndrome is approximately 1:2500 live female births.

Congenital Disorder of Glycosylation [Carbohydrate-Deficient Glycoprotein Syndrome (CDGs)] and Galactosemia

Congenital disorder of glycosylation is one of the several rare inborn errors of metabolism in which N-glycosylation of a variety of tissue proteins is deficient or defective [33]. POI occurs in approximately 60–70% of women with diagnosed galactosemia [34]. Pathomechanism is related to negative influence of galactose and its metabolites on follicle development and FSH receptor function [35].

Pseudohypoparathyroidism Type 1a (PHP1A)

Pseudohypoparathyroidism type 1a (PHP1a) also known as Albright's hereditary osteodystrophy (AHO) was first described by Albright in 1942 [36]. It is a genetic disorder caused by maternally inherited mutations of GNAS (guanine nucleotide binding protein, alpha stimulating) gene. The preferential expression of a mutant maternal allele in gonads as in other target tissues of peptide hormones acting through the same GPCR-Gsα-cAMP pathway explained the coexistence of gonadotropin resistance and POF in patients with PHP1A [37].

Autoimmune Polyglandular Syndrome Type 1

Autoimmune polyglandular syndrome type 1 (APS 1) also known as autoimmune polyendocrinopathy-candidiasis-ectodermal dystrophy (APECED) or as Whitaker syndrome was first described in 1946 [38]. This syndrome includes chronic mucocutaneous candidiasis, hypoparathyroidism, and autoimmune adrenal insufficiency. APS 1 is a disorder, with sporadic autosomal recessive inheritance [39]. Less common clinical manifestations of APS 1 could be hypergonadotropic hypogonadism, diabetes mellitus type 1, autoimmune thyroid disease (not including Graves disease), chronic active hepatitis, pernicious anemia or asplenia, and others [39].

Progressive External Ophthalmoplegia

Progressive external ophthalmoplegia (PEO) is an ocular muscles disorder. It is characterized by symmetrical inability to move the eye and is the most common manifestation of mitochondrial myopathy [40]. PEO can occur also as a part of a syndrome involving more than one part of the body, such as Kearns-Sayre syndrome. Pagnamenta et al. [41] studied that POLG mutations can segregate with POF and parkinsonism. The researchers demonstrated that the Y955C mutation can lead to mtDNA depletion.

Ovarioleukodystrophy

The "ovarioleukodystrophies" comprise a group of rare leukodystrophies associated with primary or premature ovarian failure [42]. Generally, the age of onset of neurological degeneration correlates positively with the severity of ovarian dysfunction [43].

Ataxia Teleangiectasia

A-T is caused by mutations in the ATM gene located on chromosome 11q22–23 [44]. The main characteristic features include early-onset progressive cerebral ataxia, ocular apraxia, telangiectasias, immunodeficiency, chromosomal instability, hypersensitivity to ionizing radiation, increased incidence of malignancies, and ovarian dysgenesis [45]. Mutation in ATM gene causes complete absence of mature gametes in adult gonads [46].

Demirhan Syndrome

Demirhan syndrome is an acromesomelic chondrodysplasia, which is a rare group of hereditary skeletal disorders. They are caused by homozygous mutations in growth differentiation factor 5 (GDF5), being an autosomal recessive inheritance pattern [47].

Demirhan et al. [48] presented a 16-year-old girl with homozygous mutation in BMPR1B acromesomelic manifesting chondrodysplasia, genital anomalies, amenorrhea, and hypergonadotropic hypogonadism.

Blepharophimosis, Ptosis, Epicanthus Inversus Syndrome (BPES)

BPES is an autosomal dominant eyelid malformation characterized by BPES and telecanthus associated (type I) or not (type II) to POI [49]. At present, mutations in FOXL2 are the only identified cause of BPES type I and type II. It is estimated that 2–3% of isolated POI cases have a *FOXL2* mutation [50].

3.2.2 New Suspected Genes

The latest evidence suggests impact of pathogenicity for nine genes not previously related to a POI: ELAVL2 responsible for posttranscriptional regulation, NLRP11 associated with immunity/inflammation, CENPE (regulation of cell cycle), SPATA33 (autophagy), CCDC150, CCDC185 (unknown function), as well as including DNA repair genes: C17orf53(HROB), HELQ, and SWI5 yielding high chromosomal fragility [51].

Several genes were found to be associated with POI genetic etiology in humans and animal models (SPIDR, meiosis/DNA repair; BMPR2, ovarian development and function; MSH4; MSH5, meiosis/DNA repair; GJA4, ovarian development and function; FANCM, meiosis/DNA repair; POLR2C, metabolism/protein synthesis; MRPS22, metabolism/protein synthesis; KHDRBS1, ovarian development and function; BNC1, meiosis/DNA repair; WDR62, meiosis/DNA repair; ATG7/ATG9, ovarian development and function; BRCA2, meiosis/DNA repair; NOTCH2, ovarian development; POLR3H, ovarian development and function; and TP63, meiosis/DNA repair) [52]. Association analyses comparing the POI cohort with a control cohort of 5000 individuals without POI identified 20 further POI-associated genes with a significantly higher burden of loss-of-function variants. Functional annotations of these novel 20 genes indicated their involvement in ovarian development and function, including gonadogenesis (LGR4 and PRDM1), meiosis (CPEB1, KASH5, MCMDC2, MEIOSIN, NUP43, RFWD3, SHOC1, SLX4, and STRA8), and folliculogenesis and ovulation (ALOX12, BMP6, H1–8, HMMR, HSD17B1, MST1R, PPM1B, ZAR1, and ZP3) [53]. Also new candidate genes were identified: NRIP1, XPO1, and MACF1. These genes have been linked to ovarian function in mouse, pig, and zebrafish, respectively, but never in humans [54].

3.2.3 Autoimmune Causes of POI

According to contemporary data, autoimmune disorders occur more frequently in POI patients than in general population. On the other hand, POI is more frequently presented in patients with specific autoimmune diseases.

There is significant relationship between Addison's disease and POI occurrence. Important example is autoimmune polyglandular syndrome 2 (APS2) in which Addison's disease is accompanied by autoimmune thyroid disease, autoimmune type 1 diabetes mellitus, and hypergonadotropic hypogonadism [55].

POI also is diagnosed with patients with non-adrenal disorders (thyroid diseases, hypophysitis, hypoparathyroidism).

Association between other non-endocrine disorders (rheumatoid arthritis, vitiligo, celiac disease, multiple sclerosis) and POI also can occur.

POI related to autoimmunity is associated with presence of autoantibodies which react both against steroid cells autoantibodies (SCA) in adrenal glands and gonads [56]. At present, only detection of SCA can implicate diagnosis of POI related to autoimmunity. According to ESHRE Consensus in patients with POI of unknown cause and possible immunological background, measurement of 21OH-AB should be performed. It is related also to the possible diagnosis of Addison's disease.

Thyroid autoimmunity also can be related to POI occurrence [57]. Measurements of TPO-AB antibodies should be performed in women of unknown cause or possible immunological background. Positive results of TPO-AB implicate serum TSH test every year.

3.2.4 Metabolic Disorders

Galactosemia can be referred to rare metabolic genetic disorder in which galactose is not metabolize properly. POI is a long-term consequence of this disorder. Patients with hypergonadotropic hypogonadism present primary or secondary amenorrhea. Incidence of POI in women with profound GALT deficiency is around 80% [58]. Mechanisms by which ovarian function is destroyed is not clear. The most possible mechanisms are referred to cumulation of galactose and its toxic products of metabolism (galactose-I-phosphate and galactitol) after birth can lead to direct ovarian impairment [59].

3.2.5 Infectious Causes

Different viral diseases such as HIV, cytomegalovirus, varicella, herpes zoster, malaria have been considered as a cause of POI. Among these viral infections, only mump oophoritis has been confirmed as a cause of POI [60].

According to ESHRE POI Consensus, infection screening in POI women is not recommended [1].

3.2.6 Iatrogenic Causes

Iatrogenic causes are regarded as common and increasing cause of POI.

They are related to oncological treatment and include gonadotoxic effect of chemotherapy, radiotherapy, and also surgery.

Incidence of cancer in adolescents and young women is increasing [61]. It should be stressed that abovementioned oncological treatment can cause whole spectrum of POI with leading problem as infertility.

Chemotherapy causes gonadotoxic effect on the ovary that is represented in such histological picture as apoptosis of ovarian follicles, cortical fibrosis, and vascular damage. Chemotherapy-induced POI is related to type of agent, dose of agent, and of course age of the patient. Age of the patient is important because with increasing age, the physiological follicular depletion is observed. Alkylating agents (cyclophosphamide is an example) present a strong gonadotoxic effect and in approximately 40% can cause POI. Other chemotherapeutic agents as anthracycline antibiotics, antimetabolites, and vinca alkaloids are classified as less gonadotoxic [62].

Acute POI can occur after radiation of such regions as hypothalamus, pituitary, and pelvis. The dose of the radiation is critical in the sense of ovary function. It was proved that application of dose 14.3 Gray to an ovary to the women younger than 30 years old can lead to irreversible POI [63]. When the dose is lower such as 6 Gray, the ovarian dysfunction can be reversible. Similarly to chemotherapy, the effect of irradiation depends on age of the patients. Younger patients pose higher number of follicles in early stage of development.

Type and extent of surgery can implicate POI risk. Coccia et al. [64] revealed that bilateral surgery for bilateral endometrioma can cause POI.

Oncological therapy should be discussed with the patient in the perspective of its risk for POI and POI-related infertility.

3.3 Epidemiology AP

Generally, the incidence of POI is estimated as 1% of women [65]. Specifically, it can be stated that it occurs in 1% of women younger than 40 years old and in 0.4% of women aged less than 35 years old [66]. The detailed epidemiological data regarding POI is very limited. In one large longitudinal study, ethnic differences have been reported for prevalence of POI. In comparison to Caucasian population (1.0%), some ethnicities were affected more often (African American 1.4%, Hispanic 1.4%), whereas others more seldom (Chinese 0.5%, Japanese 0.1%) [67]. The results must be interpreted cautiously since these are self-reported, and other authors found conflicting results [68].

The data regarding lifestyle and environmental risk factors for POI is also scant. Among proposed risk factors for developing following were reported: smoking, small waist-to-hip ratio, and lack of alcohol consumption [65, 69].

3.4 Definition and Clinical Presentation

3.4.1 Definition

The nomenclature of the severe decline of ovarian function before 40 years of age poses a challenge [70]. The condition was previously referred to as premature ovarian failure (POF), primary ovarian failure, premature menopause, and hypergonadotropic hypogonadism [71]. Premature ovarian insufficiency is a preferred form for the triad of amenorrhea, elevated gonadotropins, and estrogen deficiency occurring in women before the age of 40 years because the term "failure" suggests an irreversible and permanent cessation of ovarian function and the word "menopause" may be stigmatizing for some patients [72]. POI differs from menopause by its unpredictable course with intermittent resumption of function. Moreover, some women diagnosed with POI may become pregnant spontaneously albeit the likelihood is small (3–10%) [73]. The term POI encompasses both spontaneous loss of ovarian activity and ovarian function decline as a result of iatrogenic interventions.

Definition in common use applied by most authors when establishing a diagnosis of POF/POI is at least 4 months of amenorrhea in association with menopausal level of serum follicle-stimulating hormone (FSH) concentrations on two occasions (4 weeks apart) [74]. However, the duration of amenorrhea ranging from 3 to 6 months and various levels of FSH ranging from 10 to 40 IU/l have been used by different authors in the diagnosis of POF (reviewed in [75]).

European Menopause and Andropause Society (EMAS) in 2010 uses the former term premature ovarian failure (POF) and defines the condition as menopause before the age of 40, confirmed with an elevated FSH > 40 IU/L and an estradiol level below 50 pmol/l (Table 3.1) [76].

The European Society of Human Reproduction and Embryology (ESHRE) produced in 2016 guideline on management of women with POI (Table 3.1) [77]. The guideline development group agreed that the term "premature ovarian insufficiency" should be used to describe this condition in research and clinical practice. The authors define POI as a clinical syndrome with loss of ovarian activity before the age of 40 years, which is characterized by menstrual disturbance (amenorrhea or oligomenorrhea) with raised gonadotropins and low estradiol. The following diagnostic criteria were proposed: (i) oligo–/amenorrhea for at least 4 months and (ii) an elevated FSH level > 25 IU/l on two occasions >4 weeks apart. Due to unpredictable and intermittent ovarian function in POI patients, the diagnosis should be made on the basis of 4 months of disordered menses (oligomenorrhea or amenorrhea) in association with high FSH levels. This approach will allow to include larger population of patients in the group of women experiencing POI and help to avoid delayed diagnosis. It may be of paramount importance as POI is potentially associated with reduced life expectancy and accelerated health risks such as cardiovascular and neurodegenerative disorders and osteoporosis [78].

Adding to the complexity of the picture, there are conditions that represent milder forms of premature ovarian senescence termed as premature ovarian aging (POA), also called occult primary ovarian insufficiency (OPOI) or early menopause covering a group of women, whom before 45 years prematurely enter menopause [79]. It is estimated that 88% of women experience menopause over 45 years of age and 9.7% before 45 years [70].

Moreover, advanced infertility treatments identified subgroups of patients with diminished ovarian reserve (DOR) or patients with poor ovarian response (POR). There is considerable heterogeneity in the definition of DOR, including patients under the age of 40 years with regular menses and different levels of mildly elevated FSH levels (7–15 IU/l) and diminished anti-Müllerian hormone (AMH) levels (<0.5–1.1 mg/ml) [74]. In women before 40 years with regular cycles but with FSH

Table 3.1 Diagnostic criteria of premature ovarian failure/insufficiency

	EMAS	ESHRE
Nomenclature	Premature ovarian failure (POF)	Premature ovarian insufficiency (POI)
Definition	Menopause before the age of 40	Loss of ovarian activity before the age of 40 years, characterized by menstrual disturbance (amenorrhea or oligomenorrhea) with raised gonadotrophins and low estradiol
Diagnosis	Elevated FSH >40 IU/l and an estradiol level below 50 pmol/l	Oligo–/amenorrhea for at least 4 months and elevated FSH >25 UI/l on two occasions >4 weeks apart

EMAS, European Menopause and Andropause Society; ESHRE, European Society of Human Reproduction and Embryology [76, 77]

concentrations greater than 12–15 IU/l, the ovaries are unlikely to respond to the stimulating agents [4]. To define poor ovarian response, at least two of the following three features must be present: (i) advanced maternal age (≥40 years) or any other risk factor for POR (i.e., Turner syndrome, *FMRI* premutations, pelvic infection with chlamydia, chemotherapy, or endometriosis), (ii) a previous POR (≤3 oocytes with a conventional stimulation protocol), and (iii) an abnormal ovarian reserve test (i.e., AFC <5–7 follicles or AMH <0.5–1.1 ng/ml) [80]. The definition of POR covers not only the women older than 40 years that presented poor response during ovarian stimulation undergoing infertility treatment but also the POI patients with expected poor ovarian response.

3.4.2 Clinical Presentation

In patients with spontaneous POI, amenorrhea or oligomenorrhea may be accompanied by vasomotor symptoms (hot flashes and night sweats), dyspareunia related to vaginal dryness, lack of libido, sleep disturbance, and arthralgia. Symptoms of estrogen deficiency develop in many, but not all, patients. In women experiencing menopause induced by surgery or cancer treatment, the symptoms of estrogen deficiency are often more severe and longer lasting [81].

Postpubertal patients have usually established regular menstrual cycles prior to the onset of POI. Therefore, most frequently, they present with secondary amenorrhea. However, about 24–50% of women with POI have intermittent and unpredictable menses rather than complete amenorrhea [71, 82].

Ferrarini et al. [70] studied a cohort of 50 POI patients without detectable iatrogenic causes of the condition. Mean age of onset of POI in this group was 29 years. Majority of them presented normal puberty and secondary amenorrhea (94%), and only 6% normal pubertal development and primary amenorrhea. Among the studied patients, 15% had a family history of POI. Bidet et al. [82] described 358 patients with non-iatrogenic POI. The mean age at diagnosis was 26.6 years. Most of the patients (78.5%) presented secondary amenorrhea and only 21.5% primary amenorrhea.

Premature ovarian insufficiency before the age of 20 years is extremely rare. Among these young women, Turner syndrome and gonadal dysgenesis are the best known causes of early POI.

Cameron et al. [83] reviewed a cohort of adolescent patients with nonchromosomal, non-iatrogenic POI that most commonly presented primary amenorrhea (58.8%), less frequently secondary amenorrhea (23.5%), and oligomenorrhea (17.6%). Some of the patients (13.3%) were investigated due to delayed puberty.

Massin et al. [84] analyzed 63 patients with a normal karyotype and early (before the age of 20 years) onset of POI. Only 16% of the patients presented a familial history of POI. Among the studied patients, 23 were presented due to lack of pubertal development, 18 with primary amenorrhea with interrupted puberty, and 22 with secondary amenorrhea with normal puberty [84].

3.4.3 Personal and Family History

Detailed patient's personal and family history can reveal some risk factors for POI. Surgery and chemo−/radiotherapy are becoming increasingly common as a cause of iatrogenic POI. There is strong evidence that alkylating agents and radiotherapy to which the ovaries were potentially exposed increase the risk for developing POI. There are anecdotal reports of infections such as tuberculosis, mumps, malaria, varicella, or shigella followed by POI [75]. Chronic medical illnesses such as diabetes mellitus or celiac disease are also associated with POI. Patients should be queried about autoimmune disorders such as hypothyroidism, adrenal insufficiency, and hypoparathyroidism that may relate to an autoimmune polyglandular syndrome. Incidence of cases of POI, early menopause, mental retardation, and autoimmune dysfunction in the family history is important as the heritability of the age of menopause has been estimated at 30–85% and about 15–30% of cases of POI are considered to be familial [71, 81].

3.4.4 Physical Examination

Clinical features of absent, interrupted, or normal pubertal development should be observed. The signs of androgen excess or the presence of galactorrhea suggest other potential causes of secondary amenorrhea. The physical examination may reveal evidence of associated disorders such as hyperpigmentation, vitiligo, or thyroid enlargement suggesting autoimmunological involvement. Moreover, stigmata such as short statue, webbed neck, cubitus valgus, low posterior hairline, or high arched palate may suggest a Turner syndrome (Table 3.2). The height of the patients should be measured and body mass index calculated as a part of general examination.

3.4.5 Initial Laboratory Assessment

Initial assessment should confirm the POI diagnosis and exclude other common causes of oligo−/amenorrhea such as pregnancy, hypothyroidism, hyperprolactinemia, polycystic ovary syndrome, and lifestyle habits (excessive exercise, poor caloric intake, emotional stress). Therefore, appropriate tests should include follicle-stimulating hormone, luteinizing hormone, estradiol, pregnancy test, thyroid hormones, prolactin, androgen, and cortisol levels (Table 3.3). In cases of hypothalamic amenorrhea (due to eating disorders, excessive stress or exercise), the serum FSH and LH levels are in the low range. If the serum levels of FSH are at menopausal range, the test should be repeated in 1-month time.

The progesterone challenge may be misleading as half of the women will respond despite the presence of menopausal-level gonadotropins, and this may lead to delay in diagnosis [76]. Therefore, a progestin withdrawal test is not recommended in diagnosis of POI.

Table 3.2 Clinical features of Turner syndrome

Turner syndrome
Short stature
Peripheral lymphedema
Nail dysplasia
Webbed neck
Low posterior hairline
Low-set, posteriorly rotated ears
Bushy eyebrows
Shield chest
Widely spaced nipples
Cardiovascular defects
Renal anomalies
Primary ovarian failure
Delayed puberty
Infertility
Strabismus, ptosis
Recurrent otitis media
Multiple nevi
Hypothyroidism
Skeletal abnormalities
Metacarpal shortening
Madelung deformity (wrist)
Knee abnormalities
Scoliosis
Micrognathia
Cubitus valgus
High arched palate

3.4.6 Further Investigation

The etiology of POI is highly heterogeneous. It may be the consequence of iatrogenic factors such as surgery, chemotherapy, or radiotherapy. Other causes include genetic and autoimmune components. In 90% of the cases of non-iatrogenic primary ovarian insufficiency, the cause remains unknown [71].

3.4.6.1 Genetic
The association between menopausal age between sisters or mothers and daughters suggests that genetic factors play a role in the reproductive aging process. Almost half of the cases of primary amenorrhea may be associated with genetic causes, whereas in women with secondary amenorrhea as a sign of premature ovarian failure, about 13% of patients will have some genetic defects [85]. The genetic background of POI is described above.

3.4.6.2 Autoimmune
Autoimmune mechanisms are involved in pathogenesis of 4–30% of POI cases. There is lack of specific and sensitive tests to detect autoimmune pathogenesis of POI.

3 Premature Ovarian Insufficiency

Table 3.3 Investigations recommended in POI patients

	EMAS	ESHRE
Initial investigation	Endocrine screen to diagnose other causes of oligo–/amenorrhea: FSH, LH, PRL, estradiol, progesterone, testosterone, and thyroid function tests	
Genetic testing	Chromosome abnormalities, especially in women younger than 30 years	Chromosomal analysis in all women with non-iatrogenic POI Gonadectomy recommended for all women with detectable Y chromosomal material Fragile X premutation testing is indicated in POI women (the implications should be discussed before the test). Autosomal genetic testing is not at present indicated unless there is evidence suggesting a specific mutation.
Further assessment	Coexisting diseases must be detected: Hypothyroidism Diabetes mellitus Autoimmune screen for polyendocrinopathy BMD by DXA (optional) ACTH stimulation test if Addison's disease is suspected (optional).	Screening for 21 OH-Ab/ACA (if positive refer to endocrinologist) Screening for thyroid (TPO-Ab) antibodies (if positive measure TSH every year) Insufficient evidence to recommend routinely screening POI women for diabetes There is no indication for infection screening. Measurement of BMD at initial diagnosis of POI should be considered.
Ovarian biopsy	The diagnostic usefulness of ovarian biopsy outside the context of a research setting is unproven.	

EMAS, European Menopause and Andropause Society; ESHRE, European Society of Human Reproduction and Embryology; FSH, follicle-stimulating hormone; LH, luteinizing hormone; PRL, prolactin; BMD, bone mineral density; DXA, dual energy X-ray absorptiometry; ACTH, adrenocorticotropic hormone; 21-OH-Ab, 21-hydroxylase autoantibodies; ACA, adrenal cortex antibodies; TPO-Ab, antiperoxidase antibodies; TSH, thyroid-stimulating hormone [7, 8]

Antiovarian Antibodies

Several autoantibodies such as antibodies to steroid-producing cells (StCA), antibodies to gonadotropins and their receptors, granulosa cells, zona pellucida, oocyte, and corpus luteum as well as anticardiolipin and antinuclear antibodies have been proposed as the markers of ovarian autoimmunity [86]. The prevalence of antiovarian antibodies in POI women varies greatly, ranging from 3% to 66.6% [86]. Moreover, these antibodies are frequently found in significant amounts in control groups comprising women without POI. Therefore, clinical diagnosis of autoimmune POI should not be based on the presence of antiovarian antibodies.

Lymphocytic Oophoritis
Although the diagnostic usefulness of ovarian biopsy is unproven and therefore is not routinely performed, there is some insight on histological evidences of autoimmune ovarian involvement gathered by clinical research. In the cases of coexisting POI and adrenal autoimmunity, histological examination almost always shows characteristic signs of an autoimmune oophoritis: infiltration of follicles by T lymphocytes, macrophages, and natural killer cells [87]. In the whole population of nongenetic, non-iatrogenic POI patients, only 9.1–11% of the ovarian tissue samples show the histopathological evidence of autoimmune ovarian involvement [86].

Association with Other Autoimmune Disorders
The strongest evidence of autoimmune mechanisms involvement in pathology of POI comes from the high incidence of coexistence of POI with other autoimmune disorders. It is estimated that around 10–55% of patients with POI have associated autoimmune diseases. Hypothyroidism is the most common autoimmune disorder associated with POI (25–60%) [86]. Coincidence with diabetes mellitus is 2.5% [86]. The most dangerous autoimmune condition that might occur in women with POI more frequently than in controls is Addison's disease (2–10%). ESHRE guidelines include screening for antiperoxidase antibodies (TPO-Ab) and for 21-hydroxylase autoantibodies (or alternatively adrenocortical antibodies) in women with POI of unknown cause or if an immune disorder is suspected. If the tests are positive for adrenal antibodies, the patient should be referred to endocrinologist for testing of adrenal function to rule out Addison's disease. In patients with a positive TPO-Ab test, thyroid-stimulating hormone (TSH) should be measured every year [77].

Autoimmune disorders often gather into constellations grouped and named as autoimmune polyglandular syndromes. Autoimmune polyglandular syndromes (APS) comprise APS-1 (primary adrenal insufficiency, mucocutaneous candidiasis, and hypoparathyroidism) and APS-2 (primary adrenal insufficiency with autoimmune thyroid disease and/or diabetes mellitus type 1). Autoimmune polyglandular syndrome type 3 (APS-3) is defined as the coexistence of autoimmune thyroiditis with other autoimmune diseases without primary adrenal insufficiency. The fourth type of APS (APS-4) includes autoimmune adrenal insufficiency with other autoimmune disorders but does not fulfill criteria of APS-1 and APS-2.

Reato et al. [88] found that the prevalence of POI in patients with different types of APS varied: The highest prevalence was in patients with APS-1 (>40%), lower in patients with APS-4 (30%), and the lowest in APS-2 (16%). POI in APS-1 and APS-4 usually developed after Addison's disease was diagnosed, whereas POI preceded Addison's disease in patients with APS-2. Moreover, the results indicated strong relationship between POI and autoantibodies to steroid-producing cells (StCA) [88].

Around one-third of patients with APS-3 develop POI [70, 89]. Autoimmune thyroiditis without thyroid dysfunction is the most frequent presentation of autoimmunity in this group [70]. Premature ovarian insufficiency may also be associated with the dry-eye syndrome, myasthenia gravis, rheumatoid arthritis, and systemic lupus erythematosus [71].

In young patients with POI, the incidence of autoimmune comorbidities might be lower. Massin et al. [84] assessed a group of POI patients diagnosed before 20 years of age. Less than 10% of patients were found positive for antithyroid antibodies. Neither ovarian nor adrenal antibodies were found.

Concluding, for many women with POI, autoimmunity may be the pathogenic mechanism of ovarian function decline. Moreover, POI patients are at high risk of other coexisting autoimmune diseases, of which hypothyroidism is the most frequent and adrenal insufficiency the most dangerous. Therefore, women with POI should be screened for autoimmune polyendocrinopathy. At least antithyroid and anti-adrenal antibodies should be tested. Apart from research settings, there are no recommendations for assessment of ovarian antibodies or ovarian biopsy.

3.4.7 Risk Assessment for Premature Ovarian Senescence

Premature ovarian senescence frequently progresses undiagnosed until becoming clinically symptomatic in outright premature ovarian failure. Known risk factors for POI are generally known (Table 3.4). However, the statistical weight of individual predictive risk factors remains to be determined.

The risk of POI among young cancer survivors is increased and reaches approximately 8% by 40 years [90]. Compelling evidence suggests that treatment with alkylating agents and/or radiotherapy to which the ovaries are potentially exposed increases risk of POI development. Other factors such as the age of the patient at treatment, cumulative chemotherapy and radiotherapy dose, combinations of these modalities, and genetic variation may play a role in individual susceptibility to ovarian failure. Laboratory evaluation with FSH and estradiol has been recommended on the basis of clinical indication or when the patient desires assessment of potential future fertility [90].

Table 3.4 Risk factors for premature ovarian insufficiency

Risk factors for POI	
Genetic	Turner syndrome
	FMR1 mutations and premutations
	AIRE gene
	Other genetic causes
Iatrogenic	Ovarian surgery
	Chemotherapy
	Radiotherapy
Autoimmunity	Thyroid autoimmunity
	Adrenal autoimmunity
	Autoimmune polyglandular syndromes
	Other autoimmunity
Familial	POI or early menopause in mother or sibling
Other	Endometriosis

3.4.7.1 Pelvic Ultrasonography and Ovarian Biopsy

Mehta et al. [90] detected that the ovary could be identified unilaterally or bilaterally in 84% of POI patients, and follicles were observed in 41% of patients. Knauff et al. [91] in a nationwide prospective cohort study in the Netherlands conducted pelvic ultrasonography in 68 patients with normal menses and elevated FSH (IOF, incipient ovarian failure), in 79 with cycle disturbances and elevated FSH (TOF, transitional ovarian failure), and in 112 patients with amenorrhea for 4 months and FSH exceeding 40 IU/l (POI). Ovaries were not visible on ultrasound in 19% patients with IOF, in 29% patients with TOF, and in 33% in patients with POF. Antral follicle count (AFC) was defined as the total number of visible follicles with diameter between 2 and 10 mm. AFC lower than five follicles was found in 92% of patients with IOF, in 79% women with TOF, and in 81% of POF patients, compared with 29% in controls [92]. AFC ability to distinguish between various subgroups decreased significantly with increasing age. No follicles were observed in 10% of IOF, in 26.6% of TOF, and 33% of POF patients.

Massin et al. [92] performed pelvic ultrasonography in 61 patients with nongenetic POI. They calculated the surface area of the ovaries and the presence of follicles of ≥2 mm. Only 22 patients (36%) had a normal surface area (≥2 cm^2), and follicles were observed in 32 patients. The parameters observed on ultrasonography did not correlate with the presence of follicles observed at histology [92].

Ovarian biopsy has been used to differentiate the POI patients with some follicles within the ovary form those depleted of ovaries [92, 93]. Abe et al. [93] conducted minilaparoscopy and ovarian biopsy in 47 POI patients in which transvaginal ultrasonography failed to identify the ovary. They found follicles at histology in 21% of the studied patients.

However, the usefulness of ovarian biopsy has been questioned due to its invasive nature and the concern of postoperative adhesion, impairing already reduced fertility in POI patients. There is a risk that the sparse follicles may be further reduced as a result of ovarian biopsy. Moreover, there is concern over whether the minute biopsy tissue is adequate to evaluate the presence or absence of follicles in the whole ovary (reviewed in [94]). Therefore, EMAS states that the diagnostic usefulness of ovarian biopsy outside the context of a research setting is unproven [76].

3.4.7.2 AMH and Inhibin B

There are two glycoproteins of the superfamily of transforming growth factors β (TGF-β), inhibin B and anti-Müllerian hormone (AMH) reflecting the ovarian reserve. In normal ovulatory cycles, the serum concentration of inhibin B is inversely correlated with FSH levels, reaching maximum levels in the middle of the follicular phase of cycle. The use of the inhibin B as a marker of ovarian reserve has been demonstrated to correlate with antral follicular count (AFC), normal response to the test of stimulation with clomiphene citrate, and a number of oocytes obtained in in vitro fertilization programs (reviewed in [95]). However, some authors consider inhibin B more as a marker of ovarian activity rather than ovarian reserve [91]. Inhibin B has direct relationship with the amount of granulosa cells in growing small antral follicles. Compared to inhibin B, AMH is relatively stable through the menstrual cycle. Anti-Müllerian hormone represents the follicular number and ovarian age. Total ovarian reserve is made up of still unrecruited primordial follicles and smaller portion of small growing follicles. AMH represents this latter pool of small growing follicles. In the perimenopausal age, AMH levels decline earlier than FHS. Gleicher et al. [96] proposed screening paradigm for patients with POI risk factors and subsequent sequential AMH levels deviating from aging curves. Identification of high-risk females at very young ages would give the opportunity to change their pregnancy timing or pursue fertility preservation. Sensitivity of AMH in diagnosis of POI is more than that of FSH but both tests has almost equal specificity [97].

Knauff et al. [91] described the direct ovarian reserve markers AMH, inhibin B, and AFC in young women presenting with various degrees of hypergonadotropic ovarian failure. They found that AMH in POF patients are consequently below the menopausal threshold and in the vast majority even undetectable, despite fluctuations in FSH levels and incidental vaginal bleedings. Moreover, their data also suggest that AMH is more consistent than inhibin B or AFC as a measure to assess the extent of the follicle pool in young hypergonadotropic patients.

Inhibin B along with FSH and estradiol at time of POI diagnosis appeared to be predictive of resumption of ovarian activity [82]. However, AMH levels are not predictive of resumption of ovarian activity in POI patients, neither for the arrest following the resumption of ovarian function [82, 98]. Therefore, Bidet et al. [82] concluded that AMH appears to be an excellent quantitative but not good qualitative marker of ovarian reserve and seems to be more a marker than a predictor of ovarian function. Similarly, AMH and inhibin B are not good predictors of graft function or probability to achieve pregnancy after retransplantation of cryopreserved ovarian tissue.

There are several studies determining AMH levels in the specific subgroups of patients. Saglam et al. [99] showed that women with autoimmune thyroiditis have lower AMH levels compared with age-matched controls and concluded that data from the study added support to the hypothesis that women with autoimmune thyroiditis have prematurely aging ovaries.

The prognostic and predictive value of AFC and AMH for the diagnosis after childhood cancer has not been established. However, AMH may be of additive value in conjunction with FSH and estradiol for the identification of POI in at-risk survivors age > 25 years [91].

3.5 Long-Term Consequences and Follow-Up

3.5.1 Bone Health

The effect of POI-associated estrogen deficiency on bone is the most clearly established adverse consequences of POI condition although hypoestrogenism can be asymptomatic in aspect of bones for many years in most women until fracture occurs. Low bone mineral density (BMD), usually assessed by dual energy X-ray absorptiometry (DEXA), is a risk factor of fracture and widely used as a surrogate in assessing fracture risk and treatment effects. However, fracture itself is often the primary outcome of interventional trials.

DEXA can identify osteoporosis, defined as bone mineral density more than 2.5 standard deviations below peak BMD for the appropriate reference group (i.e., young women from the same population) and with the T-score used to show the difference in number of standard deviations. Osteoporosis is therefore a T-score of ≤−2.5, with osteopenia defined by a T-score ≤−1 and >−2.5. Z-scores are also frequently reported and express the number of standard deviations a patient's BMD differs from the average BMD of an age- and sex-matched control group [100].

The prevalence of osteoporosis in POI appears to be in the range of 8–14% [101].

Women with POI have reduced BMD, and this has been associated with the presence, degree, and duration of estrogen deficiency. Reduced BMD in POI has been established in many studies investigating women with POI of different etiologies, compared to reference populations.

The beneficial effects of estrogen on bone have been recognized, and likewise the adverse effect of natural menopause on bone loss, mineral density, and fracture risk [102]. Estrogen deficiency results in increased bone remodeling. Increased osteoclast activity results in increased bone resorption, and that in turn induces an increase in osteoblast activity and bone formation, however with resorption exceeding formation. The rapid remodeling of estrogen deficiency means the loss of BMD, amounting to 2–3% per year early after menopause. Additionally, the slow mineralization of new bone (over at least 6 months) causes new bone to be less mineralized than older bone. The effects on bone resorption are mediated by increased activity of the nuclear factor kappa-B ligand (RANKL) on RANK receptors on osteoclasts and their precursors. Bone resorption is also mediated by increase in pro-inflammatory cytokines such as interleukin-1 beta and tumor necrosis factor also leading to an increased bone resorption. The increased bone remodeling is reversible in the short term, but with time, the high osteoclast activity results in perforation of the cancellous bone plates so that there is a loss of the bone microarchitecture. This form of bone loss is irreversible and primarily affects trabecular rather than cortical bone. However, the rate of bone loss after the menopause slows after approximately 10 years [103].

Postmenopausal period, characterized by estrogen deficiency and its impact on bones, has been clearly established (North American Menopause Society).

The consequence of too early emerging shortage of estrogen is mainly reduction of bone mineral density (osteopenia, osteoporosis).

Even in young women with POI, osteoporosis may occur, hence the need for prescribing densitometry in such patients. Women with POI have a higher risk of bone fracture than women with osteoporosis on the other cause (hyperthyroidism, steroids, hyperparathyroidism).

Albright publications are the first to demonstrate the relationship between estrogen deficiency, menopause, and an increased incidence of fractures in women [104].

Women with POI are characterized by decreased bone density in comparison to women who regularly menstruate. Compared to Caucasians, minority of women

3 Premature Ovarian Insufficiency

with estrogen deficiency are more likely to have BMD below the expected range for age. Racial variance seems to be associated to a combined effect of several variable risk factors. Any delay in making POI diagnosis also contributes to reduced bone density by delaying proper therapy [105].

There is also the relation between the follicle-stimulating hormone (FSH) and estradiol levels with bone mineral density. It is said that serum FSH concentrations, but not estradiol, are positively associated with bone mass loss in skeletal regions (both at the lumbar spinal column and femoral neck) in patients with spontaneous POI [106]. The lumbar part of the spine was the most affected by the BMD decrease. Hormone replacement therapy should be substituted early and consistently among POI women [107].

Long-term physiological transdermal estradiol replacement therapy with oral medroxyprogesterone acetate restores mean BMD in femoral neck in women with POI. However, the addition of physiological transdermal testosterone replacement therapy did not provide additional benefit [108].

Age, reproductive age, and BMI are factors associated with the BMD of the lumbar spine. Women with the diagnosis of POI need early investigation and treatment to prevent bone loss and minimize fracture risk in the future [109].

Fracture risk in women with POI has also been discussed. Premature menopause is associated with the higher risk of fractures during lifetime. Women with premature menopause have relatively higher risks for fracture especially vertebral fracture of approximately 1.5. POI is thought to be an important predictor of fractures [110].

3.5.2 Cardiovascular Disease

The main reason of shortened life expectancy in POI patients is cardiovascular disease; therefore, some studies addressed the issue of cardiovascular risk in this group of women. To date, it has been shown that POI women present several risk factors for the development of cardiovascular disease: endothelial dysfunction, autonomic dysfunction, metabolic disturbances, and increased inflammatory factors.

Endothelial function measured as flow-mediated dilation of brachial artery has been shown to be significantly reduced in POI women. Similarly, the number of circulating endothelial progenitor cells is decreased and correlated with decreased serum estradiol concentration [111, 112]. POI women show increased carotid intima media thickness and left ventricular diastolic function [112]. Interestingly, the hormonal therapy of 6 months duration is able to improve flow-mediated dilation by 2.4-fold to the same levels as in healthy controls [111]. Goldmeier et al. [113] also showed normal endothelial dependent vasodilation in POI women under hormonal therapy. Despite this, in the same study, authors showed impaired baroreflex sensitivity and reduced heart rate variability of POI women (N = 17) in comparison to healthy controls [113].

POI patients present metabolic abnormalities, including increased incidence of dyslipidemia, insulin resistance, and elevated amount of abdominal fat [114]. Regarding the lipid profile, the results are conflicting regarding particular lipoproteins. As Knauff et al. [115] reported, POI women show significantly higher TG level and lower HDL cholesterol levels in comparison to controls after correction for age, body mass index, and smoking. This difference has not been confirmed in smaller study by Gulhan et al. [116]. This group revealed significantly higher TC and LDL levels in POI patients and a significant negative correlation between E2 and TC levels. Recently, Ates et al. [117] reported increased TC and HDL cholesterol in POI women. The analyzed population presented similar levels of glucose, insulin, HOMA-IR, low-density lipoprotein cholesterol (LDL-C), and triglyceride as the controls, but the incidence of metabolic syndrome was significantly increased. In contrary, other authors detected increased serum glucose, insulin, and homeostasis model of assessment-insulin resistance (HOMA-IR) in POI women [118]. Other reported risk factors found in POI women were increased C-reactive protein, hypertension, and impaired kidney function [114].

Even though there are conflicting data regarding lipid profile and insulin resistance indices, the overall cardiovascular risk in POI women seems to be significantly increased [119]. In recently published meta-analysis, the risk of ischemic heart disease was reported to be increased by 1.5 times in POI women in comparison to women who undergone menopause after 40 years old [120]. On the other hand, in comparison to other classical risk factors for cardiovascular disease, POI can be considered as modest risk factor for ischemic disease [121].

3.5.3 Psychological Aspects

The psychosocial aspects of POI are most often ignored in the context of the diagnosis.

POI is not a homogenous and fixed state. Distinct aspects of POI such as the absence or presence of vasomotor symptoms, as well as current treatment (e.g., fertility treatment), may impact upon different quality of life domains in distinctive ways. These effects may be mitigated by a number of variables, such as the absence or presence of a stable and satisfying relationship and/or children, and pre-POI mental health. Importantly, social and economic status is associated with access to social privileges and can powerfully influence quality of life domains so that the confounding effects of education, occupation, and income may need to be controlled for.

The decrease in the mood can be caused not only by concerns about their own health but also reproductive problems that occur in younger women who want to have children. Being diagnosed with POI can be an unexpected and upsetting diagnosis. Women with POI experience significant psychologic disturbances, such as high levels of depression and low levels of self-esteem, with negative effects on sexuality [122]. The diagnosis of POI can be an extremely devastating life experience and patients often express anger, depression, anxiety, loss, and sadness. Women after being informed of POI diagnosis can be shocked and confused. These words are describing their emotional trauma. Some of women with POI feel various emotions and caregivers should propose support regarding the unstable patient's self-image, neurocognitive decline, or sexual dysfunction.

Long-term medical conditions like POI are associated with a higher prevalence of psychological and mental health difficulties. Also, poorer psychosocial adjustment is seen in POI patients.

Poorer mental health is known to detrimentally affect capacity to self-manage health maintenance regimes and lifestyle changes leading to poorer health outcome and higher usage of healthcare services.

In women with POI, there is a higher prevalence of psychological distress. POI is said to be associated with an increased lifetime risk for major depression.

High levels of depression and perceived stress, lower levels of self-esteem, and life satisfaction are observed in women with the diagnosis of POI.

Moreover, the onset of depression frequently occurred after signs of altered ovarian function but before the diagnosis of POI.

More attention should be paid to the presence of depression in POI.

3.5.4 Mortality

Overall mortality is increased in women with POI. According to data from 19,731 women cohort from Norway, the menopause before 40 years old was linked to significantly increased mortality rate of 1.06 in comparison to women who had menopause at age 50–52 [123]. Also, early menopause has been shown to reduce the life expectancy. Data from a prospective cohort study of 68,154 US adult women showed that all-cause mortality rates were higher among women who reported that menopause occurred at age 40–44 years compared with women who reported that menopause occurred at age 50–54 years (rate ratio (RR) = 1.04, 95% confidence interval (CI): 1.00, 1.08) [124].

The increased risk of all-cause mortality is mainly dependent on higher mortality rates from coronary heart disease, respiratory disease, genitourinary disease, and external causes [114, 119].

3.6 Management

Premature ovarian insufficiency results in lifelong steroid deficiency. It is also potentially associated with accelerated health risk such as cardiovascular and cognitive disorders and osteoporosis. Moreover, the patients experience high psychological distress. Therefore, in dealing with physical and emotional needs of POI patients, multidisciplinary approach including endocrinologist, fertility specialist, oncologist, osteoporosis specialist, cardiologist, psychologist, dietician, and patient's support groups is crucial. General lifestyle modifications and dietary measures are recommended to reduce cardiovascular and osteoporosis risk. Adequate dietary intake of calcium and vitamin D as well as avoidance of smoking and maintenance of normal body weight involving weight-bearing exercise are recommended (1).

3.6.1 Hormonal Therapy

3.6.1.1 Hormonal Supplementation in Postpubertal POI Patients

Early initiated estrogen replacement is recommended in POI women to treat menopausal symptoms, maintain bone health and prevent osteoporosis, and control the future risk of cardiovascular disease (1). The treatment should be continued at least until the average age of natural menopause.

There is no agreed consensus on the optimum estrogen and progesterone replacement regimens in women with POI. Currently, combined hormone replacement therapy (HRT) is commonly prescribed. According to ESHRE recommendations, 17-β estradiol is preferred to ethinylestradiol or conjugated equine estrogens for estrogen replacement (1). Transdermal application of estrogen has theoretical advantage of delivering bio-identical estradiol directly into the systemic circulation, lowering risk of thromboembolism, and preserving sexual function by minimizing an impact on SHBG (2, 3). There is no consensus on optimal estrogen doses in women with POI. It has been suggested that transdermal administration of around 100 μg of estradiol results in serum levels equivalent to premenopausal mid-follicular concentrations (4). Cyclical progestogen should be administered in combination with estrogen therapy to protect the endometrium and to induce monthly withdrawal bleed. Many young women prefer cyclical regimen of hormonal treatment with regular monthly bleeding restoring a semblance of normality; however, a no-bleed regimen can be also adapted in some patients. There might be some metabolic and endometrial advantages associated with vaginal micronized progesterone (4, 5). However, the strongest evidence of endometrial protection is for oral cyclical combined treatment (1).

POI is associated with decrease in bone mineral density, whereas the increased risk of fracture has not been clearly demonstrated (1, 6). Beneficial effects of estrogen on bone metabolism result from reduction of osteoclastic and enhancement of osteoblastic activity as well as increase in calcium intestinal absorption and calcium renal reabsorption (7). Randomized controlled trial demonstrated that transdermal estradiol at the dose of 100 μg in regimen with oral medroxyprogesterone acetate restored bone density in 145 women with POI to that of healthy controls over 3 years (8).

Women with POI are at increased risk of cardiovascular diseases (1, 9). Although there is lack of longitudinal outcome data in POI patients, the potential beneficial effects of estrogen treatment on cardiovascular system might result from vasodilatation through endothelium and endothelium-independent mechanisms, favorable lipid and lipoprotein profile changes, as well as advantageous impact on glucose metabolism and fibrinolysis mechanisms (reviewed in 7).

Oral contraceptive pill (OCP) is an option for patients who do not desire pregnancy. Combined menopausal or bio-identical hormonal therapy is considered to be more physiological as it contains natural estrogen, whereas OCPs contain ethinylestradiol, carrying higher risk for thromboembolism, and higher doses of progestogen. However, many young women dislike the idea of treatment with specimens dedicated for menopausal women. Cartwright et al. assessed the effects of oral HRT, the OCP, and no treatment on bone density and turnover over 2 years in women with spontaneous POI (10). HRT group had significantly increased bone density at the lumbar spine compared with the OCP group. In the no-treatment group, there was a decrease in bone density at all sites compared to HRT and OCP groups (10). Crofton et al. performed similar study in POI patients comparing an impact on skeletal health of transdermal natural estradiol and vaginal micronized progesterone treatment with oral contraceptive pill over 12 months (11). The study demonstrated that physiological sex steroids replacement therapy might be more efficient in improving bone health, particularly in aspect of lumbar spine BMD, than OCP (11). Therefore, women choosing OCP as a form of hormone therapy due to POI should be informed that the effect on bone mineral density might be less favorable.

POI patients complain of worse sexual performance with more pain and poorer lubrication (12). Systemic hormonal therapy reestablishes the epithelium cells, vaginal pH, and vaginal microflora; however it might not enough effective in decreasing dyspareunia incidence (13). Local estrogen may be required to normalize sexual function. The knowledge of long-term efficacy and safety of testosterone supplementation in improving sexual function is incomplete (1).

There is strong difference in hormonal state between the patients experiencing spontaneous POI and the women in whom abrupt absence of ovarian function results from surgical treatment or chemo−/radiotherapy (14). The menopausal symptoms may be more severe in the latter group. Moreover, in spontaneous POI, the number of follicles is reduced with slow fluctuating decrease in estradiol production, but ovarian stroma still produces some androgens, whereas in iatrogenic POI, ovarian steroid production drops sharply. Therefore, patients with iatrogenic POI may require higher doses of hormone replacement therapy (3). Androgen treatment is only supported by limited data and is not routinely advocated (1).

There is no evidence that estrogen replacement in spontaneous POI increases the risk of breast cancer in comparison with normally menstruating women (15). Therefore, hormone therapy is recommended until the average age of natural menopause and there is no need to start mammographic screening early (16). It is, however, suggested that progestogen with lower potential risk should be preferentially used (17).

3.6.1.2 Puberty Induction

Young patients with primary amenorrhea due to ovarian dysgenesis or strong POI fail to initiate their ovarian function and do not manifest normal puberty. Initiation of hormonal therapy solely with estrogen is usually adopted to achieve pubertal maturation. The treatment prescribed by pediatric endocrinologists and adolescent gynecologist aims to achieve complete secondary sexual characteristics, sufficient uterine development, and adequate bone density, without an adverse effect on adequate growth.

In prepubertal girls with POI, dose and combination of hormone replacement therapy is adjusted according to the patient's height and the Tanner's stage of development to mimic puberty. European Society of Human Reproduction and Embryology recommends puberty induction with 17-β estradiol at the age of

12 years with a gradual increase over 2—3 years (1). Cyclical progestogen should be added after at least 2 years of treatment or when breakthrough bleeding occurs (1). According to these guidelines, oral contraceptive pills are contraindicated for puberty induction.

The uterine volume in women with POI might be reduced to 40% of the normal adult size, with poor blood flow and a thin endometrium (reviewed in 18). Women with primary amenorrhea are at the highest risk of decreased uterine volume. However, even girls with 5 years of menstrual cycles might not achieve a uterine development comparable with healthy peers (6). Moreover, the patients exposed to radiation may have reduced uterine volume and decreased elasticity. The optimal hormonal treatment regimen to maximize the reproductive potential for young women with POI remains unclear. Most studies that attempted to evaluate the effect of hormonal treatment on uterine cavity development were carried out in women with Turner syndrome. Better results were achieved in women with mosaic karyotype, with the earlier age of hormonal treatment commencement and with natural estrogen regimens (reviewed in 19). Some studies suggested better results with transdermal application route of natural estradiol (18, 19).

Long-lasting estrogen deprivation might have particularly deleterious effect on skeletal and cardiovascular systems in adolescents experiencing premature ovarian failure. The impact of estrogen deficiency on bone health is clearly related to the onset of ovarian impairment (6). Papagianni et al. investigated impact of hormone treatment on several endocrinologic, metabolic, and bone parameters in young women with very premature ovarian failure (7). The study group consisted of 40 women aged 14–20 years, including 12 subjects with Turner syndrome, 19 with Swyer syndrome, and 9 with very premature spontaneous ovarian insufficiency. The patients were treated for 2 years with conjugated estrogens on an oral daily dose of 0.625 mg and a daily oral dose of 5 mg medroxyprogesterone on days 17–28 of artificial cycle. Hormonal treatment resulted in adequate and stable serum estrogen levels in all patients. A significant favorable effect on HDL was noted from the first year of treatment and onward in patients with Turner syndrome and with Swyer syndrome, but not in nongenetic premature ovarian failure patients. The impact on bone density was beneficial. All patients with osteopenia recovered their z-scores after 1 year of treatment and significant gradual increase in bone density was noted during the second year of treatment.

3.6.1.3 Nonhormonal Therapies
The mainstay of POI therapy consists of different forms of HRT. Women who decline hormonal therapy or in whom it is contraindicated might benefit from nonhormonal treatment with selective serotonin reuptake inhibitors and norepinephrine reuptake inhibitors or gabapentin to control vasomotor symptoms (4). Such treatment, however, will have no benefit on future risk of osteoporosis and cardiovascular diseases.

There is no evidence for the use of complementary herbal preparations in POI patients.

Estrogen replacement is recommended to maintain bone health. If it is contraindicated or insufficient, other therapies may be considered. Bisphosphonates are not recommended in women who wish to achieve pregnancy (1).

3.6.2 Turner Syndrome Patients Management

Turner syndrome affects approximately 1 in 2000–2500 newborn females. The syndrome is caused by X-chromosome absence, structural abnormalities, or mosaicism and is characterized by an increased risk of primary or POI due to accelerated loss of germ cells before or after puberty. To some degree, the specific karyotype can predict the potential ovarian function in Turner syndrome patients. Monosomic patients (45,X) usually are born with streak gonads, whereas those with 45,X/46,XX mosaicism have the best chance of spontaneous puberty and fertility (20). Lunding et al. showed that AMH is a predictor for spontaneous puberty in prepubertal Turner syndrome girls and imminent POI in adolescents and adult Turner syndrome patients (20).

The patients with Turner syndrome need the multidisciplinary team care because of short statue, renal anomalies, heart defects, hearing problems, hypothyroidism, and delayed puberty and menstruation. Among the cardiovascular defects in Turner syndrome, the left-sided anomalies are the most common (coarctation of aorta, bicuspid aortic vessel, and aortic atresia).

The European Society of Human Reproduction and Embryology (ESHRE) gives specific recommendations for management of women with Turner syndrome (1):

1. Diagnostic workup for POI includes karyotyping for diagnosis of Turner syndrome.
2. If the test from peripheral blood lymphocytes is negative, a second analysis of the karyotype in epithelial cells is recommended in case of high clinical suspicion.
3. Women with Turner syndrome should be assessed by a cardiologist with expertise in congenital heart disease.
4. Cardiovascular risk factors such as blood pressure, smoking, weight, lipid profile, fasting plasma glucose, and HbA1c should be monitored annually.
5. Girls and women with POI due to Turner syndrome should be offered HRT throughout the normal reproductive lifespan.
6. Pregnancies in women with Turner syndrome are at very high risk of obstetric and non-obstetric complications and should be managed in an appropriate obstetric unit with cardiologist involvement.

3.6.3 Surveillance of Cancer Survivors

Recommendations for POI surveillance for female survivors of childhood, adolescent, and young adult cancer published in 2016 by International Late Effect of Childhood Cancer Guideline Harmonization Group in Collaboration with the PanCareSurFup Consortium revised already existing national guidelines and literature evidence and identified gaps in knowledge and future directions for research (21). Harmonized recommendations in cancer survivors should be based on counseling regarding the risk of POI and its implications for future fertility in the patients treated with alkylating agents and radiotherapy. After the treatment, annual monitoring of growth and pubertal development and progression (Tanner stage) is recommended for prepubertal survivors. For postpubertal survivors, a detailed history and physical examination with specific attention for POI symptoms, for example, amenorrhea or irregular cycles, is recommended. FSH and estradiol are recommended for evaluation of patients who fail to initiate or progress through puberty, in women with menstrual cycle dysfunction or who desire assessment about potential future fertility. AMH is not recommended as the primary surveillance modality. However, it may be reasonable to assess AMH in conjunction with FSH and estradiol in patients over 25 years (21).

Hormonal therapy with estrogen and progestogen is regarded contraindicated in breast cancer survivors (22). Adolescent patients experiencing acute ovarian failure after cancer treatment will not go through puberty without estrogen treatment (23). However, in the subsets of childhood cancer survivors, such as Hodgkin disease, and survivors with greater risk of breast cancer, heart disease, and stroke, hormonal therapy implementation should be individualized (24).

3.6.4 Supportive Management

The physical consequences of diminished ovarian function in women with POI have been studied extensively. However, much less is known about the repercussions of the loss of gonadal function on psychological and social factors in these women. Patients with spontaneous POI experience high level of distress at diagnosis. Nearly all the women described the diagnosis as traumatic, even when reported as having been sensitively handled (25). Clinicians have to communicate information about a sudden, unexpected diagnosis that is life alerting but not life threatening. The way it is delivered has a profound effect on patient's satisfaction, compliance to treatment, quality of life, and other health outcomes (26). In the research performed in the United States by Groff et al., assessing women's emotional responses to learning the diagnosis of POI, more than 70% were unsatisfied with the manner in which they were informed by their clinician. It is not surprising, considering that only 53% of women were informed in an office setting, and a substantial proportion (43%) was informed by a telephone call, in many cases while at work (26). Moreover, 75% of interviewed women reported that the clinician spent 15 min or less speaking about their diagnosis, with over one-third of women recalling spending 5 min or less. The majority of women got the impression that the physician had limited or very limited knowledge of POI (26). There are several steps that are important when communicating "bad news" to patient. Giving the indication that things are serious before giving the details may be helpful. After getting the physical context right, establishing how much the patient knows and how much she wants to know as well as responding to the patient's feeling is helpful in decreasing the patient's distress (27). The diagnosis and plan for management should take place during an office visit when sufficient time can be given to discuss the implications of POI (26).

Young women having POI have to deal with psychological distress, feeling of loss, anger, sadness, anxiety, fear of growing old, and low esteem (28, 29). For many women, the inability to reproduce is a profound loss. These women feel less feminine, sexually unattractive, and unproductive, exacerbating the effect of their loss of fertility (25, 28). Although no statistical differences were found in the perception of quality of life between the women with POI and those with normal ovarian function, poorer scores were identified in the physical health and psychological domains (28). Women with POI feel "less healthy" in general. POI patients report the presence of negative feelings (blue mood, despair, anxiety, depression, feeling that their life is meaningless) with the scores three times higher than control groups (28). Almost half of them request psychological support (25).

Women with idiopathic POI tend to report less support and satisfaction in their relationships compared to women with infertility resulting from known causes (28). Most patients perceive a need for clinicians to spend more time with them and provide more information about premature ovarian failure. Unfortunately, the study assessing POI patients' experience of health services in the United Kingdom disclosed that the main source of the information was the Internet. More than two-third of women affected by POI commented that insufficient information has been provided by their health professionals (25). The results of the study showed that the patients would expect information, understanding, and support at the time of the diagnosis, and regular follow-ups and psychological support later (25). Women value continuity of care, seeing the same professional on a regular basis. In those circumstances, they are more likely to feel sufficiently comfortable to ask about intimate issues as they arose such as vaginal dryness, libido, or impaired sexual well-being (25).

Informational and practical support can be provided sufficiently by specialist health professionals, the Internet, family, and friend. Emotional needs, however, are more demanding to address. For many patients, fertility concerns are associated with stigma and silence. Disclosure of the problem tends to be generally restricted to a small number of close friends or immediate family. Actual fear of rejection by a partner adds to feelings of isolation and distress. Women with POI should be offered individual and group support when dealing with their emotional needs. In the study carried out by Groff et al., only one-third of women reported seeking out professional help in dealing with the emotional and mental health aspects of POI, yet those who did most (76%) found this to be helpful (26). Only 20% of women had been involved in a support group, and most who had been found this to be helpful (85%) (26).

The emotional aspects are even more complicated in cancer survivors experiencing POI. Although most cancer patients receive the necessary information from health providers on treatment options and procedures at diagnosis, they often fail to receive support and guidance after acute treatment has completed (30). The cancer diagnosis is a shocking experience for many of patients; however, the cancer survivors have to face serious psychosocial problems after the treatment. Compared with postmenopausal women, premenopausal women with cancer may need to consider additional potential side effects of therapy. Receiving information on fertility and reproductive issues is important for younger women diagnosed with cancer. It helps to engage them in decision-making concerning treatment options. It should not be assumed that having children should not be a cancer patient's first priority. Moreover, the discussion about the treatment consequences in the future strongly indicates hope for survival and recovery. The cancer patients that have had extensive reproductive health counseling, including information on risks to fertility from cancer therapy, fertility preservation, and menopause, have a reduced distress and anxiety through cancer treatment. In general, patients who are better informed experience greater emotional well-being and report greater compliance with treatment and satisfaction with care (31).

3.6.5 Reproductive Issues

3.6.5.1 Resumption of Ovarian Function and Spontaneous Pregnancy Rate

Bidet et al. [82] assessed the incidence of resumption of ovarian function and spontaneous pregnancies in a group of 358 patients with non-iatrogenic POI (32). The authors observed intermittent ovarian function in 24% of patients and in 77% of cases within 1 year of diagnosis. Twenty-one spontaneous pregnancies (16 births, 5 miscarriages) occurred in 15 (4.4%) patients. Moreover, the authors reported on predictive factors for resumption of ovarian function in POF women. Among clinical features, age and secondary amenorrhea appeared to be critical factors for resumption of ovarian function in POF patients. Only two patients with primary amenorrhea showed resumption of ovarian activity. Familial history of POI was a good predictive factor for resumption of ovarian activity. FSH, estradiol, and inhibin B at the POI diagnosis appeared to be predictive of ovarian capacity to maintain partial activity. FSH level between 30 and 50 IU/l at diagnosis suggested a better prognosis than higher levels. Surprisingly, AMH levels were not predictive of resumption of ovarian activity in the presented study. The authors designed follow-up study of POI women after their first evaluation in a larger cohort of 507 patients (33). Among the patients with episodes of resumption of ovarian function (23%), the mean age of POI onset was 31.1 years and almost all patients (98.2%) were initially presented with secondary amenorrhea. During the follow-up period, 47% experienced an arrest of ovarian function. Higher FSH and DHEA levels were risk factors for arrest following the resumption of ovarian function. AMH level was not a predictive factor for the arrest of the resumption of ovarian function.

3.6.5.2 Fertility, Pregnancy, and Pregnancy Outcome

Premature ovarian failure in half of the affected women has intermittent and unpredictable course, and there is still 3–10% chance of spontaneous conception (17, 33).

Little progress has been made to improve reproduction with patients' own gametes. Several different interventions have been proposed to induce ovulation and achieve pregnancy in POI patients that were denied oocyte donation. The principles of proposed strategies include improvement of the ovarian responsiveness by suppression of circulating gonadotropins or immunomodulating treatment when an autoimmune origin was suspected. There are several studies evaluating the effectiveness of estrogen, standard hormonal replacement therapy, GnRH analogues, corticoids, or danazol pretreatment continued with ovarian stimulation with gonadotropins (34). Generally, ovulation and pregnancy rates for most of the strategies, assessed in systematic review performed by Robles et al. (34), were similar to the spontaneous pregnancy rates for these patients. However, some trials have reported improvements in ovulation rates when pharmacological doses of estrogen were used before gonadotropin therapy (35). Authors suggested that a threshold of FSH $\leq$ 15mIU/mL after estrogen pretreatment should be achieved for successful ovulation induction (35). The studies using immunomodulating agents would require a larger number of participating patients to have adequate power to prove influence on ovulation and pregnancy rates.

3.6.5.3 Obstetric Risks Associated with Premature Ovarian Insufficiency

According to ESHRE guidelines, women should be reassured that spontaneous pregnancies after idiopathic POI or most forms of chemotherapy do not show any higher obstetric or neonatal risk than in the general population (1).

Oocyte donation is the only proven and recommended treatment for women with POI. Cumulative pregnancy rates of oocyte donation treatment are very high and, after four cycles, reach 70–80% (34). However, such treatment is not available in some countries and not all patients would accept oocyte donation. Oocyte donation pregnancies are characterized by high rates of primiparity, advanced maternal age, and multiple gestations and are associated with increased rates of gestational complications such as gestational diabetes, hypertensive disorders, placental abnormalities, preterm delivery, and high rate of cesarean section (36). There is strong evidence that oocyte donation is a significant and independent risk factor for preeclampsia and gestational hypertension compared with pregnancies after other assisted reproductive technology methods or natural conceptions (37). The risk is independent of maternal age and multiple gestations (38).

Some other obstetric problems could be anticipated in women with premature ovarian insufficiency. Primary ovarian insufficiency manifested by primary amenorrhea and lack of normal puberty may result in inadequate uterus development despite estrogen replacement administration. Similarly, women who have received radiation to the uterus are at high risk for obstetric complications, such as early pregnancy loss, premature labor, or low birth weight.

A cardiologist should be involved in care of pregnant women with Turner syndrome and those who received anthracyclines or cardiac irradiation before gestation (1).

Turner Syndrome and Pregnancy

The Turner syndrome is caused by partial or complete loss of one of the X chromosomes. It is characterized by ovarian dysgenesis and a varying number of extragonadal abnormalities. In most of the Turner syndrome patients, accelerated follicular atresia leads to primary amenorrhea, absence of pubertal development, primary amenorrhea, and infertility. In some cases of mosaicism (45,X/46,XX), puberty and menstrual cycles occur. However, ultimately, the patients develop POI and have a limited time period during which they can become pregnant. The development of assisted reproduction technologies allowed women with Turner syndrome to achieve pregnancy through oocyte donation. Hormonal therapy in adolescents with Turner syndrome is implemented in order to achieve proper development of uterine cavity. Pregnancy rates in women with Turner syndrome after in vitro fertilization with donor oocytes are comparable to the rates achieved in women without this condition undergoing similar treatment (39). However, these pregnancies carry higher obstetric and non-obstetric risk. Therefore, women with Turner syndrome should be counseled and closely monitored. There are two large studies reviewing outcomes of almost two hundred pregnancies in women with Turner syndrome after oocyte donation (40, 41). The fetal and maternal risks in Turner syndrome patients, based mainly on mentioned two large studies, are summarized in an excellent review performed by Bouet et al. (39). There is higher risk of miscarriage (29%), perinatal fetal death (2%), small for gestational age (18–28%), prematurity (12%), and possible increased risk of fetal chromosomal abnormalities in pregnancies with autologous oocytes (39–41). Maternal risks include thyroid dysfunction (22%), gestational diabetes (4–9%), gestational hypertension (15–17%), preeclampsia (21%), and cesarean section (82%) (39–41). However, the most dangerous for the mother are cardiovascular complications: worsening of congenital heart disease (1%), heart failure (1%), aortic dissection (1–2%), and resulting maternal mortality of 2% (39–41). Therefore, in 2010, the national guidelines were published in France for the management of women with Turner syndrome (42). According to the recommendations, tests assessing thyroid, liver, and kidney function should be performed as well as blood pressure and gynecological assessment of uterine morphology need to be done. Detailed recommendations concerning check-up before pregnancy include cardiovascular examination with ultrasound examination and mandatory magnetic resonance angiography of the heart and aorta. According to these guidelines, pregnancy should be contraindicated in patients with a history of aortic surgery or dissection, when the diameter of the ascending aorta indexed for body surface area exceeds 2.5 cm/m^2 and in cases of coarctation of the aorta or resistant hypertension (42).

The American Society for Reproductive Medicine underlines that women with Turner syndrome at greatest risk of aortic dissection and rupture include those exhibiting baseline or progressive aortic root dilatation, bicuspid aortic valve, coarctation of the aorta with or without prior surgical repair, and hypertension (43). Women with Turner syndrome interested in oocyte donation should be carefully evaluated. Because of their small statue and body surface area, aortic diameter may not be an appropriate predictor of aortic dissection risk and should be adjusted by calculating the aortic size index (ASI). An ASI >2.0 cm/m^2 identifies the patients at a particularly increased risk for dissection and represents an absolute contraindication for attempting pregnancy in a woman with Turner syndrome (43). Women with Turner syndrome having a normal cardiac magnetic resonance and evaluation are still at much higher risk for associated morbidity and mortality and require careful observation throughout pregnancy and postpartum (43).

Apart from pregnancy resulted from oocyte donation, other techniques have been proposed to Turner syndrome patients in experimental settings. A spontaneous beginning of puberty occurs in 15–30% of girls with Turner syndrome, but only 2–5% reach menarche with the possibility of achieving pregnancy (44). Apparently, the dynamics of the disappearance is very individual. Borgström et al. performed laparoscopy in 57 adolescent Turner patients (44). They obtained ovarian tissue in 47 of the patients. In 15 (26%) patients, the existing follicles were identified histologically. In six of seven (86%) girls with mosaicism, follicles were found. Among the 22 girls with structural abnormalities of chromosome X, only 6 (27%) had follicles. The least chance of follicle incidence within the ovary had the girls with 45X karyotype (10.7%). Within the group of Turner girls with spontaneous onset of puberty, 58% had follicles in the tissue. In 13 girls that reached spontaneous menarche, 68% had follicles, while the girls with no signs of spontaneous puberty had only 10% of chance to have follicles identified during histological assessment. In general, five factors determinate the chances of finding remaining follicles in girls with Turner syndrome: karyotype, low FSH, high AMH, spontaneous onset of puberty, and spontaneous menarche (44). The authors of the study admitted that it was more unexpected that still some follicles were found in three girls without spontaneous puberty and in four girls with high serum concentrations of LH and FSH and low AMH levels.

Moreover, retrieval of immature oocytes from excised ovarian tissue followed by in vitro maturation and oocyte vitrification can be offered as an adjunct to ovarian tissue cryobanking (45). One important concern relates to the chromosome status of oocytes retrieved from young women with Turner syndrome. According to Borgström et al., the question cannot be neglected and possibly all women with Turner syndrome should be offered preimplantation diagnosis, chorion villous sampling, or amniocentesis if fertilization with their own oocytes is successful (44).

3.6.6 Oncofertility

There is overall increase in cancer prevalence followed by increase in long-term survival of the affected patients. The 5-year survival rate for childhood, adolescents, and young adult cancer currently exceeds 80% (21). The risk of nonsurgical POI among young cancer survivors is increased with cumulative incidence of 8% by age

40 years (21). Protection against iatrogenic infertility caused by chemotherapy, radiation therapy, or surgery assumes high priority. Evaluation of the likelihood of POI after chemotherapy or radiotherapy is often highly problematic. Individual risk of posttreatment infertility depends on the age and health status of the patient, ovarian reserve based on antral follicle count (AFC) or anti-mullerian hormone assessment, and nature of predicted treatment. The issue of possible infertility should be addressed and all oncologic patients having ahead their reproductive years. The patients should be informed of possible fertility preservation options before oncological treatment. None of the suggested methods is ideal and none guarantees future fertility in survivors. Therefore, combination of methods can be recommended for maximizing chances of future fertility (46). Fertility preservation strategies are not applicable for women with overt premature ovarian insufficiency [125].

3.6.6.1 Fertility-Sparing Surgery

It is estimated that 15–25% of women diagnosed with gynecological cancers are younger than 40 years old. Fertility-sparing surgery, after adequate counseling including oncological, fertility, and obstetrical outcomes, can be undertaken in some cases. This approach should only be discussed with women who want to be pregnant and whose chances of successful treatment of cancer would not be severely compromised by fertility-sparing surgery. The most common utilization of fertility-sparing surgery in genital tract tumors are unilateral oophorectomy in borderline and germ line ovarian cancers and radical vaginal trachelectomy in cervical cancer. Fertility-sparing surgical treatment may be considered in selected patients with stage 1A or 1C1, low-grade serous, endometrial, or mucinous ovarian cancer with expanding growth [126]. Moreover, trachelectomy may be considered in patients with HPV-related cervical squamous cell carcinomas or adenocarcinoma with <2 cm in size, with no or minimal vascular invasion and free lymph nodules [46, 122].

Diagnosis of endometrial carcinoma results in total hysterectomy with bilateral salpingo-oophorectomy. However, in premenopausal women wishing to conceive and with endometrial carcinoma with Grade 1, stage 1A without myometrial invasion and without risk factors, fertility-sparing treatment can be considered. Combined approach consists of hysteroscopic tumor resection, followed by 6–12 months treatment with progestins (oral megestrol acetate (160–320 mg/day) or medroxyprogesterone acetate (400–600 mg/day) and/or levonorgestrel intrauterine device) [127]. Pretreatment and control assessment should include hysteroscopic-guided endometrial biopsy, transvaginal US, and MRI performed by a specialized radiologist/sonographer. After completion of childbearing, definitive surgical treatment is performed.

3.6.6.2 Shielding to Reduce Radiation and Ovarian Transposition

The damage of female reproductive organs by radiation therapy is dose dependent. Age is also an important factor. Young women with high ovarian reserve may survive cancer treatment with a greater number of remaining primordial follicles and avoid POI and infertility problems. Apart from irradiation of ovaries, uterine radiation exposure may impair its growth during the pregnancy and increase risk of spontaneous abortion, premature labor, or intrauterine growth retardation. When possible, shielding to reduce radiation in young females should be applied. When shielding of the gonadal area is not possible, ovarian transposition should be considered. This procedure has been most commonly applied in gynecological cancers and in pelvic and abdominal Hodgkin's disease or sarcomas (48). Unfortunately, the procedure can be ineffective due to scattered radiation and damage of blood vessels that supply the ovaries.

3.6.6.3 Decreasing the Impact of Chemotherapy

The gonadotoxic effect of various chemotherapeutic agents is diverse. High-risk chemotherapeutic agents include alkylating agents such as cyclophosphamide, and medium-risk, platinum agents and anthracycline antibiotics, whereas low-risk chemotherapeutic agents include vinca plant alkaloids and antimetabolites. High-risk chemotherapeutic agent, cyclophosphamide, is also used to improve survival and reduce organ damage in severe connective tissue diseases and vasculitic syndromes (systemic lupus erythematosus, systemic sclerosis, Wegener's granulomatosis) with high incidence of POI, ranging from 30% to 60% (46).

The degree of ovarian follicle depletion depends also on the woman's age, chemotherapeutic regimen, and initial ovarian reserve. The reported POI rate after Hodgkin's lymphoma or breast cancer chemotherapy increases 2–3 times in women over 30 years old, compared to younger patients (46). GnRH analogues administration before and during chemotherapy treatment has been proposed to decrease POI incidence by simulating a prepubertal hormonal state. Numerous randomized trials, assessing impact of GnRH analogues (GnRHa) treatment during chemotherapy on POI incidence and fertility preservation, presented conflicting results. Therefore, the American Society of Clinical Oncology in 2013 stated that there is insufficient evidence regarding the effectiveness of ovarian suppression with GnRH analogues as a fertility preservation method, and these agents should not be relied on to preserve fertility (49). More recent meta-analyses, evaluating the efficacy of GnRHa given before and during chemotherapy in breast cancer patients in randomized controlled trials, concluded that GnRHa significantly reduces the risk of POI in young cancer patients and increases the chances for pregnancy [49, 50, 128]. Therefore, GnRH analogues are recommended only during chemotherapy in patients with breast cancer.

3.6.6.4 Oocyte and Embryo Cryopreservation

Several other methods have been proposed to preserve fertility. Cryopreservation of embryos and mature oocytes are clinically established methods (49, 52, 53). These options require controlled ovarian stimulation that will postpone cancer treatment for at least 2 weeks. Random start of the GnRh antagonist protocol is recommended. Double stimulation may be considered for optimal oocyte collection number. There are some concerns about the possible impact of exposure to high estradiol levels during ovarian stimulation in breast cancer patients. Therefore, several safer protocols can be offered, including natural cycle IVF or ovarian stimulation with letrozole or tamoxifen alone or in combination with gonadotropins (54). After oocyte retrieval, there is option to cryopreserve unfertilized oocytes or to split the oocytes to attempt both embryo and oocyte cryopreservation. Results of freezing of the mature oocytes have been improved with implementation of vitrification method, and the pregnancy rates and live births after thawing and fertilizing oocytes are currently reaching those obtained after embryo cryopreservation (around 25%) (48, 53). A study published in 2014 reported the birth of more than thousand babies resulting from vitrified-warmed oocytes, with no apparent increase in birth anomalies (55).

In 2011, a study by Kim et al. reported the birth of the first baby after oocyte vitrification in a patient with chronic myeloid leukemia (56). Following the report of Kim et al., several successful live births have been reported after oocyte vitrification in patients diagnosed with cancer. Still, it is difficult to predict the possibility of having a live birth according to the number of cryopreserved oocytes and success rates after cryopreservation of oocytes at the time of a cancer diagnosis may be lower than in women without cancer.

Remaining options such as retrieving immature oocytes aiming at maturing them later in vitro and freezing of gonadal tissue for a long time were considered experimental (49). However, ovarian tissue cryopreservation is increasingly adapted into practice in many countries and the results demonstrate that it might be highly effective technique for fertility preservation, providing a realistic chance for future pregnancy (57, 58).

3.6.6.5 Ovarian Tissue Cryopreservation

Cryopreservation of ovarian tissue is an option for prepubertal girls and women who cannot delay the start of chemotherapy. The method is also recommended for the postpubertal patients, even after a course of chemotherapy, when ovarian stimulation is no longer a viable option. Ovarian tissue is retrieved by laparoscopy and the procedure can be combined with previous ovarian stimulation or be performed at the same time as ovarian transposition. Then cortex tissue of the ovary is sliced and undergoes slow freezing procedure. Ovarian tissue cryopreservation should probably not be offered to patients with low ovarian reserve (AFC <5; AMH, 0.5 ng/ml) or with advanced age, because efficiency of the procedure is questionable above 36 years of age [111].

Once the cancer treatment is completed and the patient is disease-free, thawed ovarian tissue is reimplanted into the pelvic cavity (orthotopic site) or a heterotopic site like the forearm or abdominal wall. It takes 3.5–6.5 months after reimplantation before a rise in serum estradiol and a decrease in FSH are observed. Renewed ovarian endocrine function was reported in 95% of the women. AMH and inhibin B are not good predictors of graft function or probability to achieve pregnancy (59). Therefore, repeated measurements of FSH and estradiol levels inform about the resumption of ovarian function after transplantation. Half of the children born following ovarian tissue cryopreservation and transplantation resulted from natural conception.

Donnez et al. (58) reviewed the results of three centers (Belgium, Denmark, Spain) evaluating 60 orthotopic ovarian transplantations in women after cancer treatment (80%) and because of benign pathology (Turner syndrome, family history of POI, endometriosis, etc.). Restoration of ovarian activity was observed in a vast majority of patients (93%). Moreover, the authors showed the data of the worldwide series of 24 live births obtained by the year 2013. More than 50% of pregnancies were obtained naturally. Mean birth weight in singleton pregnancies was 3300 g and mean gestational age at time of delivery was 38–39 weeks (60).

Dittrich et al. (61) reported the results of 20 orthotropic retransplantations of cryopreserved ovarian tissue after cancer treatment. In 19 cases (95%), hormone activity in the ovary was observed at least in the form of an increase in serum estradiol levels. Initial signs of an increase in the estradiol level or follicle growth were documented on average of 3–6 months after transplantation. Seven women become pregnant. Six of these pregnancies were spontaneous and one followed IVF.

Meirow et al. (57) described the results of ovarian tissue cryopreservation and reimplantation in 20 patients by a single team. Among the patients without any ovarian activity before the transplantation, almost all (93.7%) regained their menses and half of the patients had FSH levels below 16 IU/l (57). A total of 14 patients underwent ovarian stimulation and IVF cycles with the pregnancy rates 18% per cycle and 26% per transfer. The live birth rate was 10.7% per cycle and 16% per transfer. The live birth rate per cycle was 8.8% in cases of preharvesting chemotherapy versus 13.6% in cases of no chemotherapy. In four patients, additional six pregnancies occurred spontaneously. Out of 10 live births, one newborn had a major malformation (arthrogryposis). None of the patients have experienced cancer recurrence, including the two women who had leukemia (mean time of follow-up after transplantation 3.18 years).

Jensen et al. gathered reassuring data on birth and perinatal outcome of 95 children delivered after ovarian tissue cryopreservation [129]. Half of the pregnancies resulted from natural conception and the mean birth weight was 3168 g. The findings supported ovarian cryopreservation as an established fertility preservation method.

Although there is some theoretical risk of reintroduction of cancer cells with the transplanted ovarian tissue, analysis of more than 300 transplantations revealed no such cases [130]. There appears to be no increased risk of congenital abnormalities for children born after ovarian tissue cryopreservation and transposition [111]. Specific selection criteria should be established in order to help the clinicians and their patients to make decisions [61].

3.6.6.6 Cryopreservation of Immature Oocytes

An important concern that still remains is the safety of ovarian tissue transplantation. There is the potential risk that malignant cells present in the frozen tissue may lead to recurrence of the primary disease after transplantation [60]. Retrieval of immature oocytes is performed in natural cycle and therefore can be offered to women who do not want any delay in cancer treatment or whenever a hormonal stimulation treatment is contraindicated. Immature oocytes can also be obtained from the ovarian tissue being prepared for cryopreservation giving additional strategy of fertility preservation. In vitro maturation of oocytes is still considered

3.6.6.7 Timing of the Conception After Therapy

It is not clear how much time should elapse between the end of chemotherapy and conception. Immediate pregnancy after completion of treatment is contraindicated due to the DNA toxicity of chemotherapy. If chemotherapy is administered in the first trimester of pregnancy, there is 16% incidence of fetal malformations [53]. Although "the gold standard time" has not been defined, preventing conception is recommended in the first 1–2 years after chemotherapeutic insult. Another reasons for abstaining from pregnancy are the high rate of recurrence and frequent need for tomography and other diagnostic tools during the first 2 years after treatment. Nevertheless, the risk of congenital anomalies in children born to mothers soon after completion of chemotherapy is similar to that found in the general population [53, 63]. However, data from the Swedish Medical Birth Registry concerning pregnancy course in breast cancer survivors revealed an increase in preterm births and low birth weights and delivery complications including higher rates of instrumental and cesarean section deliveries [64]. Therefore, those pregnancies should be regarded as higher risk pregnancies and carefully monitored. Historically, pregnancy after breast cancer was not recommended due to potential negative impact of increased estrogen and progesterone levels on patient's prognosis. Recent studies do not confirm the hypothesis and even show that pregnant women maintain trend toward better survival [65]. Pregnancy after breast cancer could be considered safe in terms of patient's prognosis [66].

3.6.7 Future Perspectives

3.6.7.1 In Vitro Activation (IVA)

New infertility treatment named in vitro activation (IVA) of dormant follicles has been proposed in patients with POI (68). Women with POI still have varying amounts of residual dormant follicles in ovaries. However, these follicles are difficult to grow spontaneously, and thus the patients unlikely conceive with their own oocytes. A number of intraovarian factors have been shown to be important for primordial follicle activation. IVA implements ovarian fragmentation disrupting of Hippo signaling pathway and treatment with PI3K (phosphatidylinositol-3-kinase) stimulator to activate dormant primordial and restrained secondary and preantral follicles in POF patients (68). Full cycle of IVA includes laparoscopic surgery to remove the ovary, which is subsequently cut into cortical strips and vitrified. After thawing of cryopreserved ovarian tissues, the ovarian strips are further fragmented and incubated for 2 days with PI3K stimulators. After that, the ovarian strips are autografted under laparoscopic surgery. Then the patient undergoes full protocol of ovarian stimulation and IVF procedure. Currently, two healthy babies were delivered, together with two additional pregnancies (68). The inventors of the method admit that to improve the efficiency of IVA, it is important to develop a noninvasive method to predict the presence of residual follicles before the first laparoscopy (68). Controlled studies would be required before IVA can be advocated for more widespread clinical use.

3.6.7.2 Stem Cells

Recent studies have focused on stem cell therapy of POI. Current dogma still holds that females are born with the finite pool of follicles which continue to decline until menopause. However, it has been postulated and next proved that mammalian ovary contains some ovarian stem cells that can give rise to fertilizable oocytes (69). Stimpfel et al. successfully characterized and differentiated in vitro stem cells from the adult human ovarian cortex (70).

Moreover, bone marrow mesenchymal stem cells, skin-derived mesenchymal stem cells, as well as umbilical cord blood stem cells and amniotic fluid stem cells have been used in animal models and showed some ability to prevent follicular atresia and rescue ovarian function (69).

The future application of these cells may open a new chapter in treatment of premature ovarian insufficiency.

References

1. European Society for Human Reproduction and Embryology (ESHRE) Guideline Group on POI, Webber L, Davies M, Anderson R, Bartlett J, Braat D, Cartwright B, Cifkova R, de Muinck Keizer-Schrama S, Hogervorst E, Janse F, Liao L, Vlaisavljevic V, Zillikens C, Vermeulen N. ESHRE guideline: management of women with premature ovarian insufficiency. Hum Reprod. 2016;31(5):926–37.
2. Vujovic S, et al. EMAS position statement: managing women with premature ovarian failure. Maturitas. 2010;67(1):91–3.
3. Cooper AR, Baker VL, Sterling EW, Ryan ME, Woodruff TK, Nelson LM. The time is now for a new approach to primary ovarian insufficiency. Fertil Steril. 2011;95:1890–7.
4. Kalantari H, Madani T, Zari Moradi S, Mansouri Z, Almadani N, Gourabi H, Mohseni MA. Cytogenetic analysis of 179 Iranian women with premature ovarian failure. Gynecol Endocrinol. 2013;29:588–91.
5. Meczekalski B, Podfigurna-Stopa A. Genetics of premature ovarian failure. Minerva Endocrinol. 2010;35(4):195–209.
6. Dube JL, Wang P, Elvin J, Lyons KM, Celeste AJ, Matzuk MM. The bone morphogenetic protein 15 gene is X-linked and expressed in oocytes. Mol Endocrinol. 1998;12:1809–17.
7. Di Pasquale E, Beck-Peccoz P, Persani L. Hypergonadotropic ovarian failure associated with an inherited mutation of human bone morphogenetic protein-15 (BMP15) gene. Am J Hum Genet. 2004;75:106–11.
8. Knight PG, Glister C. TGF-beta superfamily members and ovarian follicle development. Reproduction. 2006;132:191–206.
9. Laissue P, Christin-Maitre S, Touraine P, Kuttenn F, Ritvos O, Aittomaki K, Bourcigaux N, Jacquesson L, Bouchard P, Frydman R, Dewailly D, Reyss AC, Jeffery L, Bachelot A, Massin N, Fellous M, Veitia RA. Mutations and sequence variants in GDF9 and BMP15 in patients with premature ovarian failure. Eur J Endocrinol. 2006;154(5):739–44.
10. Takebayashi K, Takakura K, Wang H, Kimura F, Kasahara K, Noda Y. Mutation analysis of the growth differentiation factor-9 and -9B genes in patients with premature ovarian failure and polycystic ovary syndrome. Fertil Steril. 2000;74:976–9.

11. MacNaughton J, Banah M, McCloud P, Hee J, Burger H. Age related changes in follicle stimulating hormone, luteinizing hormone, oestradiol and immunoreactive inhibin in women of reproductive age. Clin Endocrinol. 1992;36:339–45.
12. Shelling AN, Burton KA, Chand AL, van Ee CC, France JT, Farquhar CM, et al. Inhibin: a candidate gene for premature ovarian failure. Hum Reprod. 2000;15:2644–9.
13. Marozzi A, Porta C, Vegetti W, Crosignani PG, Tibiletti MG, Dalprà L, et al. Mutation analysis of the inhibin alpha gene in a cohort of Italian women affected by ovarian failure. Hum Reprod. 2002;17:1741–5.
14. Rah H, Jeon YJ, Ko JJ, Kim JH, Kim YR, Cha SH, Choi Y, Lee WS, Kim NK. Association of inhibin α gene promoter polymorphisms with risk of idiopathic primary ovarian insufficiency in Korean women. Maturitas. 2014;77(2):163–7.
15. Verkerk AJ, Pieretti M, Sutcliffe JS, Fu YH, Kuhl DP, Pizzuti A, et al. Identification of a gene (FMR-1) containing a CGG repeat coincident with a breakpoint cluster region exhibiting length variation in fragile X syndrome. Cell. 1991;65:905–14.
16. Oostra BA, Willemsen R. FMR1: a gene with three faces. Biochim Biophys Acta. 2009;1790:467–77.
17. Murray A, Schoemaker MJ, Bennett CE, Ennis S, Macpherson JN, Jones M, Morris DH, Orr N, Ashworth A, Jacobs PA, Swerdlow AJ. Population- based estimates of the prevalence of FMR1 expansion mutations in women with early menopause and primary ovarian insufficiency. Genet Med. 2014;16:19–24.
18. Marchese A, Docherty JM, Nguyen T, Heiber M, Cheng R, Heng HH, et al. Cloning of human genes encoding novel G protein-coupled receptors. Genomics. 1994;23:609–18.
19. Mehlmann LM, Saeki Y, Tanaka S, Brennan TJ, Evsikov AV, Pendola FL, et al. The Gs-linked receptor GPR3 maintains meiotic arrest in mammalian oocytes. Science. 2004;306:1947–50.
20. Zhou S, Wang B, Ni F, Wang J, Cao Y, Ma X. GPR3 may not be a potential candidate gene for premature ovarian failure. Reprod Biomed Online. 2010 Jan;20(1):53–5.
21. Kovanci E, Simpson JL, Amato P, Rohozinski J, Heard MJ, Bishop CE, Carson SA. Oocyte-specific G-protein-coupled receptor 3 (GPR3): no perturbations found in 82 women with premature ovarian failure (first report). Fertil Steril. 2008;90(4):1269–71.
22. Köhler B, Lin L, Ferraz-de-Souza B, Wieacker P, Heidemann P, Schröder V, et al. Five novel mutations in steroidogenic factor 1 (SF1, NR5A1) in 46,XY patients with severe under androgenization but without adrenal insufficiency. Hum Mutat. 2008;29:59–64.
23. Lourenço D, Brauner R, Lin L, De Perdigo A, Weryha G, Muresan M, et al. Mutations in NR5A1 associated with ovarian insufficiency. N Engl J Med. 2009;360:1200–10.
24. Brenkman AB, Burgering BM. FoxO3a eggs on fertility and aging. Trends Mol Med. 2003;9:464–7.
25. Watkins WJ, Umbers AJ, Woad KJ, Harris SE, Winship IM, Gersak K, et al. Mutational screening of FOXO3A and FOXO1A in women with premature ovarian failure. Fertil Steril. 2006;86:1518–21.
26. Qin Y, Choi Y, Zhao H, Simpson JL, Chen ZJ, Rajkovic A. NOBOX homeobox mutation causes premature ovarian failure. Am J Hum Genet. 2007;81:576–81.
27. Qin Y, Shi Y, Zhao Y, Carson SA, Simpson JL, Chen ZJ. Mutation analysis of NOBOX homeodomain in Chinese women with premature ovarian failure. Fertil Steril. 2009;91:1507–9.
28. Bouilly J, Veitia RA, Binart N. NOBOX is a key FOXL2 partner involved in ovarian folliculogenesis. J Mol Cell Biol. 2014;6(2):175–7.
29. Soyal SM, Amleh A, Dean J. FIGalpha, a germ cell-specific transcription factor required for ovarian follicle formation. Development. 2000;127:645–54.
30. Zhao H, Chen ZJ, Qin Y, Shi Y, Wang S, Choi Y, et al. Transcription factor FIGLA is mutated in patients with premature ovarian failure. Am J Hum Genet. 2008;82:1342–8.
31. Tosh D, Rani HS, Murty US, Deenadayal A, Grover P. Mutational analysis of the FIGLA gene in women with idiopathic premature ovarian failure. Menopause. 2015 May;22(5):520–6.
32. Sybert VP, McCauley E. Turner's syndrome. N Engl J Med. 2004;351:1227–38.
33. Schachter H, Freeze HH. Glycosylation diseases: quo vadis? Biochim Biophys Acta. 2009;1792:925–30.

34. Laml T, Preyer O, Umek W, Hengstschlager M, Hanzal H. Genetic disorders in premature ovarian failure. Hum Reprod Update. 2002;8:483–91.
35. Banerjee S, Chakraborty P, Saha P, Bandyopadhyay SA, Banerjee S, Kabir SN. Ovotoxic effects of galactose involve attenuation of follicle-stimulating hormone bioactivity and up-regulation of granulosa cell p53 expression. PLoS One. 2012;2:e30709.
36. Albright F, Burnett CH, Smith PH, Parson W. Pseudohypoparathyroidism—an example of 'Seabright-Bantam Syndrome'. Endocrinology. 1942;30:922–32.
37. Giammona E, Beck-Peccoz P, Spada A. The gsalpha gene: predominant maternal origin of transcription in human thyroid gland and gonads. J Clin Endocrinol Metab. 2002;87:4736–40.
38. Alimohammadi M, Bjorklund P, Hallgren A, et al. Autoimmune polyendocrine syndrome type 1 and NALP5, a parathyroid autoantigen. N Engl J Med. 2008;358:1018–28.
39. Eisenbarth GS, Gottlieb PA. Autoimmune polyendocrine syndromes. N Engl J Med. 2004;350:2068–79.
40. Yu Wai Man CY, Smith T, Chinnery PF, Turnbull DM, Griffiths PG. Assessment of visual function in chronic progressive external ophthalmoplegia. Eye (Lond). 2006;20:564–8.
41. Pagnamenta AT, Taanman JW, Wilson CJ, Anderson NE, Marotta R, Duncan AJ, et al. Dominant inheritance of premature ovarian failure associated with mutant mitochondrial DNA polymerase gamma. Hum Reprod. 2006;21:2467–73.
42. Schiffmann R, Tedeschi G, Kinkel RP, Trapp BD, Frank JA, Kaneski CR, Brady RO, Barton NW, Nelson L, Yanovski JA. Leukodystrophy in patients with ovarian dysgenesis. Ann Neurol. 1997;41:654–61.
43. Fogli A, Schiffmann R, Bertini E, Ughetto S, Combes P, Eymard-Pierre E, et al. The effect of genotype on the natural history of eIF2B-related leukodystrophies. Neurology. 2004;62:1509–17.
44. Mavrou A, Tsangaris GT, Roma E, Kolialexi A. The ATM gene and ataxia telangiectasia. Anticancer Res. 2008;28:401–5.
45. Frappart PO, McKinnon PJ. Ataxia-telangiectasia and related diseases. NeuroMolecular Med. 2006;8:495–511.
46. Christin-Maitre S, Vasseur C, Portnoï MF, Bouchard P. Genes and premature ovarian failure. Mol Cell Endocrinol. 1998;145:75–80.
47. Kornak U, Mundlos S. Genetic disorders of the skeleton: a developmental approach. Am J Hum Genet. 2003;73:447–74.
48. Demirhan O, Türkmen S, Schwabe GC, Soyupak S, Akgül E, Tastemir D, et al. A homozygous BMPR1B mutation causes a new subtype of acromesomelic chondrodysplasia with genital anomalies. J Med Genet. 2005;42:314–7.
49. Crisponi L, Deiana M, Loi A, Chiappe F, Uda M, Amati P, et al. The putative forkhead transcription factor FOXL2 is mutated in blepharophimosis/ptosis/epicanthus inversus syndrome. Nat Genet. 2001;27:159–66.
50. De Baere E, Lemercier B, Christin-Maitre S, Durval D, Messiaen L, Fellous M, Veitia R. FOXL2 mutation screening in a large panel of POF patients and XX males. J Med Genet. 2002;8:e43.
51. Heddar A, Ogur C, Da Costa S, Braham I, Billaud-Rist L, Findikli N, Beneteau C, Reynaud R, Mahmoud K, Legrand S, Marchand M, Cedrin-Durnerin I, Cantalloube A, Peigne M, Bretault M, Dagher-Hayeck B, Perol S, Droumaguet C, Cavkaytar S, Nicolas-Bonne C, Elloumi H, Khrouf M, Rougier-LeMasle C, Fradin M, Le Boette E, Luigi F, Guerrot AM, Ginglinger E, Zampa A, Fauconnier A, Auger N, Paris F, Brischoux-Boucher E, Cabrol C, Brun A, Guyon L, Berard M, Riviere A, Gruchy N, Odent S, Gilbert-Dussardier B, Isidor B, Piard J, Lambert L, Hamamah S, Guedj AM, Brac de la Perriere A, Fernandez H, Raffin-Sanson ML, Polak M, Letur H, Epelboin S, Plu-Bureau G, Wołczyński S, Hieronimus S, Aittomaki K, Catteau-Jonard S, Misrahi M. Genetic landscape of a large cohort of primary ovarian insufficiency: new genes and pathways and implications for personalized medicine. EBioMedicine. 2022;84:104246.
52. França MM, Mendonca BB. Genetics of primary ovarian insufficiency in the next-generation sequencing era. J Endocr Soc. 2019;4(2):bvz037.

53. Ke H, Tang S, Guo T, Hou D, Jiao X, Li S, Luo W, Xu B, Zhao S, Li G, Zhang X, Xu S, Wang L, Wu Y, Wang J, Zhang F, Qin Y, Jin L, Chen ZJ. Landscape of pathogenic mutations in premature ovarian insufficiency. Nat Med. 2023;29(2):483–92.
54. Jaillard S, Bell K, Akloul L, Walton K, McElreavy K, Stocker WA, Beaumont M, Harrisson C, Jääskeläinen T, Palvimo JJ, Robevska G, Launay E, Satié AP, Listyasari N, Bendavid C, Sreenivasan R, Duros S, van den Bergen J, Henry C, Domin-Bernhard M, Cornevin L, Dejucq-Rainsford N, Belaud-Rotureau MA, Odent S, Ayers KL, Ravel C, Tucker EJ, Sinclair AH. New insights into the genetic basis of premature ovarian insufficiency: novel causative variants and candidate genes revealed by genomic sequencing. Maturitas. 2020;141:9–19.
55. Silva CA, Yamakami LY, Aikawa NE, Araujo DB, Carvalho JF, Bonfa E. Autoimmune primary ovarian insufficiency. Autoimmun Rev. 2014;13:427–30.
56. Hoek A, Schoemaker J, Drexhage HA. Premature ovarian failure and ovarian autoimmunity. Endocr Rev. 1997;18:107–34.
57. Hollowell JG, Staehling NW, Flanders WD, Hannon WH, Gunter EW, Spencer CA, Braverman LE. Serum TSH, T(4), and thyroid antibodies in the United States population (1988 to 1994): National Health and Nutrition Examination Survey (NHANES III). J Clin Endocrinol Metab. 2002;87:489–99.
58. Rubio-Gozalbo M, Gubbels C, Bakker J, Menheere P, Wodzig W, Land J. Gonadal function in male and female patients with classic galactosemia. Hum Reprod Update. 2010;16:177–88.
59. Ryan EL, Lynch ME, Taddeo E, Gleason TJ, Epstein MP, Fridovich-Keil JL. Cryptic residual GALT activity is a potential modifier of scholastic outcome in school age children with classic galactosemia. J Inherit Metab Dis. 2013;36:1049–61.
60. Kokcu A. Premature ovarian failure from current perspective. Gynecol Endocrinol. 2010;26:555–62.
61. Arora RS, Alston RD, Eden TO, Moran A, Geraci M, O'Hara C, Birch JM. Cancer at ages 15–29 years: the contrasting incidence in India and England. Pediatr Blood Cancer. 2012;58(1):55–60.
62. Chhabra S, Kutchi I. Fertility preservation in gynecological cancers. Clin Med Insights Reprod Health. 2013;21(7):49–59.
63. Ajala T, Rafi J, Larsen-Disney P, Howell R. Fertility preservation for cancer patients: a review. Obstet Gynecol Int. 2010;2010:160386.
64. Coccia ME, Rizzello F, Mariani G, Bulletti C, Palagiano A, Scarselli G. Ovarian surgery for bilateral endometriomas influences age at menopause. Hum Reprod. 2011;26(11):3000–7.
65. Haller-Kikkatalo K, Uibo R, Kurg A, Salumets A. The prevalence and phenotypic characteristics of spontaneous premature ovarian failure: a general population registry-based study. Hum Reprod. 2015;30(5):1229–38. https://doi.org/10.1093/humrep/dev021. Epub 2015 Feb 23.
66. Coulam CB, Adamson SC, Annegers JF. Incidence of premature ovarian failure. Obstet Gynecol. 1986;67:604–6.
67. Luborsky JL, Meyer P, Sowers MF, Gold EB, Santoro N. Premature menopause in a multi-ethnic population study of the menopause transition. Hum Reprod. 2003;18:199–206.
68. Wu X, Cai H, Kallianpur A, Li H, Yang G, Gao J, Xiang YB, Ji BT, Yu T, Zheng W, Shu XO. Impact of premature ovarian failure on mortality and morbidity among Chinese women. PLoS One. 2014;9:e89597.
69. Gold EB, Crawford SL, Avis NE, Crandall CJ, Matthews KA, Waetjen LE, Lee JS, Thurston R, Vuga M, Harlow SD. Factors related to age at natural menopause: longitudinal analyses from SWAN. Am J Epidemiol. 2013;178:70–83.
70. Ferrarini E, Russo L, Fruzzetti F, Agretti P, De Marco G, Dimida A, Gianetti E, Simoncini T, Simi P, Baldinotti F, Bennelli E, Pucci E, Pinchera A, Vitti P, Tonacchera M. Clinical characteristics and genetic analysis in women with premature ovarian insufficiency. Maturitas. 2013;74:61–7.
71. Nelson LM. Primary ovarian insufficiency. NEJM. 2009;360:606–14.
72. Maclaran K, Panay N. Current concepts in premature ovarian insufficiency. Womens Health. 2015;11:169–82.

73. Kovanci E, Schutt AK. Premature ovarian failure. Obstet Gynecol Clin N Am. 2015;42:153–61.
74. Cohen J, Chabbert-Buffet N, Darai E. Diminished ovarian reserve, premature ovarian failure, poor ovarian responder—a plea for universal definitions. J Assist Reprod Genet. 2015;32:1709–12.
75. Panay N, Kalu E. Management of premature ovarian failure. Best Pract Res Clin Obstet Gynaecol. 2009;23:129–40.
76. Vujovic S, Brincat M, Erel T, Gambacciani M, Lambrinoudaki I, Moen MH, Schenk-Gustafsson K, Tremollieres F, Rozenberg S, Rees M. EMAS position statement: managing women with premature ovarian failure. Maturitas. 2010;67:91–3.
77. The ESHRE Guideline Group on POI, Weber L, Davies M, Andersdon R, Bartlett J, Braat D, Cartwright B, Cifkowa R, de Muinck K-SS, Hogervorst E, Janse F, Liao L, Vlaisavljevic V, Zillikens C, Vermeulen N. ESHRE guideline: management of women with premature ovarian insufficiency. Hum Reprod. 2016;31:926–37.
78. Podfigurna-Stopa A, Czyżyk A, Grymowicz M, Smolarczyk R, Katulski K, Czajkowski K, Meczekalski B. Premature ovarian insufficiency: the context of long term effects. J Endocrinol Investig. 2016;39:983–90.
79. Gleicher N, Weghofer A, Oktay K, Barad D. Do etiologies of premature ovarian aging (POA) mimic those of premature ovarian failure (POF)? Hum Reprod. 2009;24:2395–400.
80. Ferraretti AP, La Marca A, Fauser BCJM, Tarlatzis B, Nargund G, Gianaroli L. ESHRE consensus on the definition of "poor response" to ovarian stimulation for in vitro fertilization: the Bologna criteria. Hum Reprod. 2011;26:1616–24.
81. Fenton AJ. Premature ovarian insufficiency; pathogenesis and management. J Mid-life Health. 2015;6:147–53.
82. Bidet M, Bachelot A, Bissauge E, Golmard JL, Gricourt S, Dulon J, Coussieu C, Badachi Y, Touraine P. Resumption of ovarian function and pregnancies in 358 patients with premature ovarian failure. J Clin Endocrinol Metab. 2011;96:3864–72.
83. Cameron M, Grover S, Moore P, Jayasinghe Y. Non-chromosomal, non-iatrogenic premature ovarian failure in an adolescent population: a case series. J Pediatr Adolesc Gynecol. 2008;21:3–8.
84. Massin N, Czernichow C, Thibaud E, Kutten F, Polak M, Touraine P. Idiopathic premature ovarian failure in 63 young women. Horm Res. 2006;65:89–95.
85. Dixit H, Rao L, Padmalatha V, Raseswari T, Kapu AK, Panda B, Murthy K, Tosh D, Nallari P, Deenadayal M, Gupta N, Chakrabarthy B, Singh L. Genes governing premature ovarian failure. Reprod Biomed Online. 2010;20:724–40.
86. Ebrahimi M, Asbagh FA. The role of autoimmunity in premature ovarian failure. Iran J Reprod Med. 2015;13:461–72.
87. Reato G, Morlin L, Chen S, Furmaniak J, Smith R, Masierro S, Albergoni MP, Cervato S, Zanchetta R, Betterle C. Premature ovarian failure in patients with autoimmune Addison's disease: clinical, genetic, and immunological evaluation. J Clin Endocrinol Metab. 2011;96:E1255–61.
88. Szlendak-Sauer K, Jakubik D, Kunicki M, Skórska J, Smolarczyk R. Autoimmune polyglandular syndrome type 3 (APS-3) among patients with premature ovarian insufficiency (POI). Europ J Obstet Gynecol Reprod Biol. 2016;203:61–5.
89. van Dorp W, Mulder RL, Kremer LCM, et al. Recommendations for premature ovarian insufficiency surveillance for female survivors of childhood, adolescent, and young adult cancer: a report from the international late effects of childhood cancer guideline harmonization group in collaboration with the PanCareSurFup consortium. J Clin Oncol. 2016;34:3440–50.
90. Mehta AE, Matwijiw I, Lyons EA, Faiman C. Noninvasive diagnosis of resistant ovary syndrome by ultrasonography. Fertil Steril. 1992;57:56–61.
91. Knauff EAH, Eijkemans MJC, Lambalk CB, et al. Anti-mullerian hormone, inhibin B, and antral follicle count in young women with ovarian failure. J Clin Endocrinol Metab. 2009;94:786–92.
92. Massin N, Gougeon A, Meduri G, et al. Significance of ovarian histology in the management of patients presenting a premature ovarian failure. Hum Reprod. 2004;19:2555–60.

93. Abe N, Takeuchi H, Kikuchi I, et al. Effectiveness of minilaparoscopy in the diagnosis of premature ovarian failure. J Obstet Gyneaecol Res. 2006;32:224–9.
94. Hirota Y, Ohara S, Nishizawa H, et al. Evaluation of laparoscopic management and clinical outcome in women with premature ovarian failure. Gynaecol Endosc. 2002;11:411–5.
95. de Carvalho BR, et al. Ovarian reserve evaluation: state of the art. J Assit Reprod Genet. 2008;25:311–22.
96. Gleicher N, Kushnir V, Barad D. Prospectively assessing risk for premature ovarian senescence in young females: a new paradigm. Reprod Biol Endocrinol. 2015;13:34.
97. Alipour F, Rasekhjahromi A, Maalhagh M, et al. Comparison of specificity and sensitivity of AMH and FSH in diagnosis of premature ovarian failure. Dis Markers. 2015;2015:585604.
98. Massin N, Meduri G, Bachelot A, et al. Evaluation of different markers of the ovarian reserve in patients presenting with premature ovarian failure. Mol Cell Endocrinol. 2008;282:95–100.
99. Saglam F, Onal ED, Ersoy R, et al. Anti-mullerian hormone as a marker of premature ovarian aging in autoimmune thyroid disease. Gynecol Endocrinol. 2015;31:165–8.
100. Schnatz PF. The 2010 North American Menopause Society position statement: updates on screening, prevention and management of postmenopausal osteoporosis. Conn Med. 2011;75(8):485–7.
101. Popat VB, Calis KA, Vanderhoof VH, Cizza G, Reynolds JC, Sebring N, Troendle JF, Nelson LM. Bone mineral density in estrogen-deficient young women. J Clin Endocrinol Metab. 2009;94(7):2277–83.
102. Banks E, Reeves GK, Beral V, Balkwill A, Liu B, Roddam A, Million Women Study Collaborators. Hip fracture incidence in relation to age, menopausal status, and age at menopause: prospective analysis. PLoS Med. 2009;6(11):e1000181.
103. Manolagas SC, O'Brien CA, Almeida M. The role of estrogen and androgen receptors in bone health and disease. Nat Rev Endocrinol. 2013 Dec;9(12):699–712.
104. Albright F, Smith P, Richardson AM. Post menopausal osteoporosis: its clinical features. JAMA. 1941;116:2465–74.
105. Daan NM, Muka T, Koster MP, Roeters van Lennep JE, Lambalk CB, Laven JS, Fauser CG, Meun C, de Rijke YB, Boersma E, Franco OH, Kavousi M, Fauser BC. Cardiovascular risk in women with premature ovarian insuffciency compared to premenopausal women at middle age. J Clin Endocrinol Metab. 2016;101(9):3306–15.
106. Lana MB, Straminsky V, Onetto C, Amuchastegui JM, Blanco G, Galluzzo L, Provenzano S, Nolting M. What is really responsible for bone loss in spontaneous premature ovarian failure? A new enigma. Gynecol Endocrinol. 2010;26(10):755–9.
107. Uygur D, Sengül O, Bayar D, Erdinç S, Batioğlu S, Mollamahmutoglu L. Bone loss in young women with premature ovarian failure. Arch Gynecol Obstet. 2005;273(1):17–9.
108. Popat VB, Calis KA, Kalantaridou SN, Vanderhoof VH, Koziol D, Troendle JF, Reynolds JC, Nelson LM. Bone mineral density in young women with primary ovarian insufficiency: results of a three-year randomized controlled trial of physiological transdermal estradiol and testosterone replacement. J Clin Endocrinol Metab. 2014;99(9):3418–26.
109. Leite-Silva P, Bedone A, Pinto-Neto AM, Costa JV, Costa-Paiva L. Factors associated with bone density in young women with karyotypically normal spontaneous premature ovarian failure. Arch Gynecol Obstet. 2009;280(2):177–81.
110. van Der Voort DJ, van Der Weijer PH, Barentsen R. Early menopause: increased fracture risk at older age. Osteoporos Int. 2003;14(6):525–30.
111. Yorgun H, Tokgözoğlu L, Canpolat U, Gürses KM, Bozdağ G, Yapıcı Z, Sahiner L, Kaya EB, Kabakçı G, Oto A, Tuncer M, Aytemir K. The cardiovascular effects of premature ovarian failure. Int J Cardiol. 2013;168(1):506–10.
112. Kalantaridou SN, Naka KK, Papanikolaou E, Kazakos N, Kravariti M, Calis KA, Paraskevaidis EA, Sideris DA, Tsatsoulis A, Chrousos GP, Michalis LK. Impaired endothelial function in young women with premature ovarian failure: normalization with hormone therapy. J Clin Endocrinol Metab. 2004;89(8):3907–13.

113. Goldmeier S, De Angelis K, Rabello Casali K, Vilodre C, Consolim-Colombo F, Belló Klein A, Plentz R, Spritzer P, Irigoyen MC. Cardiovascular autonomic dysfunction in primary ovarian insufficiency: clinical and experimental evidence. Am J Transl Res. 2013;6(1):91–101.
114. Daan NM, Muka T, Koster MP, Roeters van Lennep JE, Lambalk CB, Laven JS, Fauser CG, Meun C, de Rijke YB, Boersma E, Franco OH, Kavousi M, Fauser BC. Cardiovascular risk in women with premature ovarian insufficiency compared to premenopausal women at middle age. J Clin Endocrinol Metab. 2016;101(9):3306–15.
115. Knauff EA, Westerveld HE, Goverde AJ, Eijkemans MJ, Valkenburg O, van Santbrink EJ, Fauser BC, van der Schouw YT. Lipid profile of women with premature ovarian failure. Menopause. 2008;15(5):919–23.
116. Gulhan I, Bozkaya G, Uyar I, Oztekin D, Pamuk BO, Dogan E. Serum lipid levels in women with premature ovarian failure. Menopause. 2012;19(11):1231–4.
117. Ates S, Yesil G, Sevket O, Molla T, Yildiz S. Comparison of metabolic profile and abdominal fat distribution between karyotypically normal women with premature ovarian insufficiency and age matched controls. Maturitas. 2014;79(3):306–10.
118. Kulaksizoglu M, Ipekci SH, Kebapcilar L, Kebapcilar AG, Korkmaz H, Akyurek F, Baldane S, Gonen MS. Risk factors for diabetes mellitus in women with primary ovarian insufficiency. Biol Trace Elem Res. 2013;154(3):313–20.
119. Jacobsen BK, Knutsen SF, Fraser GE. Age at natural menopause and total mortality and mortality from ischemic heart disease: the Adventist health study. J Clin Epidemiol. 1999;52:303–7.
120. Tao XY, Zuo AZ, Wang JQ, Tao FB. Effect of primary ovarian insufficiency and early natural menopause on mortality: a meta-analysis. Climacteric. 2016;19(1):27–36.
121. Roeters van Lennep JE, Heida KY, Bots ML, Hoek A. Cardiovascular disease risk in women with premature ovarian insufficiency: a systematic review and meta-analysis. Eur J Prev Cardiol. 2016;23(2):178–86.
122. Schmidt PJ, Cardoso GM, Ross JL, Haq N, Rubinow DR, Bondy CA. Shyness, social anxiety, and impaired self-esteem in turner syndrome and premature ovarian failure. JAMA. 2006;295:1374–6.
123. Jacobsen BK, Heuch I, Kvåle G. Age at natural menopause and all-cause mortality: a 37-year follow-up of 19,731 Norwegian women. Am J Epidemiol. 2003;157(10):923–9.
124. Mondul AM, Rodriguez C, Jacobs EJ, Calle EE. Age at natural menopause and cause-specific mortality. Am J Epidemiol. 2005;162(11):1089–97.
125. The ESHRE Guideline Group on Female Fertility Preservation. ESHRE guideline: female fertility preservation. Hum Reprod Open. 2020;2020(4):1–17. https://doi.org/10.1093/hropen/hoaa052.
126. Kufel-Grabowska J, Łukaszuk K, Błażek M, et al. Fertility preservation during oncological treatment. Oncol Clin Pract. 2023;20:100. https://doi.org/10.5603/OCP.2023.0033.
127. Rodolakis A, Scambia G, Planchamp F, et al. ESGO/ESHRE/ESGE guidelines for the fertility-sparing treatment of patients with endometrial carcinoma. Hum Reprod Open. 2023;2023(1):hoac057. https://doi.org/10.1093/hropen/hoac057.
128. Senra JC, Roque M, Talim MCT, et al. Gonadotropin-releasing hormone agonists for ovarian protection during cancer chemotherapy: systematic review and meta-analysis. Ultrasound Obstet Gynecol. 2018;51:77–86. https://doi.org/10.1002/uog.18704.
129. Jensen AK, Macklon KT, Fedder J, et al. 86 successful births and 9 ongoing pregnancies worldwide in women transplanted with frozen-thawed ovarian tissue: focus on birth and perinatal outcome in 40 of these children. J Assist Reprod Genet. 2017;34:325–36. https://doi.org/10.1007/s10815-016-0843-9.
130. Gellert SE, Pors SE, Kristensen SG, Bay-Bjørn AM, Ernst E, Yding Andersen C. Transplantation of frozen-thawed ovarian tissue: an update on worldwide activity published in peer-reviewed papers and on the Danish cohort. J Assist Reprod Genet. 2018;35(4):561–70. https://doi.org/10.1007/s10815-018-1144-2.

Part II

Impact of Estrogen Depletion on Symptoms and Quality of Life

Clinical Symptoms and Quality of Life: Vasomotor Symptoms and Mood

4

Placido Llaneza and Cristina Llaneza-Suarez

Abstract

Hot flushes and night sweats are the predominant symptoms of menopause and usually, they are referred to as vasomotor symptoms. The mechanisms of increases in skin blood flow during hot flushes may include the withdrawal of sympathetic vasoconstrictor activity, increases in sympathetic cholinergic vasodilator activity, or a combination of both neural mechanisms and nonneural factors, with increased white matter hyperintensities suggesting that the relationship between hot flushes and cardiovascular risk observed in the periphery may extend to the brain.

The impact of vasomotor symptoms on mood and quality of life may be considerable and is often underestimated. Vasomotor symptoms were associated with decreased health-related quality of life, and baseline depression and obesity amplified this negative association. Hormonal therapy reduces the frequency and severity of hot flushes, with health benefits when started near menopause, particularly for women with early menopause. Several nonhormonal therapies including antidepressant drugs were also found effective for vasomotor symptoms over placebo. New nonhormonal neurokinin 3 receptor antagonist and dual neurokinin 1,3 receptor antagonists therapies open up a new avenue for the treatment of vasomotor symptoms with targeted therapies that do not require estrogen replacement.

P. Llaneza (✉)
Gynecological Endocrinology and Human Reproduction Unit, Hospital Central de Asturias, Universidad de Oviedo, Oviedo, Spain
e-mail: llaneza@uniovi.es

C. Llaneza-Suarez
Severo Ochoa Health Center, SESPA, Universidad de Oviedo, Oviedo, Spain
e-mail: UO290648@uniovi.es

4.1 Introduction

Hot flushes (HF) and night sweats are the predominant symptoms of menopause. These symptoms are distinct in both subjective and physiological aspects compared to other causes of flushing and blushing. The term "hot flash" typically denotes the acute sensation of heat, while the terms HF or vasomotor symptoms (VMS) encompass other sensations associated with this event. These sensations are linked to vascular reactivity characterized by initial pronounced vasodilation followed by vasoconstriction associated with estrogen withdrawal [1, 2].

The primary characteristic indicating a reduction in estrogen levels within the brain is the occurrence of VMS. Women describe these symptoms as a brief sensation of heat, accompanied by sweating and flushing that extends across the upper body, often accompanied by chills and anxiety. VMS may occur at any time of day or night and be spontaneous or triggered by a variety of common situations such as embarrassment, sudden changes in ambient temperature, stress, alcohol, caffeine, or the consumption of warm drink. The subjective features are individual and variable but typically start with a sudden sensation of heat or warmth, often accompanied by sweating, some reddening of the skin, and sometimes palpitations. Most often, this sensation begins in the upper body and spreads either upward or downward and infrequently all over the body. The perceived duration of VMS ranges from 30 s to 60 min, with an average duration typically falling between 3 and 4 min [3–5].

4.2 Prevalence

While some women report experiencing similar episodes at different stages of their reproductive life cycle, VMS typically starts before the menopause, often around the time of menstruation, and become more troublesome during the menopause transition and postmenopause stages. Approximately 75–85% of women going through natural menopause experience these symptoms, and 10–15% of women report severe and incapacitating symptoms. Notably, lower prevalence rates of VMS have been observed among Japanese and Southeast Asian women. Nevertheless, it is important to recognize that significant variability in the occurrence of VMS exists even among women from the same cultural background, and some studies have reported that Asian women who have migrated to Western countries have experienced in a manner similar to Caucasian women [6–8].

Surgical menopause or other conditions leading to an abrupt loss of ovarian function may be associated with more severe and persistent VMS. Furthermore, other factors, such as climate, diet, lifestyle, women's roles, and attitudes regarding the end of reproductive life and aging, have also been related to prevalence of VMS. Risk factors for VMS include obesity, African descent, lower socioeconomic status, the presence of premenstrual syndrome, a sedentary lifestyle, and smoking [4, 9]. The role of genetic factors has also been highlighted, and in one study evaluating single-nucleotide polymorphism (SNPs) in intronic regions of tachykinin receptor 3 gene, which codes for neurokinin B neuropeptide receptor, three SNPs (on chromosomes

3 and 11) were associated with HF, but these associations were observed exclusively within in an African American cohort [10].

4.3 Pathogenesis

Pathogenesis of VMS remains unknown. Considering that VMS are closely associated with menopause and tend to improve with estrogen therapy, estrogen deficiency seems to play a definite role in their causation. However, the precise role of estrogen deficiency remains to be fully understood. Notably, there is no significant correlation between serum estrogen levels and the frequency or severity of VMS. Furthermore, VMS tend to diminish over time after menopause, even as estrogen levels continue to decline. This suggests that the rate of decline in estrogen levels may be more critical than the actual decrease in estrogen levels itself. Another important factor is the need of a prior priming of the brain by estrogens, as women with ovarian dysgenesis only experience VMS after the withdrawal of estrogen replacement therapy [11, 12]. Peripheral estrogen levels do not differ between symptomatic and asymptomatic women, but symptomatic women have higher levels of central noradrenergic activation than asymptomatic women and elevated central noradrenergic activation narrows the thermoneutral zone, so the heat dissipation responses are triggered if the core body temperature crosses the upper threshold of the thermoneutral zone [13, 14].

The narrowing of the thermoregulatory zone is a theory proposed to explain the origin of VMS. In typically functioning women, heat loss mechanisms are activated when the core body temperature increases by 0.4 °C. However, in women experiencing HF, the vasodilatory response is initiated with a smaller increase in core body temperature. This peripheral vasodilatory response leads to profuse sweating and a sensation of intense heat. During HF, there is an increase in blood flow and hyperthermia in major parts of the body. Although the symptoms of HF are most intense in the head, neck, and upper chest, the most significant temperature increase occurs in the fingers and toes, where temperatures may rise from the normal range of 20–33 °C. The peripheral vasodilation results in heat loss, which lowers the core body temperature, as recorded in the rectum and tympanic membrane [15]. Usually, the subjective sensation of heat in the upper parts of the body seems out of proportion to the actual temperature increase, which in these areas may be only about 1 °C, and some authors have suggested that the severity of the sensation is probably related more to the rate of temperature change than to an actual temperature increase. The chills that accompany HF are a compensatory response aimed at restoring the core body temperature to normal [16–18].

An increase in heart rate coincides with the sensation of flushing during HF but typically returns to normal quickly. Multiple studies using electrocardiograph recordings did not detect changes in cardiac rhythm or in repolarization measurements during HF [17, 19], but a reduction in high-frequency heart rate variability has been also observed during HF. These changes appear to be associated with a potential increase in sympathetic activity without a discernible effect on parasympathetic activity, and a potential mechanism connecting autonomous nervous system, VMS, and cardiovascular disease (CVD) has been suggested [20–23].

In this context, some studies reported that women experiencing VMS are more likely to exhibit unfavorable CVD risk profiles compared to individuals without VMS. For instance, the SWAN study found that females with frequent VMS (at least six of the last 14 days) had a 77% higher risk of developing CVD compared with females with no or less frequent VMS [24]. Other studies employing more direct indicators of cardiovascular health detected differences between women with and without VMS. These differences include lower flow-mediated dilation (indicative of endothelial dysfunction), reduced forearm blood flow, greater aortic calcification, higher carotid intima-media thickness, and altered blood factors involved in clotting and fibrinolysis in women experiencing VMS. In the MsHeart study, VMS were linked to subclinical carotid atherosclerosis, and this connection could not be explained by CVD risk factors or sex hormone levels [25]. Lastly, according to several studies, VMS are among the strongest predictors of subclinical CVD and appears to be associated with a 50% increased risk of CVD events over the following 25 years, in the group of women with more frequent VMS reported at baseline [24, 26]. In contrast, a limited number of studies have reported either no association or even an inverse relationship between VMS and CVD [27–29].

A potential relation between hypothalamic neurons that contain luteinizing releasing hormone (LHRH) and the preoptic anterior nuclei that regulate body temperature was also suggested due to an observed surge in LH release during HF [16]. Serotonin and 5-hydrostryptamine (5-HT) has also been related to HF. Serotonin decreased by approximately 50% in postmenopause stage and the decline in estrogen levels is associated with a decrease in both 5-HT and endorphin levels. In this context, several indirect observations support the involvement of serotonin and norepinephrine in the generation of VMS. These include the increased plasma levels of the main brain metabolite of norepinephrine during HF, the favorable response of VMS to selective serotonin reuptake inhibitors (SSRIs), the reduction in VMS with clonidine (an α2 adrenergic antagonist) that decreases brain norepinephrine levels, and the potential triggering of VMS by yohimbine (an α2 adrenergic agonist) that increases brain levels of norepinephrine [17, 30]. In this sense, it must be considered that the mechanisms of increases in skin blood flow during VMS may include the withdrawal of sympathetic vasoconstrictor activity, increases in sympathetic cholinergic vasodilator activity, or a combination of both neural mechanisms and nonneural factors [31, 32].

Neuroimaging studies has shown changes in patterns of brain activity during HF in brainstem, insula, dorsal prefrontal cortex, and anterior cingulate, and there is evidence concerning the implication of central neuropeptides [33]. In the hypothalamus of postmenopausal women, there are dramatic changes in morphology and neuropeptide gene expression in the infundibular (arcuate) nucleus. Autopsy studies showed that these neurons increase in size (hypertrophy) accompanied by increased neurokinin B (NKB) and kisspeptin gene expression [34]. The hypertrophied neurons express estrogen receptor alpha and are called KNDy neurons based on the coexpression of kisspeptin, NKB, and dynorphin [35]. Nearly identical changes occur in young monkeys in response to ovariectomy and the changes are reversed by estrogen replacement. These data provide compelling evidence that hypertrophy and increased NKB and kisspeptin gene expression in postmenopausal women are due to estrogen withdrawal [36, 37]. Men and women with mutations in kisspeptin, NKB, or their receptors exhibit hypogonadotropic hypogonadism [38–40]. They do not go through puberty, are infertile, and secrete insufficient LH resulting in low levels of sex steroids. Thus, KNDy neurons express two peptides that are essential for human reproduction. Basic research in multiple species (including human) has established a role for KNDy neurons in regulating pulses of GnRH into the portal capillary system [41–44]. The close timing of LH pulses with hot flushes provides a clue that estrogen-responsive KNDy neurons could play a role in the generation of VMS [45].

To determine if KNDy neurons could play a role in thermoregulation, a series of studies were performed using a rat model (for a review, see [46]). Anatomical studies showed projections of KNDy neurons to the median preoptic nucleus (MnPO), an important component of the CNS pathway that regulates heat dissipation effectors [47, 48]. Moreover, MnPO neurons express the neurokinin 3 receptor (NK_3R), the primary receptor for NKB [34]. These data provide an anatomic framework to understand how estrogen-responsive KNDy neurons could specifically interface with hypothalamic brain areas that regulate heat dissipation effectors. Further studies using a rat model showed that KNDy neurons influence cutaneous vasodilation (flushing) via projections to NK_3R-expressing neurons in the MnPO [49–51].

Clinical studies have provided strong support for the hypothesis that KNDy neurons participate in the generation of hot flushes via NK_3R signaling. For example, infusion of NKB into the peripheral circulation induces hot flushes in women [52]. Moreover, genetic variation in the gene encoding the NK_3R receptor is associated with hot flushes in women [10]. More recently, several clinical trials have shown that treatment with an NK_3R antagonist successfully reduces the number and severity of hot flushes [53]. In the latest randomized, double-blind, placebo-controlled, phase 3 trials of nonhormonal NK_3R and dual $NK_{1,3}R$ antagonists compared to placebo, improvements in the frequency and severity of VSM were observed after 1 week and maintained over 52 weeks in the NK_3R antagonist trial [54] and after 1 week and maintained over 12 weeks in the dual $NK_{1,3}R$ antagonist trial [55]. These studies open up a new avenue for treatment of hot flushes with targeted therapies that do not require estrogen replacement.

4.4 Duration of VMS

Typically, VMS become evident within the initial 2 years following the onset of estrogen deficiency and have the potential to persist for a decade or more, with a median duration of approximately 7.4 years. Several studies on the duration of VMS suggest that women can expect VMS to continue, on average, for nearly 5 years after the final menstrual period. Around 25% of women still experience VMS 5 years after reaching menopause, and one-third continue to have VMS even a decade after menopause. Furthermore, 8% of women report the persistence of VMS even 20 years after entering menopause [3, 22].

The expected duration of menopausal VMS is important to women making decisions about possible treatments. In the Study of Women's Health Across the Nation (SWAN), conducted with a sample of 3302 women in the United States during the menopausal transition, the median total duration of VMS was found to be 7.4 years. Those who began experiencing VMS before reaching menopause had a longer duration (median 11.8 years) compared to those who were already postmenopausal when their VMS began (median of 3.4 years). Other factors as race/ethnicity, younger age, lower educational level, higher perceived stress and symptom sensitivity, as well as increased depressive symptoms and anxiety at the initial report of VMS were also associated with longer duration [9, 55]. On the contrary, Duffy et al. reported that women resilient to VMS were those who had not previously been bothered by their menstrual periods, were not experiencing somatic symptoms or night sweats, and perceived their symptoms as having a low impact on their lives [24]. Moreover, Perez-Lopez et al. in other study aimed to assess resilience, depressed mood, and menopausal symptoms in a sample of Spanish postmenopausal women have also reported that depressed mood and participation in regular exercise correlate with lower and higher resilience to menopausal symptoms. In this study, depressed mood was found to be associated with the severity of menopausal symptoms, both somatic and psychological [56]. Additionally, in a recent prospective study, a longer lifetime of lactation was associated with a decreased risk and shorter duration of frequent VMS in midlife women [57].

4.5 Vasomotor Symptoms, Depressed Mood, and Quality of Life

Health-related quality of life (HRQoL) is a subjective parameter which refers to the effects of an individual's physical state on all aspects of psychosocial functioning. It is defined as the value assigned to duration of life as modified by impairments, functional states, perceptions, and social opportunities that are influenced by disease, injury, treatment, or policy [58]. The specific domains of HRQoL include resilience or the capacity to respond to stress, health perceptions, physical functioning, and symptoms. Menopausal changes could affect HRQoL. Some domains of HRQoL may improve after menopause, but several transversal and longitudinal studies have reported negative effects of menopausal symptoms in HRQoL and the severity of menopausal symptoms is what reflects best the profile of quality-of-life dimensions [59–61].

Regardless of the frequency and severity of VMS, they are associated with a substantial impact on HRQoL [26, 62]. The impact of VMS on HRQoL may be considerable and is often underestimated. VMS may interfere with work and daily activities, as well as with sleep, causing subsequent fatigue, loss of concentration, and mood changes. All of which can interfere with family life, sexual function, and partner relationships, thereby affecting HRQoL [24, 25].

The impact of untreated VMS on HRQoL was studied in a sample of 252,000 working women with untreated VMS compared to asymptomatic age-matched women. During a 12-month period, the women with VMS showed increased work loss, 1.1 million extra medical visits, and a health insurance bill almost $400,000,000 more compared to the asymptomatic women [63]. In another recent study involving 11,452 European women, it was found that VMS had a greater impact on daily activities than on work-related activities. This impact was measured using the Work Productivity and Activity Impairment questionnaire. In this study, the prevalence of moderate-to-severe VMS among postmenopausal women aged 40–65 years was around 40% in the five European countries studied [8]. Lastly, Katon et al. [61] in a large sample of veteran and nonveteran US postmenopausal women found that any VMS was associated with decreased HRQoL and baseline depression, and obesity amplified the negative association between VMS and HRQoL.

Several studies have reported a reduction in blood flow through the middle cerebral artery during VMS, but in a recent meta-analysis study examining the effect of menopausal status on middle cerebral artery velocity, no differences were found between premenopausal and postmenopausal women [64]. However, VMS were linked to vascular and brain changes, with increased white matter hyperintensities suggesting that the relationship between VMS and CVR observed in the periphery may extend to the brain [65, 66]. These adverse brain changes observed during VMS may potentially be linked to mood swings and sleep disturbances commonly associated with VMS. Mood swings and disrupted sleep are among the most frequent complaints reported by women with VMS. Poor sleep quality often results in daytime fatigue and irritability. Sleep disruptions may occur even if the woman is not consciously aware of being awakened from sleep. Burleson et al. [67], in a study using multilevel structural equation modelling for testing whether changes in daily VMS occurrence predicted changes in occurrence of same-day sleep problems and changes in next-day positive and negative mood ratings and whether sleep problems mediated any predictive effect of symptoms on next-day mood, found, after controlling for initial depression, that daily VMS predicted same-day sleep problems and next-day positive mood although significant direct relationships between VMS and mood were found primarily only in women with initial depression scores in the low to moderate range. The authors suggested that any effect of VMS on mood may occur largely through a mechanism other than sleep disruption. However, Pinkerton et al. [68] in another placebo-controlled phase 3 trial using the Menopause-Specific Quality of Life (MSQOL) questionnaire found that frequency and severity of VMS showed approximately linear relationships with MSQOL and sleep parameters. Lastly, in a prospective study in a sample of midlife Chinese women progressing from perimenopause through natural menopause, a strong relationship between VMS bother and mood symptoms was detected [69].

Depressed mood symptoms and other depressive disorders are common among middle-aged women. Women are more vulnerable than men to depressive disorders [70] and endocrine influences have been postulated [71–73], but the effect of hormonal changes on depression and depressed mood remains unclear due to differences in coping style and response to stress or gender differences in socialization may also lead to higher rates of depression in women [74]. Notably, according to a meta-analysis, perimenopause is a phase particularly vulnerable for developing depressive symptoms and there are indications that VMS are positively related to depressive symptoms during menopausal transition [75]. Risk factors for the development of depressive symptoms and depression in the menopausal transition include the presence of VMS as well as a personal history of depression (particularly depression that is related to pregnancy or hormonal changes through the menstrual cycle), surgical menopause, adverse life events, and negative attitudes to menopause and aging [76]. Some studies have found that women with climacteric symptoms (HF, vaginal dryness, and dyspareunia) are more likely to report negative effect, anxiety, and/or depressive symptoms [77, 78]. Additionally, the risk for new-onset depression is heightened by more severe VMS [79]. Zhou et al., in a sample of Chinese women, reported an association between VMS, sleep quality, and depression [80], and Tomida et al. reported a similar association in a sample of Japanese women [81]. In another small Swedish study, anxiety and depression were significantly greater in women with surgical premature menopause [82], and Kronenberg et al. [83] reported that depressed feelings during VMS were more common in women after surgical menopause than with natural menopause and that suicidal thoughts during VMS occurred almost twice as often (10%) in these women. In a systematic review of the literature, a bidirectional association between HF and depressive symptoms has been reported in women presenting to menopause clinics [84]. However, not all studies report psychological disorders related to menopause [85] and other factors as biopsychosocial and partner factors could also have a significant influence on middle-aged women's sexuality and depressive disorders. Stress, educational level, ethnicity, socioeconomic factors, and partner status may also influence the prevalence and clinical course of both menopause symptoms and depressive disorders [72].

4.6 Vasomotor Symptoms Management with Nonhormonal Therapies

Hormonal therapy (HT) reduces the frequency and severity of VMS, with health benefits when started near menopause, particularly for women with early menopause. It carries small absolute risks and has potential health benefits on reduction of heart disease and all-cause mortality for women younger than 60 years and within 10 years of menopause [86]. However, long-term health risks in some women receiving HT for VMS were reported by the Women's Health Initiative and Million Women Study [87, 88]. Although data strongly support using HT in symptomatic women started near menopause, societal factors overwhelm the findings, and the use of HT has declined in a sustained fashion and some menopausal symptomatic women are treated with nonhormonal therapy.

Several nonhormonal therapies were found effective for VMS over placebo. NK3R antagonist or dual NK1,3R antagonist have demonstrated statistically significant reductions in VMS frequency and severity, as well as infrequent serious adverse events [54], improving sleep disorders and quality of life in women with VMS [55]. Other nonhormonal therapies as antidepressant drugs as SSRIs, serotonin norepinephrine reuptake inhibitors (SSNIs), and gabapentin have also been utilized in clinical practice. Fluoxetine, paroxetine, citalopram, escitalopram, venlafaxine, desvenlafaxine, gabapentin, and pregabalin, as well as low-dose paroxetine salt, have shown significant reductions in VMS over placebo [89, 90]. However, doses and the incidence of side effect as nauseas, dizziness, or even suicidal ideation when used in higher doses as an antidepressant must be considered. In a systematic review of articles published between 2003 and 2019, the findings regarding SSRIs indicated that escitalopram, paroxetine, and fluoxetine have demonstrated higher efficacy and safety in the treatment of menopausal HF compared to other drugs. Studies on the effectiveness of sertraline, citalopram, and fluvoxamine were either limited in number or yielded inconsistent results. Within the class of SNRIs, venlafaxine and desvenlafaxine exhibited significant efficacy in treating menopausal VMS [91, 92].

Acknowledgments The help of Prof. N. Rance from the University of Arizona College of Medicine in the implication of the KNDy neurons in hot flushes is acknowledged.

References

1. Archer DF, Sturdee DW, Baber R, de Villiers TJ, Pines A, Freedman RR, et al. Menopausal hot flushes and night sweats: where are we now? Climacteric. 2011;14(5):515–28.
2. Barlow DH. Continuing progress on vasomotor symptoms. Menopause. 2023;30(3):235–6.
3. Voda AM. Climacteric hot flash. Maturitas. 1981;3(1):73–90.
4. Freeman EW, Sammel MD, Lin H, Liu Z, Gracia CR. Duration of menopausal hot flushes and associated risk factors. Obstet Gynecol. 2011;117(5):1095–104.
5. Santoro N, Roeca C, Peters BA, Neal-Perry G. The menopause transition: signs, symptoms, and management options. J Clin Endocrinol Metab. 2021;106(1):1–15.
6. Gold EB, Colvin A, Avis N, Bromberger J, Greendale GA, Powell L, et al. Longitudinal analysis of the association between vasomotor symptoms and race/ethnicity across the menopausal transition: study of women's health across the nation. Am J Public Health. 2006;96(7):1226–35.
7. Lensen S, Archer D, Bell RJ, Carpenter JS, Christmas M, Davis SR, et al. A core outcome set for vasomotor symptoms associated with menopause: the COMMA (Core Outcomes in Menopause) global initiative. Menopause. 2021;28(8):852–8.
8. Nappi RE, Siddiqui E, Todorova L, Rea C, Gemmen E, Schultz NM. Prevalence and quality-of-life burden of vasomotor symptoms associated with menopause: a European cross-sectional survey. Maturitas. 2023;167:66–74.
9. Freeman EW, Sammel MD, Sanders RJ. Risk of long-term hot flashes after natural menopause: evidence from the Penn ovarian aging study cohort. Menopause. 2014;21(9):924–32.
10. Crandall CJ, Manson JE, Hohensee C, Horvath S, Wactawski-Wende J, LeBlanc ES, et al. Association of genetic variation in the tachykinin receptor 3 locus with hot flashes and night sweats in the women's health initiative study. Menopause. 2017;24(3):252–61.
11. Sturdee DW. The menopausal hot flush--anything new? Maturitas. 2008;60(1):42–9.
12. Bansal R, Aggarwal N. Menopausal hot flashes: a concise review. J Midlife Health. 2019;10(1):6–13.
13. Freedman RR, Woodward S. Core body temperature during menopausal hot flushes. Fertil Steril. 1996;65(6):1141–4.

14. Freedman RR, Woodward S, Sabharwal SC. Alpha 2-adrenergic mechanism in menopausal hot flushes. Obstet Gynecol. 1990;76(4):573–8.
15. Molnar GW. Body temperatures during menopausal hot flashes. J Appl Physiol. 1975;38(3):499–503.
16. Tataryn IV, Meldrum DR, Lu KH, Frumar AM, Judd HL. LH, FSH and skin temperature during the menopausal hot flash. J Clin Endocrinol Metab. 1979;49(1):152–4.
17. Sturdee DW, Hunter MS, Maki PM, Gupta P, Sassarini J, Stevenson JC, et al. The menopausal hot flush: a review. Climacteric. 2017;20(4):296–305.
18. Lobo RA. Menopause and aging. In: Yen & Jaffe's reproductive endocrinology [Internet]. Elsevier; 2014 [cited 2023 Feb 27]. p. 308–339.e8. Available from: https://linkinghub.elsevier.com/retrieve/pii/B9781455727582000159.
19. Lantto H, Mikkola TS, Tuomikoski P, Viitasalo M, Väänänen H, Sovijärvi ARA, et al. Cardiac repolarization in recently postmenopausal women with or without hot flushes. Menopause. 2016;23(5):528–34.
20. Lee JO, Kang SG, Kim SH, Park SJ, Song SW. The relationship between menopausal symptoms and heart rate variability in middle aged women. Korean J Fam Med. 2011;32(5):299–305.
21. Thurston RC, Christie IC, Matthews KA. Hot flashes and cardiac vagal control during women's daily lives. Menopause. 2012;19(4):406–12.
22. Hautamäki H, Piirilä P, Haapalahti P, Tuomikoski P, Sovijärvi ARA, Ylikorkala O, et al. Cardiovascular autonomic responsiveness in postmenopausal women with and without hot flushes. Maturitas. 2011;68(4):368–73.
23. Lee E, Anselmo M, Tahsin CT, Vanden Noven M, Stokes W, Carter JR, et al. Vasomotor symptoms of menopause, autonomic dysfunction, and cardiovascular disease. Am J Physiol Heart Circ Physiol. 2022;323(6):H1270–80.
24. Thurston RC, Aslanidou Vlachos HE, Derby CA, Jackson EA, Brooks MM, Matthews KA, et al. Menopausal vasomotor symptoms and risk of incident cardiovascular disease events in SWAN. J Am Heart Assoc. 2021;10(3):e017416.
25. Thurston RC, Chang Y, Barinas-Mitchell E, Jennings JR, Landsittel DP, Santoro N, et al. Menopausal hot flashes and carotid intima media thickness among midlife women. Stroke. 2016;47(12):2910–5.
26. Thurston RC. Vasomotor symptoms: natural history, physiology, and links with cardiovascular health. Climacteric. 2018;21(2):96–100.
27. Hitchcock CL, Elliott TG, Norman EG, Stajic V, Teede H, Prior JC. Hot flushes and night sweats differ in associations with cardiovascular markers in healthy early postmenopausal women. Menopause. 2012;19(11):1208–14.
28. Dam V, Dobson AJ, Onland-Moret NC, van der Schouw YT, Mishra GD. Vasomotor menopausal symptoms and cardiovascular disease risk in midlife: a longitudinal study. Maturitas. 2020;133:32–41.
29. Herber-Gast G, Brown WJ, Mishra GD. Hot flushes and night sweats are associated with coronary heart disease risk in midlife: a longitudinal study. BJOG. 2015;122(11):1560–7.
30. Freedman RR, Dinsay R. Clonidine raises the sweating threshold in symptomatic but not in asymptomatic postmenopausal women. Fertil Steril. 2000;74(1):20–3.
31. Berendsen HH. The role of serotonin in hot flushes. Maturitas. 2000;36(3):155–64.
32. Freedman RR, Woodward S, Mayes MM. Nonneural mediation of digital vasodilation during menopausal hot flushes. Gynecol Obstet Investig. 1994;38(3):206–9.
33. Diwadkar VA, Murphy ER, Freedman RR. Temporal sequencing of brain activations during naturally occurring thermoregulatory events. Cereb Cortex. 2014;24(11):3006–13.
34. Rance NE, Young WS. Hypertrophy and increased gene expression of neurons containing neurokinin-B and substance-P messenger ribonucleic acids in the hypothalami of postmenopausal women. Endocrinology. 1991;128(5):2239–47.
35. Goodman RL, Lehman MN, Smith JT, Coolen LM, de Oliveira CVR, Jafarzadehshirazi MR, et al. Kisspeptin neurons in the arcuate nucleus of the ewe express both dynorphin A and neurokinin B. Endocrinology. 2007;148(12):5752–60.

36. Rometo AM, Krajewski SJ, Voytko ML, Rance NE. Hypertrophy and increased kisspeptin gene expression in the hypothalamic infundibular nucleus of postmenopausal women and ovariectomized monkeys. J Clin Endocrinol Metab. 2007;92(7):2744–50.
37. Abel TW, Voytko ML, Rance NE. The effects of hormone replacement therapy on hypothalamic neuropeptide gene expression in a primate model of menopause. J Clin Endocrinol Metab. 1999;84(6):2111–8.
38. Seminara SB, Messager S, Chatzidaki EE, Thresher RR, Acierno JS, Shagoury JK, et al. The GPR54 gene as a regulator of puberty. N Engl J Med. 2003;349(17):1614–27.
39. de Roux N, Genin E, Carel JC, Matsuda F, Chaussain JL, Milgrom E. Hypogonadotropic hypogonadism due to loss of function of the KiSS1-derived peptide receptor GPR54. Proc Natl Acad Sci USA. 2003;100(19):10972–6.
40. Topaloglu AK, Reimann F, Guclu M, Yalin AS, Kotan LD, Porter KM, et al. TAC3 and TACR3 mutations in familial hypogonadotropic hypogonadism reveal a key role for Neurokinin B in the central control of reproduction. Nat Genet. 2009;41(3):354–8.
41. Rance NE, Krajewski SJ, Smith MA, Cholanian M, Dacks PA. Neurokinin B and the hypothalamic regulation of reproduction. Brain Res. 2010;1364:116–28.
42. Lehman MN, Coolen LM, Goodman RL. Minireview: kisspeptin/neurokinin B/dynorphin (KNDy) cells of the arcuate nucleus: a central node in the control of gonadotropin-releasing hormone secretion. Endocrinology. 2010;151(8):3479–89.
43. Wakabayashi Y, Nakada T, Murata K, Ohkura S, Mogi K, Navarro VM, et al. Neurokinin B and dynorphin A in kisspeptin neurons of the arcuate nucleus participate in generation of periodic oscillation of neural activity driving pulsatile gonadotropin-releasing hormone secretion in the goat. J Neurosci. 2010;30(8):3124–32.
44. Han SY, McLennan T, Czieselsky K, Herbison AE. Selective optogenetic activation of arcuate kisspeptin neurons generates pulsatile luteinizing hormone secretion. Proc Natl Acad Sci USA. 2015;112(42):13109–14.
45. Casper RF, Yen SS, Wilkes MM. Menopausal flushes: a neuroendocrine link with pulsatile luteninizing hormone secretion. Science. 1979;205(4408):823–5.
46. Rance NE, Dacks PA, Mittelman-Smith MA, Romanovsky AA, Krajewski-Hall SJ. Modulation of body temperature and LH secretion by hypothalamic KNDy (kisspeptin, neurokinin B and dynorphin) neurons: a novel hypothesis on the mechanism of hot flushes. Front Neuroendocrinol. 2013;34(3):211–27.
47. Krajewski SJ, Burke MC, Anderson MJ, McMullen NT, Rance NE. Forebrain projections of arcuate neurokinin B neurons demonstrated by anterograde tract-tracing and monosodium glutamate lesions in the rat. Neuroscience. 2010;166(2):680–97.
48. Nakamura K, Morrison SF. A thermosensory pathway mediating heat-defense responses. Proc Natl Acad Sci USA. 2010;107(19):8848–53.
49. Dacks PA, Krajewski SJ, Rance NE. Activation of neurokinin 3 receptors in the median preoptic nucleus decreases core temperature in the rat. Endocrinology. 2011;152(12):4894–905.
50. Mittelman-Smith MA, Williams H, Krajewski-Hall SJ, McMullen NT, Rance NE. Role for kisspeptin/neurokinin B/dynorphin (KNDy) neurons in cutaneous vasodilatation and the estrogen modulation of body temperature. Proc Natl Acad Sci USA. 2012;109(48):19846–51.
51. Mittelman-Smith MA, Krajewski-Hall SJ, McMullen NT, Rance NE. Neurokinin 3 receptor-expressing neurons in the median preoptic nucleus modulate heat-dissipation effectors in the female rat. Endocrinology. 2015;156(7):2552–62.
52. Jayasena CN, Comninos AN, Stefanopoulou E, Buckley A, Narayanaswamy S, Izzi-Engbeaya C, et al. Neurokinin B administration induces hot flushes in women. Sci Rep. 2015;5:8466.
53. Prague JK, Roberts RE, Comninos AN, Clarke S, Jayasena CN, Nash Z, et al. Neurokinin 3 receptor antagonism as a novel treatment for menopausal hot flushes: a phase 2, randomised, double-blind, placebo-controlled trial. Lancet. 2017;389(10081):1809–20.
54. Lederman S, Ottery FD, Cano A, Santoro N, Shapiro M, Stute P, et al. Fezolinetant for treatment of moderate-to-severe vasomotor symptoms associated with menopause (SKYLIGHT 1): a phase 3 randomised controlled study. Lancet. 2023;401(10382):1091–102.

55. Simon JA, Anderson RA, Ballantyne E, Bolognese J, Caetano C, Joffe H, et al. Efficacy and safety of elinzanetant, a selective neurokinin-1,3 receptor antagonist for vasomotor symptoms: a dose-finding clinical trial (SWITCH-1). Menopause. 2023;30(3):239–46.
56. Avis NE, Crawford SL, Greendale G, Bromberger JT, Everson-Rose SA, Gold EB, et al. Duration of menopausal vasomotor symptoms over the menopause transition. JAMA Intern Med. 2015;175(4):531–9.
57. Pérez-López FR, Pérez-Roncero G, Fernández-Iñarrea J, Fernández-Alonso AM, Chedraui P, Llaneza P, et al. Resilience, depressed mood, and menopausal symptoms in postmenopausal women. Menopause. 2014;21(2):159–64.
58. Scime NV, Shea AK, Faris PD, Brennand EA. Impact of lifetime lactation on the risk and duration of frequent vasomotor symptoms: a longitudinal dose-response analysis. BJOG. 2023;130(1):89–98.
59. Matthews KA, Bromberger JT. Does the menopausal transition affect health-related quality of life? Am J Med. 2005;118(Suppl 12B):25–36.
60. Schneider HPG. The quality of life in the post-menopausal woman. Best Pract Res Clin Obstet Gynaecol. 2002;16(3):395–409.
61. Ayers B, Hunter MS. Health-related quality of life of women with menopausal hot flushes and night sweats. Climacteric. 2013;16(2):235–9.
62. Katon JG, Gray KE, Gerber MR, Harrington LB, Woods NF, Weitlauf JC, et al. Vasomotor symptoms and quality of life among veteran and non-veteran postmenopausal women. Gerontologist. 2016;56(Suppl 1):S40–53.
63. Avis NE, Colvin A, Bromberger JT, Hess R, Matthews KA, Ory M, et al. Change in health-related quality of life over the menopausal transition in a multiethnic cohort of middle-aged women: study of women's health across the nation. Menopause. 2009;16(5):860–9.
64. Sarrel P, Portman D, Lefebvre P, Lafeuille MH, Grittner AM, Fortier J, et al. Incremental direct and indirect costs of untreated vasomotor symptoms. Menopause. 2015;22(3):260–6.
65. Ruediger SL, Koep JL, Keating SE, Pizzey FK, Coombes JS, Bailey TG. Effect of menopause on cerebral artery blood flow velocity and cerebrovascular reactivity: systematic review and meta-analysis. Maturitas. 2021;148:24–32.
66. Gordon JL, Rubinow DR, Thurston RC, Paulson J, Schmidt PJ, Girdler SS. Cardiovascular, hemodynamic, neuroendocrine, and inflammatory markers in women with and without vasomotor symptoms. Menopause. 2016;23(11):1189–98.
67. Thurston RC, Aizenstein HJ, Derby CA, Sejdić E, Maki PM. Menopausal hot flashes and white matter hyperintensities. Menopause. 2016;23(1):27–32.
68. Burleson MH, Todd M, Trevathan WR. Daily vasomotor symptoms, sleep problems, and mood: using daily data to evaluate the domino hypothesis in middle-aged women. Menopause. 2010;17(1):87–95.
69. Pinkerton JV, Abraham L, Bushmakin AG, Cappelleri JC, Komm BS. Relationship between changes in vasomotor symptoms and changes in menopause-specific quality of life and sleep parameters. Menopause. 2016;23(10):1060–6.
70. Tang R, Luo M, Li J, Peng Y, Wang Y, Liu B, et al. Relationships between vasomotor symptoms and mood in midlife urban Chinese women: observations in a prospective study. J Clin Endocrinol Metab. 2020;105(11):dgaa554.
71. Smith DJ, Kyle S, Forty L, Cooper C, Walters J, Russell E, et al. Differences in depressive symptom profile between males and females. J Affect Disord. 2008;108(3):279–84.
72. Unsal A, Tozun M, Ayranci U. Prevalence of depression among postmenopausal women and related characteristics. Climacteric. 2011;14(2):244–51.
73. Llaneza P, García-Portilla MP, Llaneza-Suárez D, Armott B, Pérez-López FR. Depressive disorders and the menopause transition. Maturitas. 2012;71(2):120–30.
74. Freeman EW. Associations of depression with the transition to menopause. Menopause. 2010;17(4):823–7.
75. Kaufert PA, Gilbert P, Tate R. The Manitoba project: a re-examination of the link between menopause and depression. Maturitas. 2008;61(1–2):54–66.

76. de Kruif M, Spijker AT, Molendijk ML. Depression during the perimenopause: a meta-analysis. J Affect Disord. 2016;206:174–80.
77. Vivian-Taylor J, Hickey M. Menopause and depression: is there a link? Maturitas. 2014;79(2):142–6.
78. Gibson CJ, Thurston RC, Bromberger JT, Kamarck T, Matthews KA. Negative affect and vasomotor symptoms in the study of women's health across the nation daily hormone study. Menopause. 2011;18(12):1270–7.
79. Seritan AL, Iosif AM, Park JH, DeatherageHand D, Sweet RL, Gold EB. Self-reported anxiety, depressive, and vasomotor symptoms: a study of perimenopausal women presenting to a specialized midlife assessment center. Menopause. 2010;17(2):410–5.
80. Cohen LS, Soares CN, Vitonis AF, Otto MW, Harlow BL. Risk for new onset of depression during the menopausal transition: the Harvard study of moods and cycles. Arch Gen Psychiatry. 2006;63(4):385–90.
81. Zhou Q, Wang B, Hua Q, Jin Q, Xie J, Ma J, et al. Investigation of the relationship between hot flashes, sweating and sleep quality in perimenopausal and postmenopausal women: the mediating effect of anxiety and depression. BMC Womens Health. 2021;21(1):293.
82. Tomida M, Otsuka R, Tange C, Nishita Y, Kimura T, Stoelzel M, et al. Vasomotor symptoms, sleep problems, and depressive symptoms in community-dwelling Japanese women. J Obstet Gynaecol Res. 2021;47(10):3677–90.
83. Nathorst-Böös J, von Schoultz B, Carlström K. Elective ovarian removal and estrogen replacement therapy--effects on sexual life, psychological well-being and androgen status. J Psychosom Obstet Gynaecol. 1993;14(4):283–93.
84. Kronenberg F. Hot flashes: epidemiology and physiology. Ann N Y Acad Sci. 1990;592:52–86. discussion 123–133.
85. Worsley R, Bell R, Kulkarni J, Davis SR. The association between vasomotor symptoms and depression during perimenopause: a systematic review. Maturitas. 2014;77(2):111–7.
86. Gibson CJ, Joffe H, Bromberger JT, Thurston RC, Lewis TT, Khalil N, et al. Mood symptoms after natural menopause and hysterectomy with and without bilateral oophorectomy among women in midlife. Obstet Gynecol. 2012;119(5):935–41.
87. Kaunitz AM, Manson JE. Management of Menopausal Symptoms. Obstet Gynecol. 2015;126(4):859–76.
88. Rossouw JE, Anderson GL, Prentice RL, LaCroix AZ, Kooperberg C, Stefanick ML, et al. Risks and benefits of estrogen plus progestin in healthy postmenopausal women: principal results from the women's health initiative randomized controlled trial. JAMA. 2002;288(3):321–33.
89. Rohan TE, Negassa A, Chlebowski RT, Habel L, McTiernan A, Ginsberg M, et al. Conjugated equine estrogen and risk of benign proliferative breast disease: a randomized controlled trial. J Natl Cancer Inst. 2008;100(8):563–71.
90. Pinkerton JV. Dose is important for nonhormonal therapy for hot flashes. BJOG. 2016;123(11):1744.
91. Wei D, Chen Y, Wu C, Wu Q, Yao L, Wang Q, et al. Effect and safety of paroxetine for vasomotor symptoms: systematic review and meta-analysis. BJOG. 2016;123(11):1735–43.
92. Azizi M, Khani S, Kamali M, Elyasi F. The efficacy and safety of selective serotonin reuptake inhibitors and serotonin-norepinephrine reuptake inhibitors in the treatment of menopausal hot flashes: a systematic review of clinical trials. Iran J Med Sci. 2022;47(3):173–93.

Clinical Symptoms and Quality of Life: Insomnia and Muscle/Joint Aches

Juan Enrique Blümel, María Soledad Vallejo, and Eugenio Arteaga

Abstract

Introduction
The variety of symptoms associated to menopause and the various forms how these symptoms affect a woman make it difficult to evaluate the impact of the estrogen deprivation on the health status. The development of the Menopause Rate Scale (MRS) has been considered a breakthrough to objectify the impact of menopause on the quality of life (QOL). Using this scale, a multinational study showed that the most prevalent menopausal symptoms were physical mental exhaustion (64.8%), joint/muscular discomfort (63%), depressive mood (60.5%), and sleep problems (59.0%); vasomotor symptoms were less frequent (54.5%). In this chapter, we will analyze only two symptoms, insomnia and muscle and joint aches.

Insomnia
Sleep disorders are highly prevalent in middle-aged women and they also deteriorate their QOL. They are closely associated with other climacteric symptoms, particularly hot flushes, suggesting a similar pathogenesis. Estrogen-related changes in serotonergic neuronal transmission, including changes in the number of serotonin transporter (SERT) binding sites, have been cited as a possible cause for changes in sleep, mood, and memory that occur during the menopausal transition. Menopause hormonal therapy (MHT) could contribute to the improvement of insomnia in women affected with menopausal symptoms.

J. E. Blümel (✉)
Medicina Interna Sur. Facultad de Medicina, Universidad de Chile, Santiago, Chile

M. S. Vallejo
Obstetricia y Ginecología, Hospital Clínico, Universidad de Chile, Santiago, Chile

E. Arteaga
Departamento de Endocrinología, Facultad de Medicina, Pontificia Universidad Católica de Chile, Santiago, Chile

Muscle and Joint Aches

They are another highly prevalent symptom in middle-aged women. As well as insomnia, this symptom has a higher prevalence in women complaining of other climacteric symptoms, particularly hot flushes. This relationship could suggest that hypoestrogenism is involved in pathogenesis of muscle and joint aches characteristic of the climacteric period. Estrogens, through glutamatergic receptors localized in dorsal horn neurons of the spinal cord, modulate pain pathways. In this regard, it is not surprising that HMT can associate to a lower risk of presenting musculoskeletal pain.

Conclusion

Hypoestrogenism characteristic of the menopausal period is not only associated with vasomotor symptoms but also with other symptoms like insomnia and joint aches, which not always is perceived as linked to menopause. MHT could have beneficial effects on all these symptoms.

5.1 Introduction

Health-related quality of life (HRQL) has been defined as the subjective assessment of a patient oriented to the exterior of himself and focused on the impact of the health status on the ability to lead a fulfilling life [1]. The multiplicity of symptoms associated to the climacteric and the subjective evaluation of the impact of this symptomatology in the welfare of a woman makes it difficult for the clinician to evaluate the potential impact of estrogen withdrawal on the woman's health.

The evaluation of the climacteric consequences on the woman's health and her HRQL has been traditionally done through clinical scores, whose main purpose is to provide a quantitative measurement of the efficacy of different medical interventions. A significant advance has been the development of the Menopause Rate Scale (MRS) [2]. This instrument is a validated questionnaire that assesses both the presence and severity of 11 symptoms divided in three subscales: (1) somatic-vegetative including VMS, cardiac disturbances, sleep difficulties, and muscular and articular discomfort or pain (items 1–3 and 11); (2) psychological: depressive mood, irritability, anxiety, and physical and mental exhaustion (items 4–7); and (3) urogenital: sexual difficulties, bladder problems, and vaginal dryness (items 8–10). Each item is rated as 0 (absent), 1 (mild), 2 (moderate), 3 (severe), and 4 (very severe). Mean and standard deviations for each item may be obtained in defined populations. The sum of means of defined items per subscale is the final value for the subscale and the sum of the three subscales corresponds to the total MRS score. The higher the score, the worse detriment in quality of life. According to this instrument, a severe impact on QOL is expected if the somatic-vegetative score is >8, the psychological is >6, the urogenital is >3, and the total MRS score is >16 [3].

Table 5.1 shows the score and the prevalence of climacteric symptoms evaluated with the Menopause Rating Scale in 8373 otherwise healthy women aged 40–59 years from 12 Latin American countries [4]. If we analyze separately each menopausal symptom, the most prevalent discomfort was joint/muscular

5 Clinical Symptoms and Quality of Life: Insomnia and Muscle/Joint Aches

Table 5.1 Scores and prevalence of climacteric symptoms (MRS) in midlife women

Domains	Score MRS (means ± SD)	% prevalence symptoms (CI 95%) Any	Severe
Somatic domain			
Hot flushes, sweating	1.02 ± 1.14	54.5 (53.5–55.6)	9.6 (9.0–10.3)
Heart discomfort	0.73 ± 0.97	43.8 (42.8–44.9)	5.0 (4.6–5.5)
Sleep problems	1.13 ± 1.18	59.0 (57.9–60.1)	13.2 (12.5–14.0)
Joint/muscular discomfort	1.25 ± 1.23	63.0 (61.9–64.0)	15.6 (14.8–16.4)
All symptoms	*4.12 ± 3.36*	*84.2 (83.4–84.9)*	*10.8 (10.1–11.4)*
Psychological domain			
4. Depressive mood	1.17 ± 1.19	60.5 (59.4–61.5)	13.7 (13.0–14.4)
5. Irritability	1.20 ± 1.13	64.6 (63.6–65.6)	12.3 (11.7–13.1)
6. Anxiety	0.99 ± 1.13	53.9 (52.8–55.0)	10.7 (10.1–11.4)
7. Physical mental exhaustion	1.24 ± 1.18	64.8 (63.7–65.8)	13.8 (13.0–14.5)
All symptoms	*4.60 ± 3.83*	*84.4 (83.6–85.2)*	*28.7 (27.7–29.7)*
Urogenital domains			
8. Sexual problems	0.90 ± 1.16	46.6 (45.6–47.7)	10.8 (10.2–11.5)
9. Bladder problems	0.76 ± 1.07	42.1 (41.0–43.1)	8.2 (7.6–8.8)
10. Dryness of vagina	0.89 ± 1.15	45.9 (44.9–47.0)	11.2 (10.5–11.9)
All symptoms	*2.54 ± 2.72*	*66.4 (65.4–67.4)*	*31.3 (30.3–32.3)*
Total	**11.27 ± 8.54**	**90.9 (90.2–91.5)**	**24.9 (24.0–25.8)**

discomfort, affecting 63% of women and reaching a severe intensity in 15.6% of them. Other prevalent symptom was physical mental exhaustion, with severe intensity in 13.8%. Other complaints of the psychological area are irritability, depressive mood, and anxiety, which globally provide 40.8% of the MRS total score, which constitutes it as the MRS domain with the greatest clinical deterioration in this report. Sleep problems affect 59.0% of women, with intense severity in 13.2% of them. The classical vasomotor symptoms, however, ranks ninth among the 11 symptoms evaluated by the MRS scale; in Europe, instead, it is the most prevalent symptom of postmenopausal women, affecting 74% of them [5]. Finally, urogenital symptoms, although ranking in the last position, reach a high intensity in 31.3% of the women. Globally, 24.9% of this population reached a total MRS score > 16, which means that these symptoms severely affect QOL [3].

The Menopause Rating Scale (MRS) is one of the most frequently used instruments to evaluate menopausal symptoms; however, no cutoff score is given that would indicate the need for treatment. One study determined, using ROC curve analysis, that the optimal cutoff score on the MRS to indicate the need for treatment would be 14. However, in clinical practice, a score of 4 for any of the MRS items could be taken to indicate the need for treatment [6].

5.2 Insomnia

In 2017–2020, US adults showed variability in sleep habits between workdays and free days, with longer sleep duration and later sleep-wake phases on free days, and high percentage of US adults experienced long-term sleep deprivation, chronic social jet lag, and frequent sleep disturbances [7]. Sleep disorders are highly prevalent in the general population mainly in females and particularly in persons with impaired physical or mental health [8, 9]. Therefore, it is not surprising that the deterioration of the QOL associated with climacteric is associated with a high risk of sleep disorders. The Study of Women's Health Across the Nation (SWAN), a multiethnic sample of 12,603 women, demonstrated that 38% of women aged 40–55 years presented with sleep disturbances and that menopause was significantly associated with sleep disorders [10]. This high percentage of insomnia in middle-aged women contrasts with prevalence of only 18% found in the general population [11].

Insomnia strongly affects the QOL. A German study, using the Short Form 36 Health Survey (SF-36), reported that only 3% of the interviewed who did not complain of insomnia had a bad QOL, but this percentage increased to 22% in those reporting insomnia [12]. Another study including three matched groups of severe insomniacs, mild insomniacs, and good sleepers recruited from the general French population, after eliminating those with DSM-IV criteria for anxiety or depression, showed that severe insomniacs had lower quality of life scores in eight dimensions of the SF-36 in comparison to mild insomniacs and good sleepers [13].

Sleep disorders not only deteriorate quality of life but also increase the risk of chronic diseases. Growing empirical evidence suggests that insomnia is strongly associated with significant medical morbidity including depression, dementia, hypertension, diabetes, and inflammatory processes [14]; however, it remains unclear whether the risk of mortality is increased for those suffering from insomnia. A meta-analysis with 17 studies, including a total of 36,938,981 individuals followed up for a mean of 11.6 years, reporting the association between mortality and frequent (≥ 3 nights/week), ongoing (≥ 1 month) insomnia, showed there was no difference in the odds of mortality for those individuals with symptoms of insomnia when compared to those without symptoms (OR = 1.06, 95%CI = 0.61–1.84, $p = 0.84$) [15].

Considering that the SWAN study showed a significant variation in the prevalence of sleep disorders among different ethnics, from 28% in Japanese women to 40% in Caucasian women [8], we intended to study the sleep disorders prevalence in Latin America [16]. On Table 5.2, it is shown that almost half of these women presented insomnia and/or bad sleep quality.

However, it is difficult to compare these results with other studies since the methodologies used are different. One of the most cited references is the Kravitz' study [8] which shows that 38% of women in the United States of America suffer "sleep difficulty," but this classification was based on a single question: "Over the past 2 weeks, have you experienced difficulty sleeping?" Another study [17], conducted in Latin America using the ISI test (Insomnia Severity Index), revealed that 41.5% of women aged 40–55 years had insomnia, almost identical to the 43.6% prevalence found when we applied the Athens scale to women of the same age. In a Japanese study, the sleep quality was self-rated by the participants in terms of sleep duration, sleep onset, sleep satisfaction, and number of awakenings per night, concluding that 50.8% of peri- and postmenopausal women presented insomnia [18]. Another study conducted in Turkey, using the Women's Health Initiative Insomnia Rating Scale,

5 Clinical Symptoms and Quality of Life: Insomnia and Muscle/Joint Aches

Table 5.2 Impact of age and climacteric status on insomnia and sleep quality

	Women 6079	Insomnia[1] % (IC 95%)	Poor sleep quality[2] % (IC 95%)
Age (years)			
40–44	1175	39.7 (36.9–42.5)	40.3 (37.4–43.1)
45–49	1692	43.1 (40.7–45.5)	45.3 (42.9–47.7)
50–54	1761	45.4 (43.0–47.7)	48.5 (46.1–50.9)
55–59	1451	45.2 (42.6–47.8)	49.3 (46.7–51.9)
p<		0.009[3]	0.0001[3]
Stage of menopause			
Premenopause 40–44 years	711	39.5 (35.9–43.2)	38.8 (35.2–42.5)
Premenopause ≥45 years	949	36.5 (33.4–39.6)	41.0 (37.9–44.2)
Perimenopause	916	41.7 (38.5–45.0)	43.7 (40.4–47.0)
Early postmenopause	1758	47.4 (45.0–49.7)	48.5 (46.1–50.8)
Late postmenopause	1745	46.3 (43.9–48.7)	51.1 (48.7–53.5)
p<		0.0001[3]	0.0001[3]

[1]Athens Insomnia Scale: score ≥6; [2]Pittsburgh Sleep Quality Index: score ≥5; [3]Square chi

the prevalence of sleep disturbance in women de 45 a 59 was 54% [19]. Summarizing, our results are in accordance with other studies conducted in different places in the world in spite of the usage of different methodologies showing that almost half of middle-aged women present sleep disorders.

Many women and their clinicians think that sleep worsens around menopause. However, there is some controversy. A well-regarded epidemiological study found that menopause does not worsen sleep quality [20]. Kalleinen, using objective methods to evaluate sleep quality as polysomnography, and specific questionnaires found that postmenopausal women had worse sleep quality than younger women (20–26 years old), but he believes that these changes may be more because of the physiology of aging than the rapid changes across menopause since similar sleep characteristics were already present in the premenopausal women [21]. We found that menopause slightly increased the risk of insomnia and it also increased somewhat more the poor quality of sleep (Table 5.2). Analyzing the different items of the Athens scale, the factor which has a greater impact in the total score was awakening during the night and the items which show the greatest increment in late postmenopause is difficulty with sleep induction. A Korean study agrees with our study showing the most common symptom of insomnia was difficulty maintaining sleep (9.7%), followed by difficulty initiating sleep (7.9%), and early morning awakening (7.5%) [22]. This last study, as well as ours, has shown that the diurnal impact of the sleep disturbances is rather low in postmenopausal women. We may conclude stating that menopause slightly deteriorates the sleep quality, mainly awakening during the night and sleep induction, disorders that have low impact on diurnal activities.

Although it seems that menopause does not severely affect the prevalence of sleep disorders, our results show that the most characteristic symptom of menopause, hot flushes, is significantly associated with a higher prevalence of insomnia (Table 5.3). Furthermore, the prevalence of sleep disorders shows a parallel increase

Table 5.3 Relationship between intensity of VMS and sleep disturbances

		Athens insomnia scale		
Intensity of VMS score (MRS)	N° Women	Score mean ± SD	Insomnia % (CI 95%)	OR (CI 95%)
0	2708	4.42 ± 4.63	32.2 (30.4–34.0)	1.00
1	2097	5.81 ± 4.49	48.1 (46.0–50.3)	1.96 (1.73–2.21)
2	934	7.13 ± 5.07	57.6 (54.4–60.8)	2.87 (2.45–3.35)
3	266	8.31 ± 4.90	67.7 (61.7–73.3)	4.41 (3.33–5.85)
4	74	9.34 ± 5.78	70.2 (58.4–80.2)	4.99 (2.92–8.57)
p<		0.0001[2]	0.0001[3]	0.0001[3]

VMS: vasomotor symptoms; MRS: menopause rating scale; p: [1]ANOVA; [2]Mann-Whitney; [3]Square chi tendency. Score SVM (MRS): 0: none, 1: mild, 2: moderate, 3: severe, 4: very severe

with vasomotor symptoms intensity, which may increase the risk of presenting insomnia in those women with severe vasomotor symptoms.

This association has been described by several authors [8, 13, 23] as well as the direct relationship between hot flushes severity and a higher prevalence of insomnia [24]. The discrepancy between studies showing no or minimal impact of the menopause on insomnia and the belief of physicians or patients concerning this topic could be due to the fact that physicians see symptomatic patients with intense hot flushes, who are those who present more insomnia. On the contrary, in the epidemiological studies, there are some women without hot flushes, which generally have lower prevalence of sleep disorders. In the same sense, insomnia was reported by 37.2% in France and Italy, 27.1% in the United States, and 6.6% in Japan [25], considering that Japanese women present with a lower prevalence of vasomotor symptoms than occidental ones [26].

Furthermore, we have observed that insomnia not only is associated to a higher risk of vasomotor symptoms but also to other climacteric-related symptoms (Table 5.4) [27]. As hot flushes do, the risk of insomnia increases with the severity of psychological symptoms, and the risk of insomnia also correlates with the severity of hot flushes. Anxiety has been associated to a four-fold increment in the risk of insomnia in the general population [28]. Depression occurs more commonly during the menopausal transition in women with vasomotor symptoms (VMS) than in those without [29], but most women with VMS do not develop depression. It has been hypothesized that VMS are associated with depression because VMS lead to repeated awakenings, which impair daytime well-being; nevertheless, sleep disturbances seen in depressed participants were not consistent with the etiology of depression secondary to VMS-associated awakenings [30]. In the same way, a study from Zervas et al. noted that mood symptoms seem to affect sleep, independent of vasomotor symptoms [31]. Therefore, we could speculate that psychological and vasomotor symptoms as well as sleep disorders in postmenopausal women are independent but related entities since all of them are triggered by a common cause:

Table 5.4 Risk factors for insomnia (Athens scale). Logistic regression analysis

Insomnia	OR	CI 95%
Troublesome drinker	5.27	1.14–24.51
Anxiety (Goldberg)	3.57	3.09–4.14
Depression (Goldberg)	2.39	2.10–2.72
VMS	2.10	1.86–2.38
Hypnotics	1.62	1.52–1.73
HT	1.41	1.18–1.68
Diabetes	1.37	1.11–1.68
Education >12 years	0.84	0.74–0.95

Logistic regression variables: depression (Goldberg), anxiety (Goldberg), smoker (>4 cigarettes/day), troublesome drinker, obesity, hypertension, diabetes, COPD, older ≥50 years, menopause, surgical menopause, VMS, HT, use of contraceptives, use of hypnotics, stable partner, education (>12 years). VSM: vasomotor symptoms; HT: hormone therapy; COPD: chronic obstructive pulmonary disease

estrogen decline [32]. The abovementioned three disorders have been linked with estrogen deficiency in the central nervous system. Therefore, changes in estradiol levels induce an elevated sympathetic activation acting through central alpha (2)-adrenergic receptors contributing to the initiation of hot flushes, possibly by narrowing the thermoneutral zone in symptomatic women; hot flushes are then triggered by small elevations in core body temperature acting within this narrowed zone [33]. The increased risk of menopause-associated depression enables us to postulate that depression is caused by the effect of fluctuations in estradiol on neurotransmitter system in the brain regions that regulate mood [34]. Anxiety has been linked to four neurotransmitter systems which are affected during menopause: gamma-aminobutyric acid, serotonin, noradrenaline, and dopamine [35]. Regarding insomnia, dopamine and serotonin are involved in sleep regulation [36]. Estrogen-related changes in serotonergic neuronal transmission, including changes in the number of serotonin transporter (SERT) binding sites, have been cited as a possible cause for changes in sleep, mood, and memory which occur during the menopausal transition [37]. Furthermore, selective serotonin depletion in the brain, a neurotransmitter classically involved in depression, is associated to insomnia in experimental animals [38].

Among the different risk factor for insomnia, in our logistic regression model, alcoholism appears as a strong independent factor. Cohn et al. had pointed out that in 57 abstinent alcoholics, 52 had sleep disorders [39]. Another factor associated with sleep disorders in our study was the use of hypnotics; however, this observation of a poor response of a proved efficacy therapy has been already reported in the literature for MHT [24] and for hypnotics themselves [40]. The possible explanation is that users of a drug to control sleep disorders are those who present the greatest symptomatology and, although the therapy improves the symptom, the irregular use of them, or the lack of adaptation of the doses to the patient needs, can cause the symptoms persistence in a greater magnitude than the average. Regarding the use of hypnotics in insomniacs, a study with peri- and postmenopausal women showed that these drugs improved the sleep disturbances [41]. MHT in that study also improved insomnia, but in our study, that situation did not happen; one explanation could be the fact that Latin American women have a high prevalence of hot flushes, a risk factor for insomnia, while the study previously mentioned was done in Asiatic women who are known to have less vasomotor symptoms [22] and in them, MHT could have better results on sleep quality considering they are less symptomatic. The logistic regression analysis also showed the high impact of depression and anxiety on the risk of sleep disorders. Finally, our study confirmed that educational level exerts a protective role against insomnia, a finding that was also detected in a Brazilian study [42]. Furthermore, other causes of sleep disorders in middle-aged women must be evaluated: poor sleep hygiene; volitional factors; environmental disturbances; alcohol intake; marital dissatisfaction; requests for care from children, grandchildren, and/or elderly parents; and financial worries. The medical conditions that may compromise sleep in this age group are common: obesity, gastroesophageal reflux, cancer, urinary incontinence and nocturia, thyroid dysfunction, chronic pain, fibromyalgia, and hypertension [43].

Classically, MHT has been considered an effective treatment for sleep disorders, but very few studies have applied specific instruments to evaluate this problem, and most of them include a rather low number of cases [44–47]. It is biologically plausible that MHT had a positive sleep effect since estrogen contributes to sleep through metabolizing norepinephrine, serotonin, and acetylcholine, which consequently increases REM cycles. Progesterone stimulates benzodiazepine receptors, causing the release of gamma-aminobutyric acid (GABA), a sedating neurotransmitter that can potentially facilitate sleep [48]. Contradicting the evidence that MHT improves sleep, the WHI study showed the opposite, i.e., that hormonal therapy had no effect on sleep disorders [49]. However, this study has a selection bias since women recruited for the study had only mild symptomatology, and for that reason, they should have had less sleep disorders. Even more, the WHI study showed that in the subgroup of woman 50–54 years of age with vasomotor symptoms at baseline, estrogen and progestin resulted beneficial effect on sleep disturbance.

Improving lifestyle can also improve sleep quality. In middle-aged women, low-mode- rate levels of exercise during 12–16 weeks significantly lower the Pittsburgh Sleep Quality Index score (improves sleep quality) compared with controls [50]. This result has been confirmed with studies that evaluate insomnia and physical activity with objective methods such as polysomnography and treadmill, respectively [51]. On the other hand, nutritional interventions may also alleviate menopause-related sleep disturbances as studies have shown that certain interventions (tart cherry juice or tryptophan-rich foods) can improve relevant aspects of sleep. An analysis of 59 studies shows that despite the large heterogeneity in the studies and choice of intervention, the majority reported that a nutritional intervention did benefit sleep in climacteric women and that it is mainly subjective sleep that is improved [52].

Another intervention that could be effective in treating sleep disorders in climacteric women is cognitive and behavioral therapies for insomnia. This therapy helps determine which thoughts and behaviors cause sleep problems or make them worse. You learn to replace these thoughts and behaviors with habits that promote deep sleep including stimulus control, sleep restriction, relaxation training, cognitive reconstruction, and sleep hygiene [53]. A meta-analysis that included 43 RCTs using cognitive behavioral therapy for insomnia found approximately 30-min increase of subjective and objective total sleep time [54].

Finally, we must mention that improving the quality of sleep, with any intervention, is important since the treatment of insomnia may reduce depressive symptoms, anxiety/worry symptoms, daytime sleepiness, fatigue, overall quality of life, daytime and social functioning, physical functioning, mental state, stress, and cognitive impairment. It could be a preventive strategy to combat the global burden of mental disorders [55].

We may conclude saying that the sleep disorders are highly prevalent in middle-aged women and affect their QOL. Hypoestrogenism is one of the factors involved in sleep quality deterioration observed in menopausal women. MHT could contribute to the improvement of insomnia in symptomatic postmenopausal women.

5.3 Muscle and Joint Aches

The International Association for the Study of Pain declared year 2010 as the "year against muscle skeletal pain," reflecting the relevance of this type of discomfort in different populations around the world. It is not surprising since these symptoms are highly prevalent in the general population, and they are a serious public health problem which strongly impaired work capacity and QOL [56], overload health systems [57], and have a high cost for companies [58]. It involves 10% of the general population but affects preferentially women, starting at the median age [59]. The SWAN study also showed this problem as the main menopausal symptom, affecting 54.3% of women 40–55 years old [60]. In Thailand, it is also the most prevalent symptom and affects 56.4% of postmenopausal, during the first year of amenorrhea [61]. In Latin American, we have found the same complain in 63% of women 40–59 years old (Table 5.1) [4]. A meta-analysis that included 16 studies estimated that overall prevalence of musculoskeletal pain among perimenopausal women was 71%. Perimenopausal women demonstrated a higher risk than premenopausal ones (OR: 1.63, 95% CI: 1.35–1.96). The odds of musculoskeletal pain increase linearly with age, from premenopause to peri- and then to postmenopause [62].

In a study whose objective was to evaluate the risk factors associated to muscle and joint aches in middle-aged women, we found that the presence of vasomotor symptoms strongly increased the risk of this symptom (Table 5.5) [63]. The association between vasomotor symptoms, a condition undoubtedly related to hypoestrogenism [64], and the presence of pain could suggest that in the pathogenesis of both symptoms could underlie common metabolic disorders. Furthermore, it has been observed that severity of muscle and joint aches correlates with a higher sympathetic activity in the CNS [65]. Coincidentally, this same disorder has been considered as a central element in the pathogenesis of vasomotor symptoms [28].

Table 5.5 Risk factors related to muscle and joint aches[1]: logistic regression analysis

Risks factors	Odds ratio	95% CI
Severe VMS[2]	6.27	5.34–7.36
History of psychiatric consulting	1.95	1.62–2.34
Premature menopause	1.73	1.13–2.65
Postmenopausal	1.20	1.11–1.29
Age ≥50 years	1.41	1.20–1.66
Use of psychotropic drugs	1.39	1.11–1.74
Current smoker	1.22	1.04–1.43
Education ≤12 years	1.16	1.01–1.34
Living at high altitude (>2500 m)	0.83	0.72–0.95
Sexually active	0.81	0.69–0.92
HT use	0.76	0.63–0.92
Access to private healthcare system	0.75	0.65–0.85
Good health (self-perception)	0.49	0.40–0.58

Taken from [63]
[1]Score MRS11 = 3or 4; [2]Score MRS1 = 3 or 4. VSM, vasomotor symptoms; HT, hormone therapy; OR, odd ratios; CI, confidence intervals. Nonsignificant variables: nulliparity, stable partner, surgical menopause, use of contraceptives, alternative therapies, use of IUD, attending church ceremonies, living in cities with average maximum temperatures ≥30 C

An elevated sympathetic activation acting through central alpha (2)-adrenergic receptors contributes to the initiation of hot flushes.

When a middle-aged woman complains of diffuse muscle and joint aches, pain or stiffness associated with tiredness, anxiety, and poor sleep, the diagnosis of fibromyalgia is postulated. In its pathogenesis, could be involved disorders in the neurotransmission linked both to pain perception as well as modulation of mood, sleep, and cognition. Cumulative evidence points to alterations in neurotransmitter systems in fibromyalgia, which is interesting because the main symptoms of fibromyalgia are closely linked to neurotransmitters. For example, central serotonin and noradrenalin are important in endogenous pain inhibitory pathways, substance P is a neuropeptide that is important for spinal nociception, and glutamate plays an important role in nociception as it has excitatory and sensitizing effects. Levels of serotonin, dopamine, and noradrenaline appear to be reduced, possibly contributing to dysfunctional descending pathways and resulting in attenuated descending inhibition. Tricyclic antidepressants, dual inhibitors of serotonin/noradrenalin reuptake, and pregabalin are treatments which could be effective to decrease pain and fatigue [66].

If we compare fibromyalgia and climacteric, we can observe that both conditions are very similar in terms of symptoms, pathogenesis, and response to treatment. Both conditions are observed in women older than 40 years; in their pathogenesis, changes in neurotransmitters and autonomic system are involved, symptomatology is almost identical, and both respond to estrogens and partially to antidepressants. Therefore, it seems to us reasonable to believe that an important percentage of fibromyalgia patients are women with climacteric symptoms, many of them even in the premenopausal period [67]. A recent article, agreeing with us, suggests that fibromyalgia can be considered a characteristic symptom of the climacteric [68].

The relationship between pain and estrogens has been suspected noting that women have 2–6 times more prevalence of pain, in comparison with men. Phylogenetically, estrogen is the first hormone that appears in the primitive living being 500 million years ago, fulfilling a role in homeostatic systems which contribute to bodily integrity, modulating intracellular signals that cause motor responses to avoid damage (nociception) [69].

Estrogen receptors alpha are observed in the dorsal horn of the spinal cord in humans, where they are also essential in nociception, reducing glutaminergic transmission and inhibiting pain perception. Furthermore, estradiol increases the expression of opioid mRNA in the spinal cord, blocking the sense of pain. But it does not only act in the nociceptive circuit in the spinal cord but also in the transmission paths to the cortex, inhibiting the sense of pain and at the CNS level, it acts in different pain-related areas such as thalamus, anterior cingulate cortex, and dorsal posterior insula [70].

Estrogens declination during climacteric, through their effects on the pain pathways, could be the cause of the increase in muscle and joint aches observed in middle-aged women. Another fact which reinforces this relationship would be the decrease in the sense of pain associated to MHT. The most important RCT done until now, related to MHT, has been the Women's Health Initiative (WHI), a trial including of 16,608 postmenopausal women, mean age 63.3 years, randomized to 0.625 mg conjugated equine estrogens plus 2.5 mg medroxyprogesterone acetate or placebo. Changes in symptoms and treatment-related effects were analyzed at year 1 in all participants. It was observed that women assigned to MHT reported relief of joint pain or stiffness and general aches or pain [71]. Another study conducted in commonwealth countries with 3721 women with a uterus randomized to combined estrogen and progestogen or placebo showed that significantly fewer women in the combined HRT group reported aching joints and muscles [72]. Similarly, another RCT using raloxifene, a Selective Estrogen Receptor Modulators (SERMs), in patients with fibromyalgia showed that this drug, which mimics estrogen action, was also associated to a greater improvement in pain and fatigue compared to placebo, produced a significant decrease of the tender points counts and sleep disturbances, and gave the possibility to reinsert in their usual activities [73]. On the contrary, it has been reported that 23% of women using aromatase inhibitors, which is associated to a profound hypoestrogenism, experience musculoskeletal symptoms [74]. Finally, a last observation in agreement with the hypothesis described above is the fact that the increase in muscle and joint aches after MHT discontinuation has been reported [75].

It seems that socioeconomic level also influences the type of climacteric symptoms that women present; thus, whereas women in higher-status work tend to regard vasomotor symptoms as their main physical symptom, women in casual work report musculoskeletal pain as more problematic [76]. Another factor that has also been related to pain is diet; a study shows increased knee pain in climacteric women with poor quality diets, a symptom that is independent of the presence of osteoarthritis [77].

We can conclude by saying that there is a high prevalence of muscle and joint aches in middle-aged women and that there is a strong parallelism between these symptoms and other variables associated with the climacteric status, mainly hot flushes. This relationship could suggest that hypoestrogenism could be involved in muscle and joint aches pathogenesis in postmenopausal women. The role of estrogens is related with the pain pathways modulation. MHT is associated to a lower risk to present musculoskeletal pain. Clinical randomized trials are required to evaluate the eventual utility of MHT in the treatment of muscle and joint aches in middle-aged women.

5.4 Conclusions

Vasomotor symptoms are not the most frequent symptom in menopause. Both insomnia and muscle and joint aches are the most prevalent symptoms and they could significantly deteriorate the QOL in middle-aged women. In its pathogenesis, different peripheral and central neural mechanisms are involved. Menopausal hormonal therapy is an alternative that may arise to treat these symptoms, particularly when menopausal symptomatology is varied and severe.

References

1. Bullinger M, Anderson R, Cella D, Aaronson N. Developing and evaluating cross-cultural instruments from minimum requirements to optimal models. Qual Life Res. 1993;2(6):451–9.
2. Heinemman K, Ruebig A, Potthof P. The menopause rating scale (MRS): a methodological review. Qual Life Res. 2004;2:45.
3. Berlin Center for epidemiology and Health Research. MRS-menopause rating scale. http://www.menopause-rating-scale.info/documents/Ref_Values_CountrGr.pdf. December, 16. 2016.
4. Blümel JE, Chedraui P, Baron G, Belzares E, Bencosme A, Calle A, et al. Menopausal symptoms appear before the menopause and persist 5 years beyond: a detailed analysis of a multinational study. Climacteric. 2012;15:542–51.
5. Genazzani AR, Schneider HP, Panay N, Nijland EA. The European menopause survey 2005: women's perceptions on the menopause and postmenopausal hormone therapy. Gynecol Endocrinol. 2006;22:369–75.
6. Blümel JE, Arteaga E, Parra J, Monsalve C, Reyes V, Vallejo MS, Chea R. Decision-making for the treatment of climacteric symptoms using the menopause rating scale. Maturitas. 2018;111:15–9.
7. Di H, Guo Y, Daghlas I, Wang L, Liu G, Pan A, Liu L, Shan Z. Evaluation of sleep habits and disturbances among US adults, 2017–2020. JAMA Netw Open. 2022;5(11):e2240788.
8. Morin CM, LeBlanc M, Bélanger L, Ivers H, Mérette C, Savard J. Prevalence of insomnia and its treatment in Canada. Can J Psychiatr. 2011;56:540–8.
9. Roy AN, Smith M. Prevalence and cost of insomnia in a state Medicaid fee-for-service population based on diagnostic codes and prescription utilization. Sleep Med. 2010;11:462–9.
10. Kravitz HM, Ganz PA, Bromberger J, Powell LH, Sutton-Tyrrell K, Meyer PM. Sleep difficulty in women at midlife: a community survey of sleep and the menopausal transition. Menopause. 2003;10:19–28.
11. Ohayon MM. Prevalence of DSM-IV diagnostic criteria of insomnia: distinguishing insomnia related to mental disorders from sleep disorders. J Psychiatr Res. 1997;31:333–46.
12. Hajak G. Epidemiology of severe insomnia and its consequences in Germany. Eur Arch Psychiatry Clin Neurosci. 2001;251:49–56.

13. Léger D, Scheuermaier K, Philip P, Paillard M, Guilleminault C. SF-36: evaluation of quality of life in severe and mild insomniacs compared with good sleepers. Psychosom Med. 2001;63:49–55.
14. Gomes S, Ramalhete C, Ferreira I, Bicho M, Valente A. Sleep patterns, eating behavior and the risk of noncommunicable diseases. Nutrients. 2023;15(11):2462.
15. Lovato N, Lack L. Insomnia and mortality: a meta-analysis. Sleep Med Rev. 2019;43:71–83.
16. Blümel JE, Cano A, Mezones-Holguín E, Barón G, Bencosme A, Benítez Z, et al. A multinational study of sleep disorders during female mid-life. Maturitas. 2012;72:359–66.
17. Arakane M, Castillo C, Rosero MF, Peñafiel R, Pérez-López FR, Chedraui P. Factors relating to insomnia during the menopausal transition as evaluated by the insomnia severity index. Maturitas. 2011;69:157–61.
18. Terauchi M, Obayashi S, Akiyoshi M, Kato K, Matsushima E, Kubota T. Insomnia in Japanese peri- and postmenopausal women. Climacteric. 2010;13:479–86.
19. Timur S, Sahin NH. Effects of sleep disturbance on the quality of life of Turkish menopausal women: a population-based study. Maturitas. 2009;64:177–81.
20. Young T, Rabago D, Zgierska A, Austin D, Laurel F. Objective and subjective sleep quality in premenopausal, perimenopausal, and postmenopausal women in the Wisconsin sleep cohort study. Sleep. 2003;26:667–72.
21. Kalleinen N, Polo-Kantola P, Himanen SL, Alhola P, Joutsen A, Urrila AS, Polo O. Sleep and the menopause—do postmenopausal women experience worse sleep than premenopausal women? Menopause Int. 2008;14:97–104.
22. Shin C, Lee S, Lee T, Shin K, Yi H, Kimm K, Cho N. Prevalence of insomnia and its relationship to menopausal status in middle-aged Korean women. Psychiatry Clin Neurosci. 2005;59:395–402.
23. Savard J, Davidson JR, Ivers H, Quesnel C, Rioux D, Dupéré V, et al. The association between nocturnal hot flashes and sleep in breast cancer survivors. J Pain Symptom Manag. 2004;27:513–22.
24. Ohayon MM. Severe hot flashes are associated with chronic insomnia. Arch Intern Med. 2006;166:1262–8.
25. Leger D, Poursain B. An international survey of insomnia: under-recognition and under-treatment of a polysymptomatic condition. Curr Med Res Opin. 2005;21:1785–92.
26. Melby MK, Lock M, Kaufert P. Culture and symptom reporting at menopause. Hum Reprod Update. 2005;11:495–512.
27. Blümel JE, Cano A, Mezones-Holguín E, Barón G, Bencosme A, Benítez Z, et al. A multinational study of sleep disorders during female mid-life. Maturitas. 2012;72(4):359–66.
28. Jansson-Fröjmark M, Lindblom K. A bidirectional relationship between anxiety and depression, and insomnia? A prospective study in the general population. J Psychosom Res. 2008;64:443–9.
29. Blümel JE, Chedraui P, Baron G, Belzares E, Bencosme A, Calle A, et al. A large multinational study of vasomotor symptom prevalence, duration, and impact on quality of life in middle-aged women. Menopause. 2011;18:778–85.
30. Joffe H, Soares CN, Thurston RC, White DP, Cohen LS, Hall JE. Depression is associated with worse objectively and subjectively measured sleep, but not more frequent awakenings, in women with vasomotor symptoms. Menopause. 2009;16:671–9.
31. Zervas IM, Lambrinoudaki I, Spyropoulou AC, Koundi KL, Voussoura E, Tzavara C, et al. Additive effect of depressed mood and vasomotor symptoms on postmenopausal insomnia. Menopause. 2009;16:837–42.
32. Bourey RE. Primary menopausal insomnia: definition, review, and practical approach. Endocr Pract. 2011;17:122–31.
33. Freedman RR. Hot flashes: behavioral treatments, mechanisms, and relation to sleep. Am J Med. 2005;118(Suppl 12B):124–30.
34. Freeman EW, Sammel MD, Lin H, Nelson DB. Associations of hormones and menopausal status with depressed mood in women with no history of depression. Arch Gen Psychiatry. 2006;63:375–82.

35. Durant C, Christmas D, Nutt D. The pharmacology of anxiety. Curr Top Behav Neurosci. 2010;2:303–30.
36. Monti JM, Jantos H. The roles of dopamine and serotonin, and of their receptors, in regulating sleep and waking. Prog Brain Res. 2008;1(72):625–46.
37. Krajnak K, Rosewell KL, Duncan MJ, Wise PM. Aging, estradiol and time of day differentially affect serotonin transporter binding in the central nervous system of female rats. Brain Res. 2003;990:87–94.
38. Delorme F, Froment JL, Jouvet M. Suppression of sleep with p-chloromethamphetamine and p-chlorophenylalanine. C R Seances Soc Biol Fil. 1966;160:2347–51.
39. Cohn TJ, Foster JH, Peters TJ. Sequential studies of sleep disturbance and quality of life in abstaining alcoholics. Addict Biol. 2003;8:455–62.
40. Englert S, Linden M. Differences in self-reported sleep complaints in elderly persons living in the community who do or do not take sleep medication. J Clin Psychiatry. 1998;59:137–44.
41. Terauchi M, Obayashi S, Akiyoshi M, Kato K, Matsushima E, Kubota T. Effects of oral estrogen and hypnotics on Japanese peri- and postmenopausal women with sleep disturbance. J Obstet Gynaecol Res. 2011;37:741–9.
42. Marchi NS, Reimão R, Tognola WA, Cordeiro JA. Analysis of the prevalence of insomnia in the adult population of São José do Rio Preto, Brazil. Arq Neuropsiquiatr. 2004;62:764–8.
43. Bonanni E, Schirru A, Di Perri MC, Bonuccelli U, Maestri M. Insomnia and hot flashes. Maturitas. 2019;126:51–4.
44. Montplaisir J, Lorrain J, Denesle R, Petit D. Sleep in menopause; differential effects of two forms of hormone replacement therapy. Menopause. 2001;8:10–6.
45. Polo-Kantola P, Ekkola R, Irjala R, Pullinen S, Virtanen I, Polo O. Effects of short-term transdermal estrogen replacement therapy on sleep: a randomized double-blind crossover trial in postmenopausal women. Fertil Steril. 1999;71:873–80.
46. Scharf MB, McDannold MD, Stoner R, ZareTsky N, Berkowitz DV. Effects of estrogen replacement therapy on rates of cyclic alternating patterns and hot-flush events during sleep in postmenopausal women a pilot study. Clin Ther. 1997;19:304–11.
47. Purdie DW, Empson JA, Crichton C, McDonald L. Hormone replacement therapy, sleep quality and psychological wellbeing. Br J Obstet Gynaecol. 1995;102:735–9.
48. Tal JZ, Suh SA, Dowdle CL, Nowakowski S. Treatment of insomnia, insomnia symptoms, and obstructive sleep apnea during and after menopause: therapeutic approaches. Curr Psychiatr Rev. 2015;11:63–83.
49. Hays J, Ockene JK, Brunner RL, Kotchen JM, Manson JE, Patterson RE, et al. Effects of estrogen plus progestin on health-related quality of life. N Engl J Med. 2003;348:1839–54.
50. Rubio-Arias JA, Marín-Cascales E, Ramos-Campo DJ, Hernandez AV, Pérez-López FR. Effect of exercise on sleep quality and insomnia in middle-aged women: a systematic review and meta-analysis of randomized controlled trials. Maturitas. 2017;100:49–56.
51. Francisco Ferreira M, Carvalho Bos S, Ferreira MA. The impact of physical activity on objective sleep of people with insomnia. Psychiatry Res. 2023;320:115019.
52. Polasek D, Santhi N, Alfonso-Miller P, Walshe IH, Haskell-Ramsay CF, Elder GJ. Nutritional interventions in treating menopause-related sleep disturbances: a systematic review. Nutr Rev. 2023;2023:nuad113.
53. Lu M, Zhang Y, Zhang J, Huang S, Huang F, Wang T, et al. Comparative effectiveness of digital cognitive behavioral therapy vs medication therapy among patients with insomnia. JAMA Netw Open. 2023;6(4):e237597.
54. Chan WS, McCrae CS, Ng AS. Is cognitive behavioral therapy for insomnia effective for improving sleep duration in individuals with insomnia? A meta-analysis of randomized controlled trials. Ann Behav Med. 2023;57(6):428–41.
55. Benz F, Knoop T, Ballesio A, Bacaro V, Johann AF, Rücker G, et al. The efficacy of cognitive and behavior therapies for insomnia on daytime symptoms: a systematic review and network meta-analysis. Clin Psychol Rev. 2020;80:101873.

56. Stubbs B, Schofield P, Patchay S. Mobility limitations and fall-related factors contribute to the reduced health-related quality of life in older adults with chronic musculoskeletal pain. Pain Pract. 2016;16(1):80–9.
57. Mäntyselkä PT, Kumpusalo EA, Ahonen RS, Takala JK. Direct and indirect costs of managing patients with musculoskeletal pain-challenge for health care. Eur J Pain. 2002;6:141–8.
58. Stewart WF, Ricci JA, Chee E, Morganstein D, Lipton R. Lost productive time and cost due to common pain conditions in the US workforce. JAMA. 2003;290:2443–54.
59. Gran JT. The epidemiology of chronic generalized musculoskeletal pain. Best Pract Res Clin Rheumatol. 2003;17:547–61.
60. Avis NE, Stellato R, Crawford S, Bromberger J, Ganz P, Cain V, Kagawa-Singer M. Is there a menopausal syndrome? Menopausal status and symptoms across racial/ethnic groups. Soc Sci Med. 2001;52:345–56.
61. Sueblinvong T, Taechakraichana N, Phupong V. Prevalence of climacteric symptoms according to years after menopause. J Med Assoc Thail. 2001;84:1681–91.
62. Lu CB, Liu PF, Zhou YS, Meng FC, Qiao TY, Yang XJ, et al. Musculoskeletal pain during the meno-pausal transition: a systematic review and meta-analysis. Neural Plast. 2020;2020:8842110.
63. Blümel JE, Chedraui P, Baron G, Belzares E, Bencosme A, Calle A, et al. Menopause could be involved in the pathogenesis of muscle and joint aches in mid-aged women. Maturitas. 2013;75:94–100.
64. NIH State of the Science Conference. Statement on management of menopause related symptoms. NIH Consens State Sci Statements. 2005;22:1–38.
65. Lerma C, Martinez A, Ruiz N, Vargas A, Infante O, Martinez-Lavin M. Nocturnal heart rate variability parameters as potential fibromyalgia biomarker: correlation with symptoms severity. Arthritis Res Ther. 2011;13(6):R185.
66. Becker S, Schweinhardt P. Dysfunctional neurotransmitter systems in fibromyalgia, their role in central stress circuitry and pharmacological actions on these systems. Pain Res Treat. 2012;2012:741–6.
67. Blümel JE, Palacios S, Legorreta D, Vallejo MS, Sarra S. Is fibromyalgia part of the climacteric syndrome? Maturitas. 2012;73:87–93.
68. Ozcivit IB, Erel CT, Durmusoglu F. Can fibromyalgia be considered a characteristic symptom of climacterium? Postgrad Med J. 2023;99(1170):244–51.
69. Lange IG. Evolution of oestrogen functions in vertebrates. J Steroid Biochem Mol Biol. 2002;83:219–26.
70. Amandusson Å, Blomqvist A. Estrogenic influences in pain processing. Front Neuroendocrinol. 2013;34:329–49.
71. Women's Health Initiative Investigators. Menopausal symptoms and treatment-related effects of estrogen and progestin in the women's health initiative. Obstet Gynecol. 2005;105(5 Pt 1):1063–73.
72. Welton AJ, Vickers MR, Kim J, Ford D, Lawton BA, MacLennan AH, et al. Health related quality of life after combined hormone replacement therapy: randomised controlled trial. BMJ. 2008;337:a1190.
73. Sadreddini S, Molaeefard M, Noshad H, Ardalan M, Asadi A. Efficacy of Raloxifen in treatment of fibromyalgia in menopausal women. Eur J Intern Med. 2008;19:350–5.
74. Park JY, Lee SK, Bae SY, Kim J, Kim MK, Kil WH, et al. Aromatase inhibitor-associated musculoskeletal symptoms: incidence and associated factors. J Korean Surg Soc. 2013;85:205–11.
75. Kahn MF. Does hormone replacement therapy discontinuation cause musculoskeletal pain? Joint Bone Spine. 2006;73:488–9.
76. Yoeli H, Macnaughton J, McLusky S. Menopausal symptoms and work: a narrative review of wo-men's experiences in casual, informal, or precarious jobs. Maturitas. 2021;150:14–21.
77. Shin WY, Kim JH. Poor diet quality is associated with self-reported knee pain in community-dwelling women aged 50 years and older. PLoS One. 2021;16(2):e0245630.

Genitourinary Syndrome of Menopause. Vaginal Health and Microbiota

María Jesús Cancelo Hidalgo and Llaura Barrera Coello

Abstract

The genitourinary syndrome of menopause (GSM) is a new term that describes various menopausal symptoms and signs including not only genital and sexual symptoms but also urinary symptoms related to a decreased estrogen level in menopause.

Since the GSM may have a negative impact on the quality of life of postmenopausal women, women should be made aware of these problems and treated with an appropriate effective therapy. Thus, in this review, we introduce new terminology and discuss the importance and the role played by the vaginal microbiota in the vaginal health, as well as available therapeutic alternatives.

6.1 Introduction

Reduced circulating estrogen levels are responsible for most anatomical cytological, bacteriological, and physiological changes that occur in female genital tract in postmenopausal women. These changes can initiate in the perimenopausal period and increase gradually.

The consequent symptoms produced by vaginal and vulva atrophy can cause vulvovaginal and urinary dysfunction that can also affect sexuality and produce changes in quality of life of menopausal women [1].

Otherwise, the term vulvovaginal atrophy related to menopause changes does not represent all symptoms. That's why in 2013, the International Society for the Study of Women's Sexual health (ISSWSH) and the North American Menopause

M. J. C. Hidalgo (✉) · L. B. Coello
Obstetrics and Gynecology Department of University Hospital of Guadalajara,
University of Alcalá, Madrid, Spain
e-mail: mjesus.cancelo@uah.es; laura.barrera@uah.es

Society (NAMS) determined the need of a new term: the genitourinary syndrome of menopause (GSM) as this will be called from now on [2].

The main objective is to integrate the big variety of signs and symptoms of vulvovaginal area, with the changes that also occur in the urethra and bladder produced because of the low estrogen levels. These symptoms, opposite of vasomotor symptoms that yield over the years, will get worse permanently if it is not diagnosed and treated. Because of that, it is needed having adequate knowledge of its physiopathology, the clinical signs, and the available treatments for the health providers.

6.2 Vaginal Health

Vaginal health term defines the vaginal state that maintains adequate physiological conditions as women age passes, which does not produce local symptoms and allow satisfactory sexual life [3]. For this to happen, it is needed the integrity of the tissue to be kept and to not disrupt the normal function of vaginal microbiota; in which both cases, estrogen levels play an important role. These factors influence each other, as represented in Fig. 6.1.

The vagina is an organ that has limited physiological functions, but besides this, it becomes a main factor for women on wellness perception and quality of life. If it gets affected during periods of low estrogen levels, it means the starting of bothering symptoms that interrupt women's sexual life.

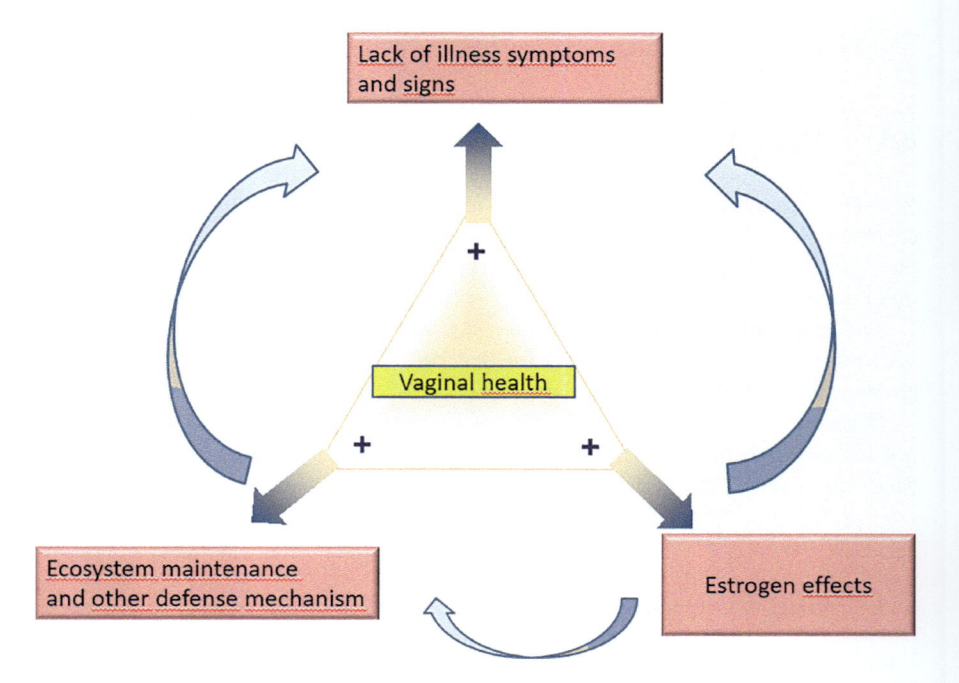

Fig. 6.1 Simple representation of factors related to vaginal health

6 Genitourinary Syndrome of Menopause. Vaginal Health and Microbiota

	New born	Childhood	Puberty	Fertil ages	Pregnancy	Menopause
Estrogens	++	- -	- +	++	+++	+ -
Epitelium	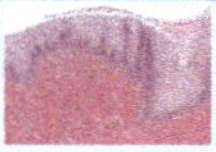	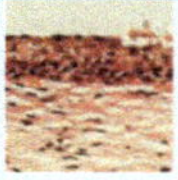	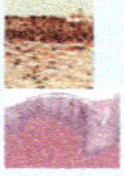	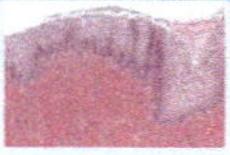	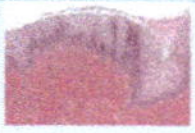	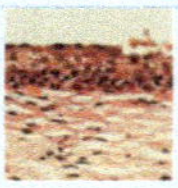
Glycogen	+	- -	- +	+	++	+ -
pH	4-5	7	7➡5	4-5	3.5-4,5	6
Microbiota	No	Low	Mixed	Lactobacilli	Lactobacilli	Mixed

Fig. 6.2 Schematic representation of the vaginal changes present in the vagina in the different vital stages of the woman

Vagina has a double embryonic origin, from Müller conduct and urogenital sinus [4]. Because of that, there is an established anatomical and clinical relation with urinary tract. It does have physiological regulating mechanisms on defensive processes. Estrogens have an important influence on this mechanism related to vaginal health and these change along the different age phases of women [5].

Figure 6.2 shows physiological changes that take place in the vagina along these different age phases.

6.3 Microbiota

Vaginal microbiota is the whole microorganisms (bacterium and yeast) that colonize vaginal site and create the balanced vaginal ecosystem. Although often dominated by lactobacilli, the vaginal microbiota is frequently composed of a collection of facultative and obligate anaerobes. The mechanisms that drive these associations have yet to be described in detail with few studies establishing causative relationships.

First studies about human vaginal microbiology, published by Döderlein in 1892 [6], described lactobacilli as the dominating organisms in vaginal habitat.

Furthermore, these other species coexist in a delicate balance in healthy women.

Disturbing this balance, because of reduction on lactobacilli levels or because of the overgrowth of other species, will introduce the presence of symptoms and signs related to vaginitis or vaginosis and it is known as dysbiosis.

Most of its components are normal in intestinal habitat, which means that gastrointestinal tract could act as a reservoir of these agents. However, related frequency of present species in the vagina and bowls is very different [7]. Vaginal microbiota is formed by different aerobic and anaerobic species, standing out lactobacilli, which are dominant in the vagina and are minority in bowls, even being exclusive in vagina in some cases. Generally, the percentage of samples of vaginal exudate that present predominance of the lactobacilli is superior to 70%, whether the processing of these samples includes cultivation [8] as if it is done by methods of genotyping [9]. On the other hand, the strict anaerobic gram-positive or gram-negative bacteria of the Clostridium-Eubacterium and Bacteroides Prevotella groups, which dominate the intestinal habitat, appear sporadically in the vagina, suggesting that in this mucosa, they are passersby rather than colonizers.

6.3.1 Lactobacilli. General Characteristics

Lactobacilli are considered to play a critical role in maintaining the vaginal ecosystem by preventing the overgrowth of other microorganisms such as Gardnerella vaginalis. They would also prevent colonization by pathogens or yeasts responsible for the production of infections.

Lactobacilli form a wide and heterogeneous group of lactic acid bacteria, characterized by being gram positive, non-sporulated, and with a strictly fermentative catabolism of sugars, in which the predominant end product is the production of this organic acid. Morphologically, they vary from elongated to short forms and from straight to curved.

In general, they are aerotolerant anaerobic bacteria. They have small genomes, so they are very nutritionally demanding. Undoubtedly, their being harmless as infectious agents is also partly due to this scarcity of genetic information; for example, genes coding for virulence factors have not been described in any of the sequenced strains.

The bacteria count in the vaginal fluid is around 100,000 per ml. With genomic sequencing techniques, about 250 species of bacteria have been identified in the vagina [10].

Table 6.1 shows a summary of the most frequent species present in the vagina of healthy women. General patterns of vaginal microbiota have been identified, which tend to differentiate between women with and without vaginosis [11].

Lactic microbiota is formed by the general Lactobacillus and Bifidobacterium, whose role is to acidify the medium and to compete with other microorganisms, some of which are potentially pathogenic, so that while they are present, they limit the overgrowth of these (vaginosis) [12].

Several species of lactobacilli have been identified. The vagina is colonized preferably by L. acidophilus, L. fermentum but L. crispatus, L. gasseri and L. jensenii, L. iners, and L. vaginalis [13].

Advances in molecular biology and DNA sequencing have enabled characterization of the taxonomic composition of the vaginal microbiota. The majority of women of reproductive age have a vaginal microbiota whose taxonomic composition resembles one of the five vaginotypes or "Community State Type (CST)" established by Ravel in 2011. This distinction is important because the vaginal microbiota of some women has been documented to vary, including shifts in CST. Changes in composition are sometimes explicable, occurring at the onset of menstruation or following vaginal intercourse due to temporarily raised vaginal pH. Other changes in the vaginal microbiota cannot be attributed to a specific factor and may be the result of

Table 6.1 Most frequent species of microorganisms present in the vagina of healthy women

Present microorganisms in the vagina of healthy women	
Cocci and bacilli gram + Optional anaerobes	Lactobacillus
	Streptococcus
	Corynebacterium
	Gardnerella
	Staphylococcus
Bacilli gram – Optional anaerobes	Escherichia
	Klebsiella
	Proteus
Cocci and bacilli gram + Strict anaerobes	Atopobium
	Peptococcus
	Peptostreptococcus
	Clostridium
	Bifidobacterium
	Propionibacterium
	Eubacterium
Bacilli gram – Strict anaerobes	Bacteroides
	Prevotella
Mycoplasma	Mycoplasma hominis

fluctuations in host physiology, competitive interactions between members of the community, ecological drift, bacteriophage activity, or some other mechanisms [14].

6.3.2 Interaction of Lactobacilli with the Vagina

Lactobacilli species is dominant in the vagina of fertile women and prevent the colonization of the muco by undesired microorganisms, generators of urogenital pathology. However, it has been found that women colonized by alternative bacteria such as Atopobium or others [15] appear to be protected as well, although lactobacilli species is still considered to be essential for the maintenance of vaginal homeostasis and it is the main candidate for use in replacement therapies during pathological conditions that affect vaginal habitat [16].

6.3.3 Mechanisms of Protection Performed by the Microbiota

Various mechanisms of action of the microbiota shows a protective effect on the vagina (Table 6.2).

6.3.4 Breakage of the Balance of the Vaginal Ecosystem. Pathophysiology of Vaginitis and Vaginosis

The rupture of the balance between lactobacilli and other microorganisms is the pathophysiological mechanism of vaginitis and vaginosis. But it is not entirely clear whether the reduction or disappearance of lactobacilli is a cause or result of the

Table 6.2 Mechanisms of protection attributed to the microbiota

Protective mechanisms performed by the microbiota
Adhesion to the vaginal epithelium and inhibition of colonization by unwanted organisms (adhesins)
Vaginal pH modification
Formation of hydrogen peroxide
Production of bacteriocins
Formation of surfactants
Production of co-aggregates
Biofilm formation

Table 6.3 Factors associated with microbiota alterations [74]

Stress	
Inflammation	
Age	
Exercise	
Use of antibiotics	
Type of diet	Reduction of carbohydrates
	Restrictive hypocaloric diets (strict vegetarian)
	Low fiber content
	High in fats and sugar

proliferation of other microorganisms. Several factors were related to alterations of the microbiota (Table 6.3).

When the concentration of lactobacilli in the vagina decreases below a critical level, this circumstance is exploited by microorganisms that are usually found in the healthy vagina or by others of exogenous origin, which will proliferate until becoming dominant, thus behaving as opportunistic pathogens [17].

Clinical symptoms that have been associated to the decrease of lactobacilli on the vaginal epithelium are:

1. Bacterial vaginosis, whose most common etiological agents are Gardnerella vaginalis, Mycoplasma hominis, Prevotella, and Peptostreptococcus.
2. Candidiasis, produced by Candida albicans in 85% of cases; C. glabrata; and C. tropicalis.
3. Trichomoniasis, a consequence of the proliferation of Trichomonas vaginalis.
4. Lower urinary tract infections, mainly caused by Enterobacteriaceae of intestinal origin such as Escherichia coli which is responsible for at least 80% of the cases, although sometimes gram-positive cocci are isolated like Enterococcus faecalis.

Although lower urinary tract infections (UTIs) are not specifically genitals, their presence and relapse have been linked to alterations in the vaginal ecosystem. It has been determined that the urinary tract infection is practically always preceded by vaginal colonization by the urinary pathogens [18].

The frequency of UTI is inversely proportional to the presence of a normal microbiota, dominated by lactobacilli, in the vagina of healthy women. A compelling hypothesis is to consider that the anatomical proximity and functional interrelations

Table 6.4 Factors that can modify the vaginal microbiota

Exogenous factors	Endogenous factors
Sexual activity	Menstruation
Use of antibiotics	Variation of hormone levels
Use of soaps, deodorants, etc.	Local and systemic immunity
Vaginal showers	Systemic diseases
DIU	Cofactors: Tobacco
Gynecological interventions	

of the urinary, gynecological, and digestive systems makes the evaluation of perineal symptoms (urinary, vaginal, and digestive) of the woman and should be considered in an integral way. The microbiota is a clear example of this, being verified how modifications of the intestinal, vaginal, or urinary habitat can affect each other [19].

Table 6.4 summarizes the exogenous and endogenous factors that can modify the vaginal microbiota.

6.3.5 Estrogens and Vagina

Vaginal atrophy is caused primarily by estrogen deficiency. It acts on the vagina, vulva, urethra, and trigone of the bladder via estrogen receptors on these structures. Estrogens help to maintain the collagen content of epithelium and thus effects on thickness and elasticity; it helps to maintain acid mucopolysaccharides and hyaluronic acid, which keep epithelial surfaces moist. Estrogens maintain optimal vaginal blood flow.

The vaginal epithelium becomes dry and atrophic and loses elasticity which may cause inflammation, itching, burning, dryness, bleeding, spotting, dysuria, dyspareunia, urinary incontinence, and recurrent urinary tract infections. The vulvar skin can become thinner; the labia flatten and shrink; and the clitoris, uterus, and ovaries decrease in size.

The bladder, urethra, pelvic floor musculature, and endopelvic fascia are affected by a hypoestrogenic state because of estrogen receptors [20]. Possible consequences of advanced atrophy of the urinary tract include urethral discomfort, frequency, hematuria, and dysuria. Urinary tract infection is more common. The laxity from estrogen loss causes pelvic floor and organ prolapsed.

Anatomic and histologic changes occur in female genital tissues, including reduction in the content of collagen and hyaluronic acid and in the levels of elastin, thinning of the epithelium, alterations in the function of smooth muscle cells, increase in the density of connective tissue, and fewer blood vessels. These changes reduce elasticity of the vagina, increase vaginal pH, lead to changes in vaginal flora, diminish lubrication, and increase vulnerability to physical irritation and trauma.

Glycogen is the substrate for Döderlein's lactobacilli, which convert glucose into lactic acid, thereby creating an acidic vaginal environment. The pH of an estrogen-primed vagina ranges from 3.5 to 5.0. This acidic range helps protect the urogenital area from vaginal and urinary tract infections. The low glycogen content of the thinned epithelium leads to a reduction in lactic acid production by lactobacilli, resulting in an increase in vaginal pH that encourages the overgrowth of coliforms and other pathogen agents such as Candida, bacterial vaginosis, and Trichomonas. The vaginal environment becomes more susceptible to inflammation or infection and easily traumatized.

About the lower urinary tract, the urethra of a woman is covered to the full extent by a thick, nonkeratinized squamous epithelium similar to that of the vagina. Also like the vagina, the epithelium of the female urethra, although not the subepithelial layer, expresses abundant estrogen receptors, which are completely absent in the contiguous urothelium of the bladder except in the part of the trigone [21].

Lack of awareness of the association between recurrent UTIs and GSM may result in multiple unnecessary courses of antibiotic therapy, antibiotic prophylaxis, and altered patterns of antimicrobial drug resistance [22], hence the importance of the new terminology adopted to refer to the genitourinary menopause syndrome, integrating both systems into one unit.

6.4 Genitourinary Syndrome of Menopause. Justification of Terminology

The GSM describes various symptoms and signs associated with physical changes of the vulva, vagina, and lower urinary tract related with menopausal estrogen deficiency. It includes not only genital symptoms (dryness, burning, and irritation) and sexual symptoms (lack of lubrication, discomfort or pain) but also urinary symptoms (urgency, dysuria, and recurrent urinary tract infections).

The terms *vulvovaginal atrophy* or *atrophic vaginitis* have been considered to be inadequate for referring to the constellation of symptoms and signs associated with estrogen deficiency because they imply a state of inflammation or infection and they do not take into account the symptoms of the lower urinary tract. For these reasons, the board of directors of the International Society for the Study of Women's Sexual Health (ISSWSH) and the Board of the North American Menopause Society (NAMS) held a terminology consensus conference in 2013.

The genitourinary symptoms related to an abrupt menopause in these patients tend to present in relatively younger women usually in induced hypoestrogenic states including surgical menopause, use of gonadotropin-releasing hormone (GnRH) agonists, hypothalamic amenorrhea, or because of cancer treatments like chemotherapy, pelvic radiation, or endocrine therapy [23].

6.4.1 Prevalence

Vulvovaginal symptoms are directly related to the reduced circulating estrogen levels after menopause [24]. It can affect—depending on the series—45% to 63% of postmenopausal women [25], the most common symptom being vaginal dryness; other symptoms include dyspareunia, vaginal irritation, itching sensation, vaginal tenderness, and vaginal bleeding or spotting during intercourse. Cultural, religious, and social influences may play a role in making women feel uncomfortable discussing concerns related to the genitourinary system. Moderate or severe symptoms can contribute to sexual dysfunction and loss of sexual intimacy and may have a negative impact on overall quality of life [26]. Dyspareunia leads to decreased interest in coitus and as the frequency of coitus diminishes, vaginal lubrication declines further. They make lifestyle changes stop such as sexual activity to avoid dyspareunia caused by vaginal dryness and pain.

In Spain, data from an online survey (REVIVE) shows that the most troublesome symptom is dyspareunia (80%). Vulvovaginal atrophy symptoms significantly impact ability to achieve sexual enjoyment (75%), relationship with partner (67%), and sexual spontaneity (66%) [27].

Estrogen deficiency after menopause causes the lower urinary tract symptoms such as dysuria, urgency, frequency, nocturia, urinary incontinence (UI), and recurrent urinary tract infection (UTI).

The incidence of UTI rises in elderly women. Studies have shown that 15–20% of women aged 65–70 years and 20–50% of women aged >80 years have bacteriuria [28]. Postmenopausal and premenopausal women may have different risk factors for UTI. Sexual intercourse is the most common cause among younger women. In older women, anatomic changes such as a cystocele and diabetes are the more frequent risk factors for recurrent UTI [29].

6.4.2 Diagnosis

The diagnosis is based on history and findings and physical examination [30] (Table 6.5). Physical examination shows that atrophic epithelium appears pale, dry vaginal epithelium that is smooth and shiny with loss of most rugae. Often, inflammation may be present with erythema, petechiae, increased friability, and bleeding. Ecchymoses and minor lacerations peri-introital may also occur after coitus or during a speculum examination, resulting in vaginal bleeding and spotting [31]. The vagina may be shortened, narrowed, and poorly distensible. The vaginal fornices become obliterated. The external genitalia show reduced elasticity; the skin appears less turgor; there is scarcity of pubic hair, dry lips, vulvar dermatoses, vulvar lesions, and fusion of the labia minora. This friable and insufficiently rugated vaginal epithelium is more prone to traumatic damage. Similar symptoms can be caused by

Table 6.5 Symptoms and signs of GSM

Symptoms	Signs
Decreased lubrication	Decreased elasticity
Genital dryness	Loss of moisture
Irritation, burning, or itching	Loss of vaginal rugae
Dysuria, urinary frequency, and urgency	Labia resorption
Discomfort or dyspareunia	Tissue fragility and petechias
	ITUs

infective processes, desquamative inflammatory vaginitis, inflammatory conditions, or allergic reactions due to environmental agents such as soaps, perfumes, deodorants, pads, spermicides, lubricants, or synthetic clothing [32]. Papanicolaou smear that can confirm the presence of urogenital atrophy shows an increased proportion of parabasal cells and a decreased percentage of superficial cells (a high maturation index value) and can be similar to those observed in women with squamous intraepithelial neoplasia. Vaginal pH of ≥5 of the vaginal vault in the absence of other causes, such as infection or semen, can be considered an indicator of vaginal atrophy due to estrogen deficiency.

Laboratory tests are unnecessary and not diagnostic.

Different validated indices have been designed with the aim of having objective measures of impact. The most common assessment tools for GSM diagnosis are the visual analog scale (VAS) of vulvovaginal atrophy (VVA) symptoms and the female sexual function index (FSFI) [33]. While the VAS score is a progressive 10-point measure through which patients are asked to record their disturbances, the FSFI analyzes dyspareunia and general sexual disturbances with a six-domain structure form that includes questions about sexual desire, orgasm, satisfaction, subjective arousal, lubrication, and pain [34]. They both consider subjective outcomes and are influenced by patient perception of the symptoms.

A quantitative assessment of vaginal health can be performed by using the Vaginal Health Index [35] (Table 6.6). This system is used to evaluate vaginal elasticity, fluid volume, pH, epithelial integrity, and moisture on a scale of 1–5.

6.4.3 Treatment

GSM is a chronic and progressive condition that does not resolve spontaneously and often worsens without treatment due to its pathogenesis and correlation with age progression and menopause state [36]. Treatment is indicated for relief of symptoms and recovery of physiological urogenital function.

Table 6.6 Vaginal Health Index Score [36]

Score	1	2	3	4	5
Elasticity	None	Poor	Fair	Good	Excellent
Fluid volume (pooling of secretion)	None	Scant amount; vault not entirely covered	Superficial amount; vault entirely covered	Moderate amount of dryness (small areas of dryness on cotton tip applicator)	Normal amount (fully saturates on cotton tip applicator)
pH	≥ 6.1	5.6–6.0	5.1–5.5	4.7–5.0	≤ 4.6
Epithelial integrity	Petechiae noted before contact	Bleeds with light contact	Bleeds with scraping	Not friable-thin epithelium	Normal
Moisture (coating)	None; surface inflamed	None; surface not inflamed	Minimal	Moderate	Normal

6.4.3.1 Nonhormonal Vaginal Therapy
Nonhormonal vaginal lubricants and moisturizers as first-line therapies for women with vaginal atrophy. A combination of vaginal moisturizing agents used on a regular basis and lubricants to intercourse can alleviate symptoms of vaginal dryness. These compounds do not reverse the atrophic vaginal changes but improve coital comfort and maintain vaginal secretions. Such drugs are indicated for women with mild symptoms [37].

Mucoadhesive and controlled release formulations consisting of aqueous solutions containing 0.05–5% by weight of a natural purified polymer having xyloglucan structure and 10–70% by weight of glycerol are suitable for the application on human mucous membranes, such as vaginal mucous membranes, as moisturizing and softening agents or as pharmaceutical release system. The composition is contacted with the vaginal mucous membrane to be moisturized, and that contact is maintained for a time period sufficient to moisturize the contacted area.

Vaginal administration of hyaluronic acid also acts as a protective macromolecule for the vaginal mucosa that penetrates into deeper vaginal layers [38].

Through the topical remodeling of connective tissue and the production of new collagen, elastic fibers, and other components of the extracellular matrix, laser CO_2 effects appear to significantly relieve related symptoms [39].

Other point is the administration of lactobacilli or probiotics as vaginal soft-gel capsule that comprises a quantity of lactobacilli in a solid form that is preserved during insertion into the vagina and released in the warm and moist vaginal environment, considering the potential of probiotics to reinstate vaginal homeostasis following menopause [40]. Oral and vaginal probiotics hold great promise and initial studies complement the findings of previous research efforts concerning menopause and the vaginal microbiome; however, additional trials are required to determine the efficacy of bacterial therapeutics to modulate or restore vaginal homeostasis [41].

Promising results from studies reporting the efficacy of vaginal microbiota transplants as a potential approach to treat recurrent bacterial vaginosis [42]. The concept involves sampling vaginal secretions from an individual with a *Lactobacillus*-dominant vaginal microbiota and introduce it into the vagina with recurrent bacterial vaginosis. Each donation requires extensive testing for vaginal pathogens and viruses (e.g., HSV or HPV) and contains a relatively small bacterial load.

Sexual activity plays a role in maintaining a healthy vaginal epithelium by preserving vaginal elasticity and preventing introital stenosis. Sexual activity, including masturbation, leads to fewer symptoms of atrophic vaginitis [43].

6.4.3.2 Vaginal and Systemic Hormone Therapy
Estrogen is the most effective treatment for women with moderate to severe symptoms of vaginal atrophy, given that atrophy is a direct consequence of a low estrogen level.

Estrogen therapy reverses vaginal atrophy by decreasing vaginal pH and vaginal dryness, thickening and revascularizing the vaginal epithelium, increasing vaginal secretions and the number of superficial cells, and producing reduction in recurrent urinary tract infection and restoring normal vaginal microbiota [44].

Estrogen or combined hormone (estrogen-progestin) therapy is highly efficacious for managing the signs and symptoms of urogenital atrophy. All routes are effective, both systemic and local estrogen replacement. Various forms of estrogen-based therapies have been shown to effectively manage menopausal signs and symptoms. The dose and duration of the treatment should be individualized to the woman's specific needs and her degree of vaginal atrophy symptoms. Treatment can be continued indefinitely although safety data for treatment beyond 1 year have not been established [45].

Lower-dose estrogen therapy provides therapeutic efficacy while minimizing adverse effects. Literature supports the use of low dosages of estrogen therapy for effectively relieving symptoms and restoring healthy vaginal cytology in postmenopausal women with vaginal atrophy.

A meta-analysis shows that local, low-dose vaginal therapy is preferred because lower drug doses can be administered to achieve comparable changes in the vulvovaginal epithelium while minimizing estrogen exposure to other organs. Lower drug doses are associated with fewer systemic side effects, such as breast tenderness, withdrawal bleeding, and endometrial stimulation. However, the low estrogen doses recommended for vaginal therapy usually do not achieve serum estrogen levels sufficient for relief of hot flushes or prevention of bone loss [46].

The systemic absorption of vaginal estrogen is conditioned to the vaginal epithelium and the estrogen dose. When the vaginal mucosa becomes atrophic, the cornification of the vaginal epithelium decreases, leading to increased absorption.

With the low-dose vaginal estrogen regimens, systemic absorption is minimal; thus, serum estradiol concentrations remain within the normal postmenopausal range and no significant increases in endometrial thickness were observed.

A progestin is probably not necessary to protect against endometrial hyperplasia in women receiving low-dose local estrogen therapy.

A Cochrane review shows that creams, pessaries, tablets, and the estradiol vaginal ring appeared to be equally effective for the symptoms of vaginal atrophy [47].

Vaginal tablets with 25 mcg and 10 mcg E2 provided relief of vaginal symptoms, improved urogenital atrophy, decreased vaginal pH, and increased maturation of the vaginal and urethral epithelium. Those improvements were greater with 25 mcg than with 10 mcg E2. Both doses were effective in the treatment of atrophic vaginitis [48].

The choice of modality for local estrogen administration should be guided by patient preference. A systematic review of 16 randomized trials investigating local estrogen treatment of vaginal atrophy found that creams, pessaries, and rings were all similarly effective in relieving the symptoms.

Vaginal ring is a device consisting of a silastic ring impregnated with estradiol and it is the lowest dose option for delivering estrogen locally to the vagina, 6–9 mcg of estradiol to the vagina daily for a period of 3 months. It is estimated that only 10% is absorbed systemically; thus, the systemic effects would be expected to be minimal [49].The efficacy of this method was similar to that of orally administered estrogen.

Vaginal tablets: A low-dose tablet containing 25 mcg of estradiol is available and is inserted into the vagina daily for 2 weeks and then twice per week thereafter. Estradiol levels in plasma minimally increase during use of these tablets, although not to premenopausal levels. An ultra-low-dose 10 mcg tablet of estradiol for vaginal use is effective for relief of vaginal symptoms [50].

Creams: Vaginal treatment with 0.625 g cream of conjugated estrogen cream daily for 21 days of two consecutive 28-day cycles resulted in beneficial changes in the vaginal tissues and induced an overall genital health pattern more characteristic of the premenopausal state. Promestriene used vaginally to relieve vaginal atrophy is a locally effective estrogen that has not shown systemic estrogenic effects. Thus, it could be a first-line option for those who necessitate a minimal or ideally no vaginal absorption, particularly in symptomatic cancer patients. After a long-term market experience (almost 40 years), in 34 countries, and millions of pieces prescribed, the side effects were very rarely reported in pharmacovigilance data, whereas the effectiveness to relieve atrophy was good [51].

Crystalline estradiol can also be given by vaginal applicator at a dose of one-eighth of an applicator or 0.5 g (which contains 50 mcg of estradiol). It should be noted that the maximal doses indicated on the package insert (2.0 g) produce premenopausal plasma levels of estradiol and should not be used long term.

In order to obtain a prompt improvement in relieving urogenital symptoms, the association of local therapy acting on the genital epithelium to the systemic treatment should be considered. Adding vaginal estriol to HRT may shorten the latency period for urinary symptoms [52].

Among women with a history of estrogen-dependent breast cancer who are experiencing urogenital symptoms, vaginal estrogen should be reserved for those patients who are unresponsive to nonhormonal remedies. The decision to use vaginal estrogen may be made in coordination with the patient's oncologist. Additionally, it should be preceded by an informed decision-making and consent process in which the woman has the information and resources to consider the benefits and potential risks of low-dose vaginal estrogen. Data do not show an increased risk of cancer recurrence among women currently undergoing treatment for breast cancer or those with a personal history of breast cancer who use vaginal estrogen to relieve urogenital symptoms [53].

Tibolone

Tibolone is a synthetic steroid that has estrogenic, androgenic, and progestogenic properties. Tibolone itself has no biological activity; its effects are the results of the activity of its metabolites on various tissues. The concentrations of tibolone metabolites and the metabolic regulation of hormonal activities vary depending on tissue type. Tibolone has estrogenic effects on bone and vaginal tissue. In endometrial tissue, the Δ4-isomer functions as a progestogen, whereas in the brain and liver, it has androgenic effects. In breast tissue, the main actions of tibolone are strong inhibition of sulfatase activity and weak inhibition of 17ß-hydroxysteroid dehydrogenase activity, which results in blocking the conversion of estrone sulfate to E2. Tibolone significantly reduces hot flushes and sweating and genital atrophy in postmenopausal women.

Tibolone has estrogenic effects on the vagina but not on the uterus. This drug has been associated with significant improvements in sexual function in postmenopausal women, reflecting both its estrogenic and androgenic properties. There were significantly greater increases in vaginal blood flow with tibolone in response to erotic fantasy but not film, suggesting two possible pathways of female sexual response.

A menopausal atrophic symptom questionnaire revealed that tibolone 2.5 mg significantly reduced nocturia compared with placebo and urinary urgency and increased the vaginal maturation value from baseline [54].

Dehydroepiandrosterone (DHE), Prasterone
It is an intermediate steroid hormone in the biosynthesis of androgens and estrogens and has been demonstrated to be effective in improving VVA symptoms and vaginal pH without causing endometrial stimulation [55].

Vaginal dehydroepiandrosterone (DHEA) is a steroid prohormone with the ability to transform into testosterone and estradiol. It induces local effects in tissues due to its intracrine or intracellular transformation to reproductive steroids and theoretically provides a nonsystemic hormonal approach. The recommended dose is one 6.5 mg suppository per day administered vaginally before going to bed. There is no limit on the duration of use.

Compared with placebo, prasterone produces significant improvements in vaginal cell maturation, pH, and dyspareunia [56] and in all domains of sexual function on the Female Sexual Function Index (FSFI) [57]. Intravaginal prasterone exerts biological activity on the androgenic endodermal vestibule, resulting in amelioration of pain associated with sexual activity [58]. Prasterone has been studied as a treatment for GSM in cancer survivors. They concluded that DHEA resulted in increased hormone concentrations although the levels were still within the lowest half or quartile of the postmenopausal range. Prasterone label includes a warning against this use in breast cancer survivors [59].

The limitations for its use, included in the technical information sheet, are the same as for local estrogen therapy.

6.4.3.3 Alternative and Complementary Medicine
Alternative and complementary therapies have been proposed for the treatment of atrophic vaginitis, but data are not in agreement regarding efficacy.

Administration of the phytoestrogen genistein (54 mg/d) found no significant difference in maturation value score compared to placebo, either at baseline or after 12 months [60].

Black cohosh, used alone or as part of a multi-botanical product with or without soy dietary changes, had no effects on vaginal epithelium, endometrium, or reproductive hormones.

There is not enough information for its recommendation.

6.4.3.4 Selective Estrogen Receptor Modulator (SERM)

Ospemifene

Selectively targeted SERMs against VVA underlying physiopathology could be an alternative to local estrogen or systemic hormone therapy in the management of symptoms, apart from moisturizers and lubricants.

Ospemifene (a toremifene derivative) has an estrogenic agonist activity on the vaginal epithelium already noted in the first nonclinical studies and phase I, II, and III studies [61]. This singular tissue selectiveness seems to be molecular structure related. It is the first nonhormonal selective modulator with multiple tissue-specific actions and, contrary to other SERMs, with an antagonist function in endometrial and breast tissue [62].

Ospemifene demonstrated efficiency in vaginal dryness and dyspareunia, regenerating vaginal cells, improving lubrication, and reducing pain during sexual intercourse. Symptoms improved in the first 4 weeks and endured for up to 1 year. Additionally, it demonstrated a good endometrial, cardiovascular system, and breast safety profile [63].

Ospemifene is the only marketed SERM that has demonstrated an estrogen agonist effect in the vaginal epithelium. It is the first nonhormonal, non-estrogenic drug indicated for moderate to severe VVA treatment in women not eligible for vaginal estrogen therapy [64].

Ospemifene treats the underlying cause of vaginal dryness and dyspareunia, regenerating vaginal cells, improving lubrication, and reducing pain during sexual intercourse [65]. VVA symptoms improve in most women receiving ospemifene, and they begin to revert following the first 4 weeks.

Physiological improvements endure for up to 1 year of daily ospemifene use, as well as those related to all sexual function aspects. Apart from its proven safety profile in the endometrium and the bone and cardiovascular systems, its safety in the breast makes it the first VVA oral treatment not contraindicated in women with a previous history of breast cancer who have completed treatment [66].

The association of SERM with estrogens (bazedoxifene and conjugated equine estrogens), although it has shown to have beneficial effect on the vaginal symptoms, would not have this as the genitourinary symptoms only indication of use.

Table 6.7 shows the different therapeutic alternatives available for the treatment of the genitourinary syndrome of the menopause with available evidence level.

6.4.3.5 Regenerative Therapy

Recently, more specifically in the last decade, new therapies encompassed within the concept of regenerative therapies have been developed for the treatment of GSM with very good results. These therapies are based not on the treatment of the

Table 6.7 Evidence level of treatments for vaginal atrophy

Treatment		Level evidence
Lifestyle	Sexual activity	II-2B
	Avoiding obesity	III-C
	Exercise	III-C
	Quit smoking	II-3B
Vaginal hydrating	Regular use 2–3 times/week	I-A
	Recovery of symptoms	I-A
Vaginal lubricants	Use during sex relations	II-2B
Alternative and complementary medicine	Homeopathy	III-D
	Phytotherapy	III-D
	Phytoestrogens	II-3D
Systemic HT	Improvement of symptoms and trophism	I-A
Local HT	Improvement of symptoms and trophism	I-A
Ospemifene	Improvement of symptoms and trophism	I-A
Prasterone	Improvement of symptoms and dyspareunia	I-A
Regenerative therapies	Improvement of symptoms and trophism	I-A

symptoms but instead aim to reestablish the basal conditions of the vagina in terms of elasticity, lubrication, and hormonal functioning with the repair, replacement, or regeneration of cells [67]. These therapies are as follows.

Vaginal Laser

It is based on the stimulation of the body's natural mechanisms to produce tissue repair and regeneration. The laser concept comes from the abbreviation in English: "light amplification by stimulated emission of radiation." The emitted electromagnetic radiation is produced by stimulated emissions. The resulting light is monochromatic and coherent, meaning it is emitted at a single wavelength and in phase. The characterization of each type of laser is carried out through its specific wavelength and the active medium where the energy is stimulated. Two of the most researched lasers to address GSM are:

- The CO_2 gas micro-ablative fractional laser.
- The non-ablative YAG (Yttrium, Aluminum, Garnet) crystal laser with Erbium (Er:YAG).

Both are effective in the treatment of GMS since they have repairing, remodeling, and regenerating properties of collagen.

Laser therapy is characterized by its minimally invasive nature, typically consisting of three treatment sessions over a specific period. Generally, these sessions are performed on an outpatient basis, without requiring anesthesia, and are spaced at intervals of 4–6 weeks between each one. The sum of the applied energy interactions resulting from the application of thermal energy to the tissue leads to the activation of the key cell, i.e., the fibroblast.

The CO_2 laser emits a specific pulse that first produces an initial acute thermosablative effect, which leads to the ablation of the epithelial layer of the atrophic vaginal mucosa and then generates a prolonged thermal effect that promotes the proliferation of collagen and connective tissue [68]. In the case of the Erbium:YAG laser, its action is based on heating. It breaks up the water molecules present in the tissue mucosa by emitting short laser micropulses separated by short intervals, which allows the treated surface to be refreshed and prevents its ablation [69].

Other Energy-Based Treatments

- Radiofrequency: The release of thermal energy causes the contraction of collagen, the stimulation of the formation of new collagen (neocollagenesis), and the generation of new blood vessels (neovascularization). All of these responses contribute to restoring the elasticity and hydration of the vaginal mucosa.
- Photobiomodulation: This modality uses nonthermal energy, which lacks cytotoxic effects and is not coherent. It consists of exposing the target tissue to light sources that use light-emitting diodes (LED) in the visible spectrum and near the infrared zone. It has been shown that this technique has a restorative effect on tissues.

Hyaluronic Acid Infiltration

It is the main component of connective tissue and plays a fundamental role in maintaining the tone, tropism, and flexibility of the skin and mucous membranes. In addition, it plays a prominent role in the wound healing process and has a notable moisturizing capacity, being used in various vulvovaginal creams and gels.

The application of hyaluronic acid in the form of injectable vials for intradermal administration raised the possibility of its use in the treatment of genitourinary menopausal syndrome (GMS). Injectable hyaluronic acid is available for the purpose of rehydrating and biostimulating the skin and genital mucosa. Although the average duration of the effect has not been established, it is known that hyaluronic acid gradually degrades, and its effect diminishes over time.

Scientific evidence on the use of hyaluronic acid in this context is limited. Although there are small case series reporting positive results, the absence of a control group limits the ability to draw solid conclusions to establish clinical recommendations. Adverse effects are few and mostly local [70].

Platelet-Rich Plasma (PRP)

It consists of a portion of autologous plasma with a platelet concentration higher than the basal level. It contains more than 30 bioactive proteins that contribute to cellular immunomodulation, promote the synthesis of extracellular matrix, promote neovascularization, and participate in the regeneration of specific cells of each tissue. PRP can improve dyspareunia by releasing growth factors and cytokines that play an essential role in angiogenesis, differentiation, and release of pluripotent stem cells in areas close to the injection site, thus improving vaginal vascularization [71].

Carboxytherapy

Subcutaneous administration of carbon dioxide (CO_2) results in an increase in tissue oxygenation (PO_2) through the Bohr effect. This process also increases vascular endothelial growth factor (VEGF), promotes blood flow, shows a high diffusion capacity in tissues, stimulates connective tissue, and restores tissue microcirculation [72].

Nanofat

Intradermal infiltration of emulsified autologous fat, known as Nanofat, is used for skin regeneration. This procedure takes advantage of the activity of stem cells, which play a crucial role in tissue regeneration.

Botulinum Toxin

Botulinum toxin stands out for its application in patients with GSM who experience spasm in the external third of the vagina. The loss of elasticity, turgor, hydration, and lubrication associated with hypoestrogenism can lead to secondary vaginismus. Botulinum toxin is presented as a complementary treatment to the conventional approach in cases that do not respond adequately [73].

6.4.4 Importance of Adherence to Treatment

GMS is a chronic disorder and requires adequate, long-term treatment where a proactive attitude on the part of healthcare professionals is essential since treatment abandonments are frequent. In a study with more than 30,000 participants with GMS treated with local estrogens, 85–90% of cream users and about 60% of tablet users abandoned treatment in the first months. The lack of adhesion generalizes to other treatments such as lubricants and moisturizers.

In the event of a lack of response to a treatment, it is necessary to evaluate adherence. If the woman does not accept the treatment, she is uncomfortable with it, or it causes great discomfort, it is easier for her to abandon it. Good communication between doctor and patient is important for adherence because the treatment can be chosen taking into account the preferences of the woman with GMS. In this way, it will be easier to achieve continuity in treatment.

6.5 Final Comment

Over the past decade, we have learned a great deal about the vaginal microbiome and how it relates to host health. Unfortunately, most of the information derives from observational studies that propose hypotheses about the mechanisms of interrelation of the vaginal microbiota with each other and with the host.

These observational studies have generated innumerable hypotheses that must be tested in the laboratory for it to have a proper evidence level.

Recent in vitro work has characterized aspects of the biology of individual bacteria, but these studies often do not include the microbiota and/or the host. For clinicians, information on the relationships of the vaginal microbiota with the host is essential.

One of the barriers to obtaining this knowledge is the development of unified research models that include pathophysiological aspects of the vagina and its alterations, such as GSM. In this, multi-omics research will have enormous relevance as integration of metagenomic, metatranscriptomic, metabolomic, and immunology datasets could afford a detailed look into the biology of the microbiota-host relationship as it exists in vivo.

Results from such in vitro and in vivo studies, along with interventional clinical trials, will likely drive the development of advanced and innovative treatment options and preventative measures for the adverse health outcomes that impact vaginal health and quality of life and remain unaddressed.

References

1. Palacios S, Sánchez-Borrego R, Suárez Álvarez B, Lugo Salcedo F, González Calvo AJ, Quijano Martín JJ, Cancelo MJ, Fasero M. Impact of vulvovaginal atrophy therapies on postmenopausal women's quality of life in the CRETA study measured by the Cervantes scale. Maturitas. 2023;172:46–51. https://doi.org/10.1016/j.maturitas.2023.03.007.
2. Portman DJ, Gass ML, Vulvovaginal Atrophy Terminology Consensus Conference Panel. Genitourinary syndrome of menopause: new terminology for vulvovaginal atrophy from the International Society for the Study of Women's Sexual Health and the North American Menopause Society. Maturitas. 2014;79(3):349–54. https://doi.org/10.1016/j.maturitas.2014.07.013.
3. Menoguia Salud vaginal. Asociación Española para el Estudio de la Menopausia. 2014. ISBN: 978-84-940319-5-3.
4. Robinson D, Cardozo LD. The role of estrogens in female lower urinary tract dysfunction. Urology. 2003;62(4 Suppl 1):45–51. https://doi.org/10.1016/s0090-4295(03)00676-9.
5. Cancelo MJ, Beltrán D, Calaf J, Campillo F, Cano A, Guerra JA, Neyro JL. Protocolo Sociedad Española de Ginecología y Obstetricia de diagnóstico y tratamiento de las infecciones vulvovaginales. Prog Obst Gynecol. 2013;56(5):278–84.
6. Döderlein ASG. Das Scheidensekret und seine bedeutung für das puerperalfieber. Leipzig: O. Durr; 1892.
7. Miller EA, Beasley DE, Dunn RR, Archie EA. Lactobacilli dominance and vaginal pH: why is the human vaginal microbiome unique? Front Microbiol. 2016;7:1936. https://doi.org/10.3389/fmicb.2016.01936.
8. Alvarez-Olmos MI, Barousse MM, Rajan L, Van Der Pol BJ, Fortenberry D, Orr D, Fidel PL Jr. Vaginal lactobacilli in adolescents: presence and relationship to local and systemic immunity, and to bacterial vaginosis. Sex Transm Dis. 2004;31(7):393–400. https://doi.org/10.1097/01.olq.0000130454.83883.e9.
9. Zhou X, Bent SJ, Schneider MG, Davis CC, Islam MR, Forney LJ. Characterization of vaginal microbial communities in adult healthy women using cultivation-independent methods. Microbiol (Reading). 2004;150(Pt 8):2565–73. https://doi.org/10.1099/mic.0.26905-0.

10. Gudnadottir U, Debelius JW, Du J, Hugerth LW, Danielsson H, Schuppe-Koistinen I, Fransson E, Brusselaers N. The vaginal microbiome and the risk of preterm birth: a systematic review and network meta-analysis. Sci Rep. 2022;12(1):7926. https://doi.org/10.1038/s41598-022-12007-9.
11. Gajer P, Brotman RM, Bai G, Sakamoto J, Schütte UM, Zhong X, Koenig SS, Fu L, Ma ZS, Zhou X, Abdo Z, Forney LJ, Ravel J. Temporal dynamics of the human vaginal microbiota. Sci Transl Med. 2012;4(132):132ra52. https://doi.org/10.1126/scitranslmed.3003605.
12. Nurainiwati SA, Ma'roef M, Pravitasari DN, Putra PYP. Effectivity and efficacy probiotics for bacterial vaginosis treatments: meta-analysis. Infect Dis Model. 2022;7(4):597–604. https://doi.org/10.1016/j.idm.2022.09.001.
13. Boyd MA, Antonio MA, Hillier SL. Comparison of API 50 CH strips to whole-chromosomal DNA probes for identification of lactobacillus species. J Clin Microbiol. 2005;43(10):5309–11. https://doi.org/10.1128/JCM.43.10.5309-5311.2005. PMID: 16208005; PMCID: PMC1248469.
14. Lev-Sagie A, De Seta F, Verstraelen H, Ventolini G, Lonnee-Hoffmann R, Vieira-Baptista P. The vaginal microbiome: II. Vaginal Dysbiotic conditions. J Low Genit Tract Dis. 2022;26(1):79–84. https://doi.org/10.1097/LGT.0000000000000644.
15. Hyman RW, Fukushima M, Diamond L, Kumm J, Giudice LC, Davis RW. Microbes on the human vaginal epithelium. Proc Natl Acad Sci USA. 2005;102(22):7952–7. https://doi.org/10.1073/pnas.0503236102.
16. Reid G, Burton J, Devillard E. The rationale for probiotics in female urogenital healthcare. MedGenMed. 2004;6(1):49. PMID: 15208560.
17. Kenyon CR, Osbak K. Recent progress in understanding the epidemiology of bacterial vaginosis. Curr Opin Obstet Gynecol. 2014;26(6):448–54. https://doi.org/10.1097/GCO.0000000000000112.
18. Stamey TA. The role of introital enterobacteria in recurrent urinary infections. J Urol. 1973;109(3):467–72. https://doi.org/10.1016/s0022-5347(17)60454-3.
19. Cancelo Hidalgo MJ, de la Fuente P. Perception ans attitude of spanish gynaecologists towards women with integral perineal symptomatology (IPS). 8th European Congress on MenoReid G, Bruce AW. Urogenital infections in women: can probiotics help? World J Urol. 2003;24:28–32. pause (EMAS) London UK 16–20 May 2009.
20. Hodgins MB, Spike RC, Mackie RM, MacLean AB. An immunohistochemical study of androgen, oestrogen and progesterone receptors in the vulva and vagina. Br J Obstet Gynaecol. 1998;105(2):216–22. https://doi.org/10.1111/j.1471-0528.1998.tb10056.x.
21. Blakeman PJ, Hilton P, Bulmer JN. Oestrogen and progesterone receptor expression in the female lower urinary tract, with reference to oestrogen status. BJU Int. 2000;86(1):32–8. https://doi.org/10.1046/j.1464-410x.2000.00724.x.
22. Kwok M, McGeorge S, Mayer-Coverdale J, Graves B, Paterson DL, Harris PNA, Esler R, Dowling C, Britton S, Roberts MJ. Guideline of guidelines: management of recurrent urinary tract infections in women. BJU Int. 2022;130(Suppl 3):11–22. https://doi.org/10.1111/bju.15756.
23. The NAMS 2020 GSM Position Statement Editorial Panel. The 2020 genitourinary syndrome of menopause position statement of The North American Menopause Society. Menopause. 2020;27(9):976–92. https://doi.org/10.1097/GME.0000000000001609.
24. Nappi RE, Palacios S. Impact of vulvovaginal atrophy on sexual health and quality of life at postmenopause. Climacteric. 2014;17(1):3–9. https://doi.org/10.3109/13697137.2013.871696.
25. Nappi RE, Kokot-Kierepa M. Women's voices in the menopause: results from an international survey on vaginal atrophy. Maturitas. 2010;67(3):233–8. https://doi.org/10.1016/j.maturitas.2010.08.001.
26. Freedman MA. Quality of life and menopause: the role of estrogen. J Womens Health (Larchmt). 2002;11(8):703–18. https://doi.org/10.1089/15409990260363661.

27. Palacios S, Cancelo MJ, Branco CC, Llaneza P, Molero F, Borrego RS. Vulvar and vaginal atrophy as viewed by the Spanish REVIVE participants: symptoms, management and treatment perception. Climacteric. 2017;20(1):55–61. https://doi.org/10.1080/13697137.2016.1262840.
28. Raz R, Colodner R, Rohana Y, Battino S, Rottensterich E, Wasser I, Stamm W. Effectiveness of estriol-containing vaginal pessaries and nitrofurantoin macrocrystal therapy in the prevention of recurrent urinary tract infection in postmenopausal women. Clin Infect Dis. 2003;36(11):1362–8. https://doi.org/10.1086/374341.
29. Goldstein I, Dicks B, Kim NN, Hartzell R. Multidisciplinary overview of vaginal atrophy and associated genitourinary symptoms in postmenopausal women. Sex Med. 2013;1(2):44–53. https://doi.org/10.1002/sm2.17.
30. Palacios S, Cancelo MJ. Guía práctica de asistencia del síndrome urogenital de la menopausia (SEGO). Actualización 2015. Ed: SEGO (Junio 2015). Madrid. España.
31. Johnston SL, Farrell SA, Bouchard C, Farrell SA, Beckerson LA, Comeau M, Johnston SL, Lefebvre G, Papaioannou A, SOGC Joint Committee-Clinical Practice Gynaecology and Urogynaecology. The detection and management of vaginal atrophy. J Obstet Gynaecol Can. 2004;26(5):503–15. https://doi.org/10.1016/s1701-2163(16)30662-4.
32. O'Connell TX, Nathan LS, Satmary WA, Goldstein AT. Non-neoplastic epithelial disorders of the vulva. Am Fam Physician. 2008;77(3):321–6. PMID: 18297956.
33. Mension E, Alonso I, Tortajada M, Matas I, Gómez S, Ribera L, Ros C, Anglès-Acedo S, Castelo-Branco C. Genitourinary syndrome of menopause assessment tools. J Midlife Health. 2021;12(2):99–102. https://doi.org/10.4103/jmh.jmh_93_21.
34. Rosen R, Brown C, Heiman J, Leiblum S, Meston C, Shabsigh R, Ferguson D, D'Agostino R Jr. The Female Sexual Function Index (FSFI): a multidimensional self-report instrument for the assessment of female sexual function. J Sex Marital Ther. 2000;26(2):191–208. https://doi.org/10.1080/009262300278597.
35. Bachmann GA, Notelovitz M, Kelly SJ, et al. Long-term nonhormonal treatment of vaginal dryness. Clin Pract Sex. 1992;8:12.
36. Palacios S, Cancelo MJ, González S, Manubens M, Sanchez BR. Genitourinary syndrome of menopause: recommendations from the Spanish Society of Obstetrics and Gynecology. Prog Obstet Ginecol. 2019;62(2):141–8. https://doi.org/10.20960/j.pog.00182.
37. Palacios S, Mejias A. An update on drugs for the treatment of menopausal symptoms. Expert Opin Pharmacother. 2015;16(16):2437–47. https://doi.org/10.1517/14656566.2015.1085508.
38. Origoni M, Cimmino C, Carminati G, Iachini E, Stefani C, Girardelli S, Salvatore S, Candiani M. Postmenopausal vulvovaginal atrophy (VVA) is positively improved by topical hyaluronic acid application. A prospective, observational study. Eur Rev Med Pharmacol Sci. 2016;20(20):4190–5. PMID: 27831658.
39. Salvatore S, Nappi RE, Zerbinati N, Calligaro A, Ferrero S, Origoni M, Candiani M, Leone Roberti Maggiore U. A 12-week treatment with fractional CO_2 laser for vulvovaginal atrophy: a pilot study. Climacteric. 2014;17(4):363–9. https://doi.org/10.3109/13697137.2014.899347. Epub 2014 Jun 5. PMID: 24605832.
40. Mei Z, Li D. The role of probiotics in vaginal health. Front Cell Infect Microbiol. 2022;12:963868. https://doi.org/10.3389/fcimb.2022.963868.
41. Muhleisen AL, Herbst-Kralovetz MM. Menopause and the vaginal microbiome. Maturitas. 2016;91:42–50. https://doi.org/10.1016/j.maturitas.2016.05.015.
42. Tuniyazi M, Zhang N. Possible therapeutic mechanisms and future perspectives of vaginal microbiota transplantation. Microorganisms. 2023;11(6):1427. https://doi.org/10.3390/microorganisms11061427.
43. Leiblum S, Bachmann G, Kemmann E, Colburn D, Swartzman L. Vaginal atrophy in the postmenopausal woman. The importance of sexual activity and hormones. JAMA. 1983;249(16):2195–8. PMID: 6834616.
44. Palacios S, Coronado PJ. New options for menopausal symptoms after 15 years of WHI study. Minerva Ginecol. 2017;69(2):160–70. https://doi.org/10.23736/S0026-4784.16.04007-7.

45. Lethaby A, Ayeleke RO, Roberts H. Local oestrogen for vaginal atrophy in postmenopausal women. Cochrane Database Syst Rev. 2016;2016(8):CD001500. https://doi.org/10.1002/14651858.CD001500.pub3.
46. Cardozo L, Bachmann G, McClish D, Fonda D, Birgerson L. Meta-analysis of estrogen therapy in the management of urogenital atrophy in postmenopausal women: second report of the Hormones and Urogenital Therapy Committee. Obstet Gynecol. 1998;92(4 Pt 2):722–7. https://doi.org/10.1016/s0029-7844(98)00175-6.
47. Suckling J, Lethaby A, Kennedy R. Local oestrogen for vaginal atrophy in postmenopausal women. Cochrane Database Syst Rev. 2006;18(4):CD001500. https://doi.org/10.1002/14651858.CD001500.pub2. Update in: Cochrane Database Syst Rev. 2016;8:CD001500.
48. Bachmann G, Lobo RA, Gut R, Nachtigall L, Notelovitz M. Efficacy of low-dose estradiol vaginal tablets in the treatment of atrophic vaginitis: a randomized controlled trial. Obstet Gynecol. 2008;111(1):67–76. https://doi.org/10.1097/01.AOG.0000296714.12226.0f.
49. Santen RJ. Vaginal administration of estradiol: effects of dose, preparation and timing on plasma estradiol levels. Climacteric. 2015;18(2):121–34. https://doi.org/10.3109/13697137.2014.947254.
50. Simon JA, Maamari RV. Ultra-low-dose vaginal estrogen tablets for the treatment of postmenopausal vaginal atrophy. Climacteric. 2013;16(Suppl 1):37–43. https://doi.org/10.3109/13697137.2013.807606.
51. Del Pup L, Di Francia R, Cavaliere C, Facchini G, Giorda G, De Paoli P, Berretta M. Promestriene, a specific topic estrogen. Review of 40 years of vaginal atrophy treatment: is it safe even in cancer patients? Anticancer Drugs. 2013;24(10):989–98. https://doi.org/10.1097/CAD.0b013e328365288e.
52. Palacios S, Castelo-Branco C, Cancelo MJ, Vázquez F. Low-dose, vaginally administered estrogens may enhance local benefits of systemic therapy in the treatment of urogenital atrophy in postmenopausal women on hormone therapy. Maturitas. 2005;50(2):98–104. https://doi.org/10.1016/j.maturitas.2004.04.007.
53. American College of Obstetricians and Gynecologists' Committee on Gynecologic Practice, Farrell R. ACOG Committee Opinion No. 659: the use of vaginal estrogen in women with a history of estrogen-dependent breast cancer. Obstet Gynecol. 2016;27(3):e93–6. https://doi.org/10.1097/AOG.0000000000001351.
54. Mendoza N, Abad P, Baró F, Cancelo MJ, Llaneza P, Manubens M, Quereda F, Sánchez-Borrego R. Spanish Menopause Society position statement: use of tibolone in postmenopausal women. Menopause. 2013;20(7):754–60. https://doi.org/10.1097/GME.0b013e31827b18c5.
55. Portman DJ, Labrie F, Archer DF, Bouchard C, Cusan L, Girard G, Ayotte N, Koltun W, Blouin F, Young D, Wade A, Martel C, Dubé R, Other Participating Members of VVA Prasterone Group. Lack of effect of intravaginal dehydroepiandrosterone (DHEA, prasterone) on the endometrium in postmenopausal women. Menopause. 2015;22(12):1289–95. https://doi.org/10.1097/GME.0000000000000470.
56. Labrie F, Archer DF, Koltun W, Vachon A, Young D, Frenette L, Portman D, Montesino M, Côté I, Parent J, Lavoie L, Beauregard A, Martel C, Vaillancourt M, Balser J, Moyneur É, Members of the VVA Prasterone Research Group. Efficacy of intravaginal dehydroepiandrosterone (DHEA) on moderate to severe dyspareunia and vaginal dryness, symptoms of vulvovaginal atrophy, and of the genitourinary syndrome of menopause. Menopause. 2018;25(11):1339–53. https://doi.org/10.1097/GME.0000000000001238.
57. Bouchard C, Labrie F, Derogatis L, Girard G, Ayotte N, Gallagher J, Cusan L, Archer DF, Portman D, Lavoie L, Beauregard A, Côté I, Martel C, Vaillancourt M, Balser J, Moyneur E, VVA Prasterone Group. Effect of intravaginal dehydroepiandrosterone (DHEA) on the female sexual function in postmenopausal women: ERC-230 open-label study. Horm Mol Biol Clin Investig. 2016;25(3):181–90. https://doi.org/10.1515/hmbci-2015-0044. PMID: 26725467.
58. Goldstein SW, Goldstein I, Kim NN. Vestibular tissue changes following administration of intravaginal prasterone: a vulvoscopic open-label pilot study in menopausal women with dyspareunia. Sex Med. 2023;11(3):qfad028. https://doi.org/10.1093/sexmed/qfad028.

59. Lubián López DM. Management of genitourinary syndrome of menopause in breast cancer survivors: an update. World J Clin Oncol. 2022;13(2):71–100. https://doi.org/10.5306/wjco.v13.i2.71.
60. D'Anna R, Cannata ML, Atteritano M, Cancellieri F, Corrado F, Baviera G, Triolo O, Antico F, Gaudio A, Frisina N, Bitto A, Polito F, Minutoli L, Altavilla D, Marini H, Squadrito F. Effects of the phytoestrogen genistein on hot flushes, endometrium, and vaginal epithelium in postmenopausal women: a 1-year randomized, double-blind, placebo-controlled study. Menopause. 2007;14(4):648–55. https://doi.org/10.1097/01.gme.0000248708.60698.98.
61. Cui Y, Zong H, Yan H, Li N, Zhang Y. The efficacy and safety of ospemifene in treating dyspareunia associated with postmenopausal vulvar and vaginal atrophy: a systematic review and meta-analysis. J Sex Med. 2014;11(2):487–97. https://doi.org/10.1111/jsm.12377.
62. Taras TL, Wurz GT, DeGregorio MW. In vitro and in vivo biologic effects of Ospemifene (FC-1271a) in breast cancer. J Steroid Biochem Mol Biol. 2001;77(4–5):271–9. https://doi.org/10.1016/s0960-0760(01)00066-8.
63. Palacios S, Cancelo MJ. Clinical update on the use of ospemifene in the treatment of severe symptomatic vulvar and vaginal atrophy. Int J Women's Health. 2016;8:617–26. https://doi.org/10.2147/IJWH.S110035.
64. DeGregorio MW, Zerbe RL, Wurz GT. Ospemifene: a first-in-class, non-hormonal selective estrogen receptor modulator approved for the treatment of dyspareunia associated with vulvar and vaginal atrophy. Steroids. 2014;90:82–93. https://doi.org/10.1016/j.steroids.2014.07.012.
65. Constantine G, Graham S, Portman DJ, Rosen RC, Kingsberg SA. Female sexual function improved with ospemifene in postmenopausal women with vulvar and vaginal atrophy: results of a randomized, placebo-controlled trial. Climacteric. 2015;18(2):226–32. https://doi.org/10.3109/13697137.2014.954996.
66. European Medicines Agency. Senshio Summary of Product Characteristics. EMA; 2015. Available from: http://www.ema.europa.eu/docs/en_GB/document_library/EPAR_-_Product_Information/human/002780/WC500182775.pdf. Accessed December 1, 2016.
67. Palacios S, Mejía A, Neyro JL. Treatment of the genitourinary syndrome of menopause. Climacteric. 2015;18(Suppl 1):23–9. https://doi.org/10.3109/13697137.2015.1079100. PMID: 26366797.
68. Gambacciani M, Palacios S. Laser therapy for the restoration of vaginal function. Maturitas. 2017;99:10–5. https://doi.org/10.1016/j.maturitas.2017.01.012. Epub 2017 Feb 4. PMID: 28364861.
69. Gaspar A, Brandi H, Gomez V, Luque D. Efficacy of Erbium:YAG laser treatment compared to topical estriol treatment for symptoms of genitourinary syndrome of menopause. Lasers Surg Med. 2017;49(2):160–8. https://doi.org/10.1002/lsm.22569. Epub 2016 Aug 22. PMID: 27546524; PMCID: PMC5347840.
70. Dos Santos CCM, Uggioni MLR, Colonetti T, Colonetti L, Grande AJ, Da Rosa MI. Hyaluronic acid in postmenopause vaginal atrophy: a systematic review. J Sex Med. 2021;18(1):156–66. https://doi.org/10.1016/j.jsxm.2020.10.016. Epub 2020 Dec 5. PMID: 33293236.
71. Hersant B, SidAhmed-Mezi M, Belkacemi Y, Darmon F, Bastuji-Garin S, Werkoff G, Bosc R, Niddam J, Hermeziu O, La Padula S, Meningaud JP. Efficacy of injecting platelet concentrate combined with hyaluronic acid for the treatment of vulvovaginal atrophy in postmenopausal women with history of breast cancer: a phase 2 pilot study. Menopause. 2018;25(10):1124–30. https://doi.org/10.1097/GME.0000000000001122. PMID: 29738415.
72. Hartmann BR, Bassenge E, Pittler M. Effect of carbon dioxide-enriched water and fresh water on the cutaneous microcirculation and oxygen tension in the skin of the foot. Angiology. 1997;48(4):337–43. https://doi.org/10.1177/000331979704800406. PMID: 9112881.
73. Abbott JA, Jarvis SK, Lyons SD, Thomson A, Vancaille TG. Botulinum toxin type a for chronic pain and pelvic floor spasm in women: a randomized controlled trial. Obstet Gynecol. 2006;108(4):915–23. https://doi.org/10.1097/01.AOG.0000237100.29870.cc. PMID: 17012454.
74. Costello EK, Stagaman K, Dethlefsen L, Bohannan BJ, Relman DA. The application of ecological theory toward an understanding of the human microbiome. Science. 2012;336(6086):1255–62. https://doi.org/10.1126/science.1224203.

Sexual Health

7

Nicolás Mendoza Ladrón de Guevara, Ana Rosa Jurado, and Loreto Mendoza Huertas

Abstract

Menopause is an opportunity for sexuality to become more intimate and relaxed. Acceptance of physical changes and a previous history of good sexual health positively influence sexual health over the years. At any age, especially in long-term relationships, the quality of the relationship remains the most important factor influencing sexual health and desire. Pharmacological treatments may be reserved for cases where couples therapy or lifestyle changes have not been effective in improving sexual health.

7.1 Introduction

Sexual health can be defined as a state of physical, emotional, mental and social wellbeing that is related to sexuality and not merely the absence of disease, dysfunction or infirmity. The sexual health of individuals requires them to have a positive and respectful attitude towards sexuality and sexual relations and the possibility of having sexual experiences that are pleasurable, safe and free of coercion, discrimination and violence. Therefore, sexual health is not exclusive to the prevention of sexually transmitted diseases; it also entails a broader approach that is related to the full development of a person's welfare, health, education and love [1].

N. M. L. de Guevara (✉) · L. M. Huertas
Department of Obstetrics and Gynecology, University of Granada, Granada, Spain
e-mail: nicomendoza@ugr.es

A. R. Jurado
Department of Obstetrics and Gynecology, University of Granada, Granada, Spain

Instituto Europeo de Sexologia, Marbella, Málaga, Spain

© The Author(s), under exclusive license to Springer Nature Switzerland AG 2025
A. Cano (ed.), *Menopause*, https://doi.org/10.1007/978-3-031-83979-5_7

7.2 Changes in Sexuality Related to Menopause

The physical, psychological and sociocultural changes that occur in peri- and postmenopausal women people may favour sexual intercourse, but it is more common for them to harm or even completely interrupt sexual activity. Sexuality at this age is conditioned by previous sexual experiences and is often affected by health problems and the treatment of these problems with medications. Age and disease most often affect sexual desire in women (hypoactive sexual desire disorder), and erection most often affects men (erectile dysfunction) [2].

Age should not be considered a factor that is responsible for impaired sexual function. In the postmenopausal women, certain factors affect sexual desire:

7.2.1 Hormonal Factors

The serum levels of certain hormones, including testosterone, oestrogen, oxytocin, beta-endorphins and prolactin, influence sexual activity. Testosterone is a hormone that stimulates sexual desire in both men and women, but from 40 years of age, testosterone levels decrease in the blood. Women of childbearing age have a peak secretion of testosterone and androstenedione for half of the ovarian cycle that coincides with ovulation that has been associated with an increase in spontaneous desire. Oestrogens help to maintain tropism and vaginal lubrication. Hence, they indirectly enable pleasurable sex. In postmenopausal women, a decrease in oestrogen levels results in atrophy and decreased vaginal lubrication. These changes may be responsible for less pleasurable or painful intercourse in women (dyspareunia), which could adversely affect their motivation and sexual desire [2].

Additionally, a progressive decrease in testosterone levels has been associated with decreased sexual activity. However, hormonal factors do not fully explain the changes that are observed in sexuality with increasing age.

Age fundamentally modifies the sexual response, just as it affects multiple other physical abilities in humans. Women are more likely than men to experience specific hormonal changes throughout their life that temporarily alter their sexual responses [3]. However, strong evidence has shown that neither age nor hormonal changes themselves are solely responsible for the decline of sexual health observed in individuals over 50. Rather, this decline is thought to occur in response to a number of other factors that are psychological, relational or sociocultural in nature [4].

7.2.2 Psychological and Relationship Factors

Different psychological problems can lead to decreased sexual desire. These include depressive syndrome or anxiety disorders. During menopause, changes in mood or sleep disturbances can influence desire in women. Additionally, decreased self-esteem or changes in body images that occur as a result of a disease or its treatment may lead to a deterioration in sexual health.

Relationship problems with partners can lead to decreased libido, especially in women. A good relationship is fundamental because a stable and harmonious relationship promotes the prompt and satisfactory resolution of any sexual conflicts that may arise. Conversely, a bad relationship itself can cause problems in a couple's sexual life [5]. Additionally, drugs can affect sexual experiences and lead to risky sexual behaviour and social conflicts within the couple [2].

Continued stressful situations facilitate the production of prolactin, and increases in serum prolactin levels decrease sexual desire [6].

In our society, models of education that do not encourage the acceptance of sexuality can have negative effects on sexual desire. Additionally, the false belief that older women do not have sex can unconsciously cause a loss of motivation and desire [2].

The sexual response of men progresses linearly and usually begins with desire. This desire can be triggered by sexual thoughts and fantasies or the urgency to experience sexual satisfaction. However, the female sexual response resembles that of males only occasionally, in particular at the beginning of romantic relationships, after which women require more stimulation. In general, spontaneous sexual desire decreases with women's increasing age [2].

According to Rosemary Basson, the progression of the sexual response in women is cyclical, and the phases of the female sexual response (desire, arousal, plateau, orgasm and resolution) do not necessarily follow this order but can overlap with each other or progress in an order that can vary according to the situation. Therefore, desire does not usually mark the start of the female sexual response. This entire cycle can be influenced by emotional intimacy, sexual stimulation and the woman's satisfaction with the relationship [7].

The human sexual response to exciting stimuli involves a cycle of motivation that is based on incentives and that comprises the physiological changes and subjective experiences of the individual. Psychological and biological factors influence the processing of sexual stimuli in the brain, causing it to allow or not allow the activation of the next phase of sexual response. The results obtained during both sexual and non-sexual intercourse influence an individual's future motivation to seek intimacy [8].

7.2.3 Cultural Factors

In our society, the belief that people do not have sex after a certain age is pervasive. This can unconsciously lead older adults to consider it to be normal to not have sexual relationships, motivation or desire. This myth is negated by studies showing that over 80% of people over 60 years of age continue having sex.

The cultural perception of sexuality in young people as a fiery and intense activity and attempts to enforce the social standards of youth and power could influence the sexual activity of the elderly. They leave no opportunity for a more leisurely and intimate sexuality, which could be the ideal type of sexuality for this population.

On the other hand, the physical factors and physiological changes that occur with ageing do not determine the sexual activity of older people because there are other factors that determine this behaviour, including the following:

- Previous sexual history: The level of sexual activity of each person during earlier life stages is very important to sexual activity in the second part of his or her life.
- The interest and existence of a partner in addition to the health of this partner have special importance in these stages of life. Older people discontinue sexual activities more as a result of a lack of available partners than a lack of interest.
- Physical and psychological health: Health problems can hinder sexual activity. If necessary and to avoid complications related to health problems, changing the usual recommended positions to perform sexual activity using a side or rear position may be advised. The use of a support pillow might also be advised.

7.3 Changes in Sexuality Related to Chronic Diseases

The existence of organic disease can decrease sexual desire although it rarely fully prevents sexual activity. However, genitourinary diseases that require surgical treatment or are cancer-based have a greater impact on people's sexual health. At this age, a frequent consumption of drugs may be responsible for decreased desire, including antihypertensives, antidepressants and opioid analgesics [2].

Sexual health can deteriorate because of a variety of medical or psychiatric problems that become increasingly frequent over an individual's lifespan. This deterioration in sexual health results not only from the primary effects of the disease and its treatment on sexual responses but also from the negative psychological consequences that occur secondary to the development and pharmacological management of disease (i.e., decreased self-esteem, changes in body image or depression) [9]. However, evidence is scarce regarding the impact of disease on sexual health. Furthermore, much of the evidence that is available is heterogeneous and of low quality. Even the guidelines for clinical practice rarely mention sexual health unless the course of treatment directly targets sexual dysfunction.

Genitourinary pathology deserves special mention, especially if its treatment is surgical or the basis of the pathology is oncological, in which case sexual health can be compromised by alterations in the anatomy, physiology and psychology of the individual suffering the disease [10, 11]. The same can be said regarding breast cancer: Even if a condition does not directly affect the genital area, female sexual health can be greatly impaired due to the physical and psychological pain that results directly from the disease process itself or as an indirect consequence of various treatment regimens. For example, drugs with anti-oestrogen activity can compromise sexual health by greatly increasing vaginal atrophy [12].

7.4 Changes in Sexuality Related to Surgical Menopause

The uterus has historically been considered a regulator and controller of important physiological functions in addition to a sexual organ and a source of energy, vitality and maintenance of youthfulness and attractiveness in women. It is therefore not surprising that some women may feel that their sex life could be affected by the removal of the organ [13].

Female sexual responses are complex because they are influenced by physical and emotional factors and women's sexual experiences. Unlike what occurs in men, desire is not usually the beginning of the female sexual response. The female orgasm is also a complex process that is characterized by intermittent and rhythmic muscle contractions of the pelvic floor and the outermost portion of the vagina, anus and sometimes the uterus, which results in a more pleasurable feeling [14].

Women in stable relationships may be more concerned about emotional intimacy with their partners, and although in some cases the frequency of sexual intercourse can be related to a better sex life, female sexual functions are more a matter of quality than quantity. Thus, the sexual wellbeing of women should not be defined as the mere absence of sexual dysfunction.

A hysterectomy may be necessary to treat tumours of cervix or body of the uterus or advanced endometriosis or prolapse, among other conditions. These conditions may be responsible for pelvic pain, painful intercourse (dyspareunia) or vaginal bleeding unrelated to menstruation, all of which can negatively influence the sexual health of women. Therefore, removing the uterus may improve the sexual relations of women who are affected by these problems.

When a subtotal or total hysterectomy is performed, it may affect the ligaments, blood vessels and nerves that are involved in sexual function. Moreover, following a total hysterectomy, the shortening of the dome of the vagina could be responsible for dyspareunia. However, there are currently conservative surgical techniques that can preserve the nerves that innervate the pelvic organs [15].

A hysterectomy does not adversely affect sexual health. Most women who have only their uterus removed will have equal or better sexual function after the surgery than before, probably because their symptoms and previous problems are relieved. In this sense, some authors claim that after a subtotal or total hysterectomy, women experience a decrease in abdominal pain and increased desire, excitability and the frequency of intercourse. However, in women whose previous sexual experiences were not good, their sexual health is often worse after surgery [16].

In addition to hysterectomies, the removal of the ovaries may be necessary for the treatment of some benign, premalignant or malignant diseases of the internal genitalia [17]. In postmenopausal women, the removal of the ovaries causes no symptoms or major changes to their sexual health, but in premenopausal woman, it causes surgical menopause, with sudden and intense hormonal changes and subsequent consequences, mainly climacteric syndrome (hot flashes, sweating, psychological problems, insomnia, etc.) and impaired sexual function [18]. In this sense, women with surgical menopause show an increased risk of developing hypoactive sexual desire disorder and more emotional involvement than premenopausal women who experience natural menopause [19]. Additionally, a lower frequency of sexual intercourse, difficulty in lubrication, reduced sexual satisfaction, dyspareunia and difficulty achieving orgasm have been observed in women with surgical menopause [20].

The bilateral removal of the ovaries in premenopausal women causes a significant decrease in the levels of oestrogen and testosterone in the blood [17], which may explain some of the changes observed in these patients. Lower levels of oestrogen cause atrophy and decreased vaginal lubrication, which can cause less pleasurable or even painful sex in women, and this could negatively influence their sexual motivations and desire. The hypothesis in which a decline in blood testosterone causes hypoactive sexual desire disorder and sexual dysfunction in women with surgical menopause has not been supported. In all hysterectomy cases, it is recommended that women practice sexual self-stimulation 2 weeks after surgery because it allows them to experience pleasure without the pressure that can be exerted when in a relationship [6].

Some problems related to surgical menopause can be treated by oestrogen hormone therapy, which mitigates hot flashes and vaginal dryness and reduces dyspareunia, but it is less clear what effect this therapy may have on improving sexual function [21]. Testosterone replacement therapy patches seem to improve sexual desire and the frequency of intercourse and orgasms. In our experience, the use of tibolone has proved more effective in improving the sexual health of these women [2].

Moreover, psycho-educational therapy has been proposed to help women with surgical menopause to manage their sexual health problems. Short educational sessions on sexual health, body awareness and relaxation techniques seem to have a positive effect. Preoperative knowledge of the possible side effects decreased sexual distress after surgery [22].

In conclusion, removing the uterus does not adversely affect the sexual health of women. In most cases, the relief of symptoms and previous problems leads equal to or better sexual performance than they experienced before the surgery. In postmenopausal woman, removing the ovaries does not cause major changes. However, in premenopausal woman, it induces surgical menopause, which leads to sudden hormonal changes and impaired sexual functions and can be treated with hormone therapy and psycho-educational methods.

7.5 Hormonal Treatments

According to a Cochrane review, menopause hormone therapy (MHT) improves postmenopausal sexual function when used during the 5 years immediately following menopause [23]. The use of tibolone, a synthetic steroid with diverse actions in different tissues, has proven effective in the treatment of female sexual dysfunction, and its effectiveness is similar to that described for androgens. In some cases, tibolone is considered the best option for postmenopausal women with impaired sexual health [24].

Low-dose oestrogens are highly effective treatments for dyspareunia, low interest in sex and sexual dissatisfaction in women with atrophic vaginitis. Local oestrogen therapy is the treatment of choice for women with vaginal atrophy who do not have any other postmenopausal symptoms. In Spain, the most widely used product is the topical cream of promestriene [25].

Oestrogens and androgens can also be used in women with surgical menopause and HSDD. Women treated with 300 mcg of transdermal testosterone per day had a statistically significant increase of the sexual events, the orgasms and sexual desire, as well as a decrease in distress compared with women receiving placebo, although some of these values are not clinically meaningful [26]. However, considering the full hormonal deficit of these patients, the use of tibolone has been proven superior to promote improvements in the sexual health of women with surgical menopause [27].

Ospemifene is a selective oestrogen receptor modulator (SERM) with oestrogen agonist action in the vagina. It has been approved for the treatment of moderate-to-severe dyspareunia secondary to atrophic vaginitis. A recent meta-analysis indicates that ospemifene is an effective and safe treatment for dyspareunia associated with postmenopausal vulvar and vaginal atrophy [28].

Although preclinical data and those from animal experiments suggest that ospemifene has a neutral or inhibitory effect on mammary carcinogenesis, further studies are necessary to evaluate its safety in women with breast cancer. No thrombotic events have been reported either, although more data are necessary to rule out the complication that occurs with other SERMs. However, ospemifene use is contraindicated in women with breast cancer, endometrial cancer, venous thromboembolism, stroke or myocardial infarction [29].

Below, we summarize the recommendations of the Spanish Menopause Society on these THM [2]:

- Pharmacological treatments should be restricted to women with sexual dysfunctions for whom non-pharmacological interventions have proven ineffective.
- A low dose of vaginal oestrogen is recommended for postmenopausal women with dyspareunia due to atrophic vaginitis (Grade 1A).
- The use of aqueous lubricants before or during intercourse is suggested for women with contraindications for oestrogen (Grade 2B).
- For postmenopausal women with sexual dysfunctions and vasomotor symptoms, the use of MHT is recommended (Grade 1A). Tibolone can be an alternative to MHT in the treatment of postmenopausal women with impaired sexuality (Grade 2B) and appears to be more effective than MHT in women with surgical menopause (Grade 2C).
- For postmenopausal women with HSDD in whom pharmacological treatments have been unsuccessful, treatment with testosterone is suggested (Grade 2B). However, testosterone is not recommended for premenopausal women with sexual dysfunction (Grade 1B).
- The first line of treatment for vaginal atrophy symptoms in women with breast cancer includes non-hormonal options (i.e., lubricants or hydrating creams).

Using vaginal oestrogen therapy is not recommended for women using aromatase inhibitors for breast cancer (Grade 2C). However, low-dose oestrogen therapy is a reasonable option for those who do not receive aromatase inhibitors or who present a low risk of recurrence.
- For women with arousal or orgasm disorders associated with SSRI use, discontinuing the SSRI or changing to another antidepressant is not advisable; it is recommended to add a PDE-5 inhibitor (Grade 2B).
- Bupropion may be an effective treatment for sexual dysfunction in women with or without associated depression. However, no published data have proven the safety and effectiveness of phytotherapy in sexual dysfunction.

7.6 Sexual Dysfunctions in Menopause

We should not talk about a general sexual dysfunction in menopausal women, but it would be more appropriate if we consider different affections in the sexual response that can turn into abnormal sexual drive. It is very typical to have some difficulty, or variations, in the normal sexual response, due to ageing, hormonal changes, chronic diseases, medications and surgeries, not turning into dysfunction. These are simply predisposing factors, which if the patient cannot adapt to could become pathological. Adaptability is related to attitudes, education, social myths, quality of the relationship and several other factors that doctors should explore to help women during menopausal transition [2].

It is also typical that people cannot recognize what part of the sexual response was first affected. Main reason for consultation is low sexual desire, but if we diagnose correctly, it will be presumably different. When a person suffers lack of sexual arousal (erection, lubrication), he or she uses to think that it is due to low desire, but it is more frequent that low desire is a consequence of repeated frustrations because of dissatisfaction during intercourse due to lack of sexual arousal.

Doctors should provide a correct diagnosis to prescribe the most optimum treatment and explore all involved factors to procure the best individual sexual counselling. The following pages will try to describe the diagnosis and therapeutic approach of the most frequent sexual dysfunctions around menopause.

7.6.1 Low Sexual Desire

There are different concepts of low sexual desire for women and men since DSM-V publication [30]. DSM criteria for sexual dysfunctions reflect new theoretical approach trying to explain sexual behaviour in women after linear model of sexual response proposed by Masters and Johnson was found to be inadequate [31].

Male Hypoactive Sexual Desire Disorder (MHSDD) remains similar to the prior concept for men and women hypoactive sexual desire disorder (HSDD), meaning lack or absence of sexual fantasies and desire for sexual activity, causing marked distress or interpersonal difficulties, and not being better accounted for by another mental disorder, a drug or some other medical condition [30].

New concept for women amalgamates female disorders of desire and arousal into a single diagnosis called Female Sexual Interest/Arousal Disorder. This disorder is defined by a complete lack of or significant reduction of an interest in sexual activity, absence of fantasies or erotic thoughts, decline to initiate sexual encounters and no sense of pleasure during sexual acts. Three or more of these symptoms decide the diagnosis, if they persist more than 6 months, result in distress and are not better explained by drugs or another physical, biological and/or relational condition [30].

This new diagnosis approach has often been discussed, but in postmenopausal women, it could be adequate because one of the main reasons for low sexual desire in these women comes from inadequate arousal due to age and hormonal physiological changes.

Knowledge about low desire after decades of research is based on prior HSDD. Thus, we know that prevalence of HSDD remains constant across age because low desire can increase but related distress decreases. This sexual dysfunction is present in 8,9% of women ages 18 to 44, 12,3% aged 45 to 64 and 7,4% over 65. Common associated factors to low desire are poor health-related quality of life, lower general happiness and satisfaction with relationship, and negative emotional states [32].

Around menopause, researchers find several specific factors to explain low desire in women [33]. They find general poor sexual function in older women or those affected by menopausal symptoms, suffering anxiety/depress disorder or sharing sexual life with alcoholic partner or with a man suffering erectile dysfunction. Among women with low desire, inadequate intimacy, context or sexual stimulation are found to contribute to diagnosis in 85%, while hormonal-related changes contributed only in 25% [34].

From a physiologic point of view, researchers have found 87% postmenopausal women believed vaginal dryness a factor causing reduced libido, but only 46% had discussed it with health professionals and only half of them had received treatment [35].

However, it is rare to find a single cause for low sexual desire. So with a view to be successful with the treatment, doctors need to help patient to initiate discussions and identify all associated factors. The correct treatment approach requires biological information to patients, psychotherapeutic and pharmacological interventions.

There is not too much approved medication for use in female low desire. We had a label indication for testosterone patch for surgical postmenopausal women, and the new recently approved is flibanserin. Testosterone has demonstrated in several studies, not only for the development of the patches, that it can be a good option for improving sexual drive in peri- and postmenopausal women, and when added to HRT, it has a beneficial effect on sexual function [36].

Flibanserin is indicated for the treatment of premenopausal women with acquired generalized HSDD. It works as a serotonin 1A receptor agonist and serotonin 2A receptor antagonist, but its mechanism of action in the treatment of this sexual dysfunction remains unknown [37]. It has demonstrated an increase in the number of satisfying sexual events and sexual desire (FSFI desire domain score) over 28 days of use. In addition, it reduces distress associated with total sexual dysfunction and associated with low desire [38].

Other medical products have demonstrated slight improvement in sexual function, for example, DHEA, probably because its conversion into oestrogen and testosterone in postmenopausal women [39], or phytoestrogens (soya, red-clover, black cohosh), perhaps by enhancing quality of life. But they all still have an "out of label" indication for sexual desire.

By individualizing every treatment, most of the options could be considered and should be used adding sexual education about how to optimize sexual response, ways to enhance intimacy with partner and recommendations for couples [2].

7.6.2 Sexual Pain

Before DSM-V publication, we used to talk about dyspareunia (genital pain associated with sexual intercourse, either a male or a female) and the most related to psychosomatic concerns, vaginismus (involuntary spasm of the musculature of the outer third of the vagina that interferes with sexual intercourse). They are both amalgamated into a new diagnosis called genitopelvic pain/penetration disorder [30]. Male dyspareunia is very infrequent and has been erased from the nomenclature.

To establish the diagnosis of genitopelvic pain/penetration disorder (GPPPD), one of these four conditions should persistently or recurrently occur:

Difficulty in vaginal penetration
Marked vulvovaginal or pelvic pain during penetration or attempt at penetration
Fear or anxiety about pain in anticipation of, during or after penetration
Tightening or tensing of pelvic floor muscles during attempted penetration

It could be difficult to evaluate if a patient is suffering pain because threat or threat because pain. Stronger automatic threat associations are related to lowered sexual arousal [40], but doctors need to be attentive during menopausal transition because it is well known the relationship between low hormonal level and changes in sexual response (vaginal dryness, low lubrication, different vulvovaginal senses, delayed orgasm) [2]. Difficulty in penetration, dyspareunia and vestibulodynia are also frequent symptoms of the genitourinary syndrome of menopause (GSM), due to lack of oestrogen, and these conditions could cause sex-related threats and avoidance [40].

Around menopause, the most frequent reason for sexual pain is, in different degrees, GSM. A correct examination should be enough to make the diagnosis (pale aspect of genital tissues, loss of vaginal folds, etc.) and sometimes just the clinical interview about changes in sexual response. We often find the patient experiences less pain during examination than intercourse. It is due to psychological factors (threats used to be sexual related).

First-line treatment for this condition should be low dose of oestrogens applied locally because this improves genital tissues irrigation, vaginal ph, dryness and lubrication. The efficacy does not differ between pharmacological presentations (pessaries, vaginal ring, creams, gels), but there is a consensus about using low dose of oestrogens in order to avoid high absorption to minimize side effects [41]. Low dose of oestrogens applied locally does not need to add progestin neither control endometrium and can be used in long term.

HRT, and tibolone, are also indicated, but women feel them less safe if vaginal problems are the only reason for their indication, and several studies have found symptoms of vaginal atrophy even when using them. If this happens in women on HRT or tibolone, we can add vaginal treatment.

Conjugated oestrogens/bazedoxifene development has demonstrated the effect of this TSEC (tissue selective oestrogen complex) on GSM. It improves vaginal epithelium cells maturation index, vaginal ph and dryness [42].

The same effects have been found during the development of the medication ospemifene. It is the first selective hormone receptor modulator with label indication in vulvovaginal atrophy and dyspareunia treatment because it has demonstrated a benefit in dyspareunia by improving FSFI scale [43, 44].

Non-hormonal treatments have also shown to be effective. For example, intra-vaginal soya gel reduces vaginal dryness, ph and dyspareunia by increasing epithelium maturation and thickness and oestrogen receptor expression in postmenopausal women [29]. A topically and intravaginally administered gel containing another phytoestrogen (8-prenynaringenin) from *Humulus lupulus L.* reduces symptomatology in postmenopausal women with genital atrophy [45], and we have got some scientific evidence about another phytotherapeutics giving benefits over sexual arousal, such as *Centella asiatica* (with a large traditional use) [46], *Panax ginseng* [47], *Tribulus terrestris L* [48], *Turnera diffusa* [49] and *Ginkgo biloba* [50].

The latest proposal is to treat GSM with laser, but we need more evidence to have guidelines for using it and to know the duration of its effect over epithelial tissues.

Personalized treatment leads us to provide sexual counsel to address psychological and couple issues and to inform about physical changes, to use sex therapy if needed to help women to see penetration in a more positive way, to add pelvic floor physical therapy to relax musculature if necessary, to recommend lubricants and moisturizers to be used as a part of sexual play and to design strategies using combined or sequential options [51].

7.6.3 Female Orgasmic Disorder

This frequent dysfunction (prevalence 11–41%) [52] is diagnosed when some significant change occurs in orgasm, such as delay, reduction of intensity or cessation. Female orgasmic disorder (FOD) could appear after a period of normal sexual activity but affect 75–100% of sexual attempts, during more than 6 months, and cause distress and/or relational problems [30].

No single cause is used to be identified, but it is common to be associated with partner problems (health or sexual matters), relationship problems (poor intimacy or communication, abuse, etc.), life stressors and personal vulnerabilities (self-esteem, body image, anxiety, attitude about sex, sexual education, sexual history, etc.) [2, 52, 53].

Medical conditions can also be the cause of cardiovascular diseases; thyroid problems; chronic conditions affecting neurological aspect of sexual response, such as diabetes or multiple sclerosis; or use of several drugs that can inhibit the orgasm (antidepressants, antipsychotics, cancer treatment, etc.) [2].

It is common the association to other sexual dysfunctions, such as desire or arousal problems, and it is probably the most common reason for FOD during menopause. Hormonal changes can modify senses in genital tissues and hinder sexual arousal and orgasm. These variations can produce less sensation or even hypersensitivity, leading women to adapt their abilities for sexual stimulation.

Apart from the address of the found etiological factors, all hormonal and non-hormonal treatments proposed for arousal problems can help menopausal women with FOD, but this sexual dysfunction is specifically well treated with sexual therapy. Psychological interventions have the best results in desire and orgasmic disorders [54] and consists mainly in cognitive behavioural therapy to reduce stress and promote relaxation, direct masturbation training (in which women are exposed to genital stimulation and gradually incorporate sexual fantasies, role play and sexual toys to facilitate orgasm), couple therapy if necessary and/or cooperation of the partner during the training.

Thus, in menopausal women affected by FOD, the best option for treatment is to associate hormonal treatment to sexual therapy [55].

7.7 Sexual Violence and Menopause

Violence against women (VAW) has become a global sexual health issue for women. Although we still lack accurate data on the number of women who have been victims of VAW, it is estimated that at least one in four women reaching menopause has been a victim of some form of VAW [55, 56].

Although VAW may be recognized as a critical problem for women's overall health, we continue to experience a lack of prospective studies on its influence on women's sexual health when they reach menopause. Similarly, we draw on estimation data to assume that for every woman who loses her life to VAW, more than 400 suffer varying degrees of severe disability, including severe sexual problems and worse menopausal symptoms [57, 58]. Neurobiological and epigenetic mechanisms have been proposed to explain the worsening of menopausal symptomatology with VAW, which are equally justified in sexual health. On the one hand hypoestrogenism, but also alterations of the serotonergic pathways, of the sympathetic nervous system, or of the hypothalamic-pituitary-adrenal or hypothalamic-pituitary-adrenal pathways after VAW [59, 60].

In addition, psychiatric problems, which are much more frequent in women who have suffered VAW at any time in their lives, not only influence the perception of pain or emotions. It is likely that there are other hitherto unknown brain pathways that link VAW to menopausal and sexual symptoms, opening up interesting avenues for future research [61].

In a recent study, experiencing any form of VAW at any point in a women's life will have a detrimental impact on her overall health, particularly during midlife and postmenopausal stages [62].

7.8 Conclusions

In conclusion, even though sex may be constrained by the physical, psychological and social changes that accompany age, this should not disrupt sexual activity. Maturity can be an opportunity for a more intimate or relaxed type of sex. The acceptance of physical changes and a history of good sexual experiences can positively influence the maintenance of sexual health as the years pass. At any age, especially in long-term relationships, a good relationship is the most important factor that influences desire and sexual health. Pharmacological treatments could be reserved for cases in which couple therapy or changing lifestyles have not been effective at improving sexual health.

Acknowledgments This chapter has been translated and corrected by Patricia R. Mollahan and American Journal Experts.

References

1. World Health Organization. Defining sexual health: report of a technical consultation on sexual health, 28–31 January 2002. Geneva: WHO; 2006.
2. Spanish Association for the Study of Menopause (AEEM). Menoguía: perimenopause [Internet]. Madrid: AEEM; 2021 [cited 2024 Jun 17]. Available from: https://www.aeem.es/menoguia-perimenopausia.
3. Mendoza N, Sánchez-Borrego R, Cancelo MJ, Calvo A, Checa MA, Cortés J, et al. Position of the Spanish menopause society regarding the management of perimenopause. Maturitas. 2013;74(3):283–90.
4. Lambrinoudaki I, Armeni E, Goulis D, Bretz S, Ceausu I, Durmusoglu F, Erkkola R, Fistonic I, Gambacciani M, Geukes M, Hamoda H, Hartley C, Hirschberg AL, Meczekalski B, Mendoza N, Mueck A, Smetnik A, Stute P, van Trotsenburg M, Rees M. Menopause, wellbeing and health: a care pathway from the European Menopause and Andropause Society. Maturitas. 2022;163:1–14.
5. Parish SJ, Simon JA, Davis SR, Giraldi A, Goldstein I, Goldstein SW, Kim NN, Kingsberg SA, Morgentaler A, Nappi RE, Park K, Stuenkel CA, Traish AM, Vignozzi L. International Society for the Study of Women's Sexual Health Clinical Practice Guideline for the Use of Systemic Testosterone for Hypoactive Sexual Desire Disorder in Women. J Sex Med. 2021;18(5):849–67. https://doi.org/10.1016/j.jsxm.2020.10.009.
6. Cabello SF. Aspectos psicosociales del manejo de la disfunción eréctil. Hábitos tóxicos y estilo de vida. La pareja en la disfunción eréctil. Psicoterapia y terapia de pareja ArchEspUrol. 2010;63(8):693–702.

7. Basson R, Wierman ME, van Lankveld J, Brotto L. Summary of the recommendations on sexual dysfunctions in women. J Sex Med. 2010;7(1 Pt 2):314–26. https://doi.org/10.1111/j.1743-6109.2009.01617.x.
8. Basson R. Human sexual response. Handb Clin Neurol. 2015;130:11–8.
9. Atlantis E, Sullivan T. Bidirectional association between depression and sexual dysfunction: a systematic review and meta-analysis. J Sex Med. 2012;9(6):1497–507.
10. Coyne KS, Sexton CC, Thompson C, Kopp ZS, Milsom I, Kaplan SA. The impact of OAB on sexual health in men and women: results from EpiLUTS. J Sex Med. 2011;8(6):1603–15.
11. Sousa Rodrigues Guedes T, Barbosa Otoni Gonçalves Guedes M, de Castro Santana R, Costa da Silva JF, Almeida Gomes Dantas A, Ochandorena-Acha M, Terradas-Monllor M, Jerez-Roig J, Bezerra de Souza DL. Sexual dysfunction in women with cancer: A systematic review of longitudinal studies. Int J Environ Res Public Health. 2022;19(19):11921. https://doi.org/10.3390/ijerph191911921.
12. Sánchez-Borrego R, Mendoza N, Beltrán E, Comino R, Allué J, Castelo-Branco C, et al. Position of the Spanish Menopause Society regarding the management of menopausal symptoms in breast cancer patients. Maturitas. 2013;75(3):294–300.
13. Thakar R. Is the uterus a sexual organ? Sexual function following hysterectomy. Sex Med Rev. 2015;3:264–78.
14. Arias-Castillo L, García L, García-Perdomo HA. The complexity of female orgasm and ejaculation. Arch Gynecol Obstet. 2023;308(2):427–34. https://doi.org/10.1007/s00404-022-06810-y.
15. Mikhail E, Cain MA, Shah M, Solnik MJ, Sobolewski CJ, Hart S. Does laparoscopic hysterectomy increase the risk of vaginal cuff dehiscence? An analysis of outcomes from multiple academic centers and a review of the literature. Surg Technol Int. 2015;27:157–62.
16. Peterson ZD, Rothenberg JM, Bilbrey S, Heiman JR. Sexual functioning following elective hysterectomy: the role of surgical and psychosocial variables. J Sex Res. 2010 Nov;47(6):513–27. https://doi.org/10.1080/00224490903151366.
17. ACOG. Practice Bulletin no. 89. Elective and risk-reducing salpingo-oophorectomy. Obstet Gynecol. 2008;111:231–41.
18. Finch A, Metcalfe KA, Chiang JK, Elit L, McLaughlin J, Springate C, et al. The impact of prophylactic salpingo-oophorectomy on menopausal symptoms and sexual function in women who carry a BRCA mutation. Gynecol Oncol. 2011;121:163–8.
19. Parish SJ, Hahn SR. Hypoactive sexual desire disorder: A review of epidemiology, biopsychology, diagnosis, and treatment. Sex Med Rev. 2016;4(2):103–20. https://doi.org/10.1016/j.sxmr.2015.11.009.
20. Bober SL, Recklitis CJ, Bakan J, Garber JE, Patenaude AF. Addressing sexual dysfunction after risk-reducing salpingo-oophorectomy: effects of a brief, psychosexual intervention. J Sex Med. 2015;12:189–97.
21. Tucker PE, Bulsara MK, Salfinger SG, Jit-Sun Tan J, Green H, Cohen PA. Prevalence of sexual dysfunction after risk-reducing salpingo-oophorectomy. Gynecol Oncol. 2016;140:95–100.
22. Brotto LA, Branco N, Dunkley C, McCullum M, McAlpine JN. Risk-reducing bilateral salpingo-oophorectomy and sexual health: a qualitative study. J Obstet Gynaecol Can. 2012;34(2):172–8.
23. Nastri CO, Lara LA, Ferriani RA, Rosa-E-Silva AC, Figueiredo JB, Martins WP. Hormone therapy for sexual function in perimenopausal and postmenopausal women. Cochrane Database Syst Rev. 2013;4(6):CD009672.
24. Mendoza N, Abad P, Baró F, Cancelo MJ, Llaneza P, Manubens M, et al. Spanish Menopause Society position statement: use of tibolone in postmenopausal women. Menopause. 2013;20(7):754–60.
25. Nappi RE, Kokot-Kierepa M. Women's voices in the menopause: results from an international survey on vaginal atrophy. Maturitas. 2010;67:233–8.
26. Wylie K, Rees M, Hackett G, Anderson R, Bouloux PM, Cust M, Goldmeier D, Kell P, Terry T, Trinick T, Wu F. Androgens, health and sexuality in women and men. Maturitas. 2010;67(3):275–89.

27. Mendoza N, Suárez AM, Álamo F, Bartual E, Vergara F, Herruzo A. Lipid effects, effectiveness and acceptability of tibolone versus transdermic 17ß-estradiol for hormonal replacement therapy in women with surgical menopause. Maturitas. 2000;37(1):37–43.
28. Cui Y, Zong H, Yan H, Li N, Zhang Y. The efficacy and safety of ospemifene in treating dyspareunia associated with postmenopausal vulvar and vaginal atrophy: a systematic review and meta-analysis. J Sex Med. 2014;11(2):487–97.
29. Sánchez S, Baquedano L, Cancelo MJ, Jurado AR, Molero F, Nohales F, Mendoza N, Palacios S. Managing vulvar and vestibular pain in postmenopausal women: recommendations from the Spanish Menopause Society, Sociedad Española de Ginecología y Obstetricia, Sociedad Española de Medicos de Atención Primaria y Federación Española de Sociedades de Sexología. Gynecol Endocrinol. 2021;14:1–4. https://doi.org/10.1080/09513590.2021.1963954.
30. American Psychiatric Association. Diagnostic and statistical manual of mental disorders. 5th ed. Arlington, VA: American Psychiatric Publishing; 2013.
31. Basson R. The female sexual response: a different model. J Sex Marital Ther. 2000;26(1):51–65.
32. Parish SJ, Hahn SR. Hypoactive sexual desire disorder: a review of epidemiology, biosychology, diagnosis, and treatment. Sex Med Rev. 2016;4(2):103–20.
33. Pérez-López FR, Fernández-Alonso AM, Trabalón-Pastor M, Vara C, Chedraui P, Menopause Risk Assessment (MARIA) Research Group. Assessment of sexual function and related factors in mid-aged sexually active Spanish women with the sex-item Female Function Index. Menopause. 2012;19(11):1224–30.
34. Basson R. Using a different model for female sexual response to address women's problematic low sexual desire. J Sex Marithal Ther. 2001;27(5):395–403.
35. Cumming GP, Currie HD, Moncur R, Lee AJ. Web-based survey on the effect of menopause on women's libido in a computer-literature population. Menopause Int. 2009;15(1):8–12.
36. Somboonporn W, Davis S, Seif MW, Bell R. Testosterone for peri- and postmenopausal women. Cochrane Database Syst Rev. 2005;4:CD004509.
37. Gohil K. Pharmaceutical Approval Update. Flibanserine (Addyi). P T. 2015;40(10):649–89.
38. Katz M, DeRogatis LR, Ackerman R, Hedges P, Lesko L, García M Jr, Sand M. BEGONIA trial investigators. J Sex Med. 2013;10(7):1807–15.
39. Scheffers CS, Armstrong S, Cantineau AE, Farquhar C, Jordan V. Dehydroepiandrosterone for women in the peri- or postmenopausal phase. Cochrane Database Syst Rev. 2015;1:CD0011066.
40. Sanchez S, Baquedano L, Mendoza N. Treatment of vulvar pain caused by atrophy: a systematic review of clinical studies. Clin Exp Obstet Gynecol. 2021;48(4):800–5.
41. Kagan R, Williams RS, Pan K, Mirkin S, Pickar JH. A randomized, placebo- and active-controlled trial of bazedoxifene/conjugated estrogens for treatment of moderate to severe vulvar atrophy in postmenopausal women. Menopause. 2010;17(2):281–9.
42. Portman DJ, Bachmann GA, Simon JA, Ospemifene Study Group. Ospemifene, a novel selective estrogen receptor modulator for treating dyspareunia associated with postmenopausal vulvar and vaginal atrophy. Menopause. 2013;20(6):623–30.
43. Constantine G, Graham S, Portman DJ, Rosen RC, Kinsberg SA. Female sexual function improved with ospemifene in postmenopausal women with vuvlar and vaginal atrophy: results of a randomized, placebo-controlled trial. Climacteric. 2015;18:226–32.
44. Lima SM, Bernardo BF, Yamada SS, Reis BF, da Silva GM, Galvao MA. Effects of glycine mas (I.) Merr. Soy isoflavone vaginal gel on epithelium morphology and estrogen receptor expression in postmenopausal women: a 12-week, randomized, double-blind, placebo-controlled trial. Maturitas. 2014;78(3):205–11.
45. Markowska J, Markowska A, Madry R. Evaluation of Cicatridine efficacy in healing and repairing process of uterine cervix, vagina and vulva –open no randomized clinical study. Gineckol Pol. 2008;79(7):494–8.
46. Kim MS, Lim HJ, Yang HJ, Lee MS, Shin BC, Ernst E. Ginseng for managing menopause symptoms: a systematic review of randomized clinical trials. J Ginseng Res. 2013;37(1):30–6.
47. Postigo S, Lima SM, Yamada SS, dos Reis BF, da Silva GM, Aoki T. Assessment of the effects of Tribulus terrestris on sexual function of menopausal women. Rev Bras Ginecol Obstet. 2016;38(3):140–6.

48. Yto TY, Trant AS, Polan ML. A doublé-blind placebo-controlled study of ArginMax, a nutritional supplement for enhancement of female sexual function. J Sex Marital Ther. 2001;27(5):541–9.
49. Meston CM, Rellini AH, Telch MJ. Short and long-term effects of Ginkgo biloba extract on sexual dysfunction in women. Arch Sex Behav. 2008;37(4):530–47.
50. Jurado AR, Sánchez F. Salud Sexual en Atención Primaria (Curso de Formación on line en Internet). Madrid: Science Tools; 2012. Disponible en: http://www.dpcap.es. acceso 30 de septiembre de 2012.
51. Rellini AH, Clifton J. Female orgasmic disorder. Adv Psychosom Med. 2011;31:35–56.
52. Ishak WW, Bokarius A, Jeffrey JK, Davis MC, Bakhta Y. Disorders of orgasm in women: a literature review of etiology and current treatments. J Sex Med. 2010;7(10):3254–68.
53. Frühauf S, Gerger H, Schmidt HM, Munder T, Barth J. Efficacy of psychological interventions for sexual dysfunction: a systematic review and meta-analysis. Arch Sex Behav. 2013;42(6):915–33. https://doi.org/10.1007/s10508-012-0062-0.
54. Laan E, Rellini AH, Barnes T. International Society for Sexual Medicine. Standard operating procedures for female orgasmic disorder: consensus of the International Society for Sexual Medicine. J Sex Med. 2013;10(1):74–82.
55. Kapoor E, Okuno M, Miller VM, Rocca LG, Rocca WA, Kling JM, Kuhle CL, Mara KC, Enders FT, Faubion SS. Association of adverse childhood experiences with menopausal symptoms: Results from the Data Registry on Experiences of Aging, Menopause and Sexuality (DREAMS). Maturitas. 2021;143:209–15. https://doi.org/10.1016/j.maturitas.2020.10.006.
56. Mendoza-Huertas L, Garcia Jabalera I, Mendoza N. Effects of violence against women on health during menopause: a systematic review and metanalysis. Clin Exp Obstet Gynecol. 2021;48(6):1292–9. https://doi.org/10.31083/j.ceog4806205.
57. Mendoza-Huertas L, Mendoza N. Impact of violence against women on sexual and reproductive health: research protocol and results from a pilot study. Clin Exp Obstet Gynecol. 2022;49(7):145. https://doi.org/10.31083/j.ceog4907145.
58. Carson MY, Thurston RC. Childhood abuse and vasomotor symptoms among midlife women. Menopause. 2019;26(10):1093–9. https://doi.org/10.1097/GME.0000000000001366.
59. McCrory E, De Brito SA, Viding E. Research review: the neurobiology and genetics of maltreatment and adversity. J Child Psychol Psychiatry. 2010;51(10):1079–95. https://doi.org/10.1111/j.1469-7610.2010.02271.x.
60. Shanmugan S, Loughead J, Cao W, Sammel MD, Satterthwaite TD, Ruparel K, Gur RC, Epperson CN. Impact of tryptophan depletion on executive system function during menopause is moderated by childhood adversity. Neuropsychopharmacology. 2017;42(12):2398–406. https://doi.org/10.1038/npp.2017.64.
61. McCrory E, De Brito SA, Viding E. The link between child abuse and psychopathology: a review of neurobiological and genetic research. J R Soc Med. 2012;105(4):151–6. https://doi.org/10.1258/jrsm.2011.110222.
62. Mendoza-Huertas L, Mendoza N, Godoy D. Impact of violence against women on quality of life and menopause-related disorders. Maturitas. 2024;180:107899.

Part III

The Impact of Estrogen Depletion on Disease Susceptibility

Postmenopausal Osteoporosis

Amparo Carrasco-Catena, Aitana Monllor-Tormos, Nicolás Mendoza Ladrón de Guevara, Miguel Ángel García-Pérez, and Antonio Cano

Abstract

Bone cell metabolism is strongly regulated by estrogens and therefore the risk of osteoporosis is favored by menopause. Fragility fractures define the outcome to be prevented in osteoporosis. Since age adds to menopause as a risk factor, and menopause occurs at a relatively early age, preventive measures during the early postmenopausal period are desirable. Physical activity, balanced nutrition, and restriction of toxics, smoking, and excess alcohol should be universally encouraged. Attention to osteoporosis risk factors should be part of any basic clinical evaluation of menopausal women. Identification of strong risk factors, such as the presence of previous fragility fracture, identification of fracture in first-degree relatives, or age over 65 years, mandates further evaluation, including bone densitometry. When pharmacological treatment is necessary, the range of antiresorptives includes menopausal hormone therapy, which adds further

---

A. Carrasco-Catena
Clinical Area Women's Health, Hospital Universitario y Politécnico La Fe, Valencia, Spain
e-mail: carrasco_ampcat@gva.es

A. Monllor-Tormos
Women's Health Research Group, INCLIVA – Hospital Clínico Universitario, Valencia, Spain
e-mail: monllor_ait@gva.es

N. M. L. de Guevara
Department of Obstetrics and Gynecology, University of Granada, Granada, Spain
e-mail: nicomendoza@ugr.es

M. Á. García-Pérez
Faculty of Biological Sciences, Department of Cellular Biology, Functional Biology and Physical Anthropology, University of Valencia, Valencia, Spain
e-mail: Miguel.garcia@uv.es

A. Cano (✉)
Full Professor of Obstetrics and Gynecology, Salus Vitae Women's Health Clinical Center, Valencia, Spain
e-mail: Antonio.cano@uv.es

© The Author(s), under exclusive license to Springer Nature Switzerland AG 2025
A. Cano (ed.), *Menopause*, https://doi.org/10.1007/978-3-031-83979-5_8

benefits in case of menopausal symptoms affecting quality of life. Selective estrogen receptor modulators (SERMs), bisphosphonates, and denosumab may follow in a strategy resulting from a rational sequence based on the specific profile of each therapeutic option. SERMs add breast cancer risk reduction (raloxifene and perhaps bazedoxifene) and protection against vertebral fractures. Hip fracture risk reduction requires bisphosphonates or denosumab. More recently, anabolic drugs have opened a new field and are now proposed as a first step in the treatment sequence in women at high or very high risk of fragility fracture.

8.1 Osteoporosis and Women

Osteoporosis is a disease in which reduced bone mass and microarchitectural deterioration of bone tissue increase the risk for fragility fracture. Osteoporosis, which affects 500 million men and women worldwide [1], is one of the noncommunicable diseases (NCDs) with the greatest impact on the aging population. Those figures were found by using the World Health Organization (WHO) bone mineral density (BMD) as diagnostic criterion [2], which in women establishes osteoporosis when reaching 2.5 standard deviations or more below the average value for young healthy population [3].

The more recent evidence that BMD is a strong, but insufficient, parameter to assess risk for fragility fracture in many subjects has uncovered the role of clinical traits, like age or others, which have emerged as strong risk factors (Fig. 8.1). Moreover, the availability of osteoporotic fracture data from cohorts at different

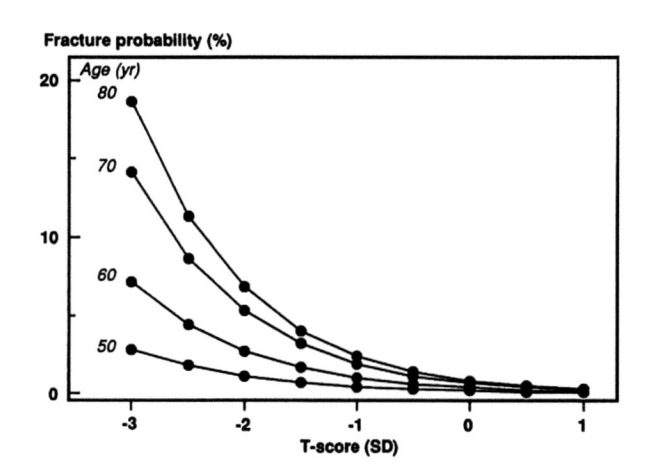

Fig. 8.1 Age is a strong risk factor for fragility fracture. The figure shows the 10-year hip fracture probability in a Swedish population according to age and bone mineral density (BMD) at the hip, which is presented as T-score. It is obvious that the lower the bone density (lower T value), the higher the risk for hip fracture. However, for a given T value, and particularly in ranges below −1 (osteopenia), age imposes dramatic differences in risk. (With permission of Springer Verlag from Kanis et al. Osteoporos Int. 2001; 12:989–95. Permission obtained through Copyright Clearance Center, Inc.)

geographical settings has made possible the integration of clinical parameters into the prediction of risk for fracture. New tools have been designed in which both clinical and densitometric factors are integrated and provide an absolute risk for fracture. It has been again the WHO that has issued the Fracture Risk Assessment Tool (FRAX) [4]. FRAX provides a 10-year absolute individual risk for fragility fracture and is sensitive to the varying conditions of different populations in the world.

The emphasis on fracture is a most-needed approach to better identify those individuals who will suffer the up to 37 million fragility fractures occurring annually worldwide in people aged ≥55 years. Indeed, the lifetime risk for osteoporotic fracture, which moves between 30% and 40% in developed countries, approaches that for coronary heart disease. Complications of osteoporotic fractures include both increased morbidity and mortality, which translate into 2.8 million disability-adjusted life years (DALYs) annually. These figures are above those accounted by hypertension and rheumatoid arthritis [5].

One strong risk factor for osteoporosis is gender. Women have an increased vulnerability since 1 in 3 women over age 50 will suffer an osteoporotic facture vs 1 in 5 men [1]. A more fragile habitus, with thinner bone constitution, is a variable influencing the higher risk of women. Another important variable is menopause, one unique endocrinological phenomenon of women. Albright already observed the impact of the abrupt fall in ovarian hormonal production on the risk for fragility fractures in women with surgical menopause [6]. The arrival of reliable densitometers confirmed that the fall in the circulating level of estrogens at menopause was associated with an accelerated loss of bone density [7].

8.2 The Biological Basis

8.2.1 Structure of Bone

Bone is the system that maintains the body in an erect position. Against its static aspect, bone is a live tissue subjected to continuous change. The composition of bone includes cells and inert material. Three main cellular types, osteoblasts, osteoclasts and osteocytes, distribute according to a framework provided by mineral, a calcium salt called hydroxyapatite, and a net of intertwined collagen fibers [8].

Two different forms of structures may be found in bone. Trabecular bone is a spongelike design that fills up the vertebral bodies, where a network of trabecular plates determines a porous texture occupied by bone marrow. The transmission of tension through the trabeculae facilitates the flexibility required for energy absorption while maintaining a quite light fabric. Cortical bone, instead, is the basic component of long bones. Layers of bone are tightly overlapped to produce a thick structure most optimized to support loading. Cortical bone results from massive overlapping of osteons, structures composed of concentric layers of compact bone (lamellae) that surround a central canal (Haversian canal). The composition of lamellae is that of compact bone, i.e., the net of collagen fibers immersed into the hydroxyapatite mineral matrix [8].

8.2.2 Bone Cells

Osteoclasts, osteoblasts, and osteocytes inhabit and exert regulatory functions in this seemingly inhospitable environment. Both osteoclasts and osteoblasts are cells deriving from progenitors at the bone marrow, which occupies spaces close to the surface of mineralized bone. Their role is crucial for bone renovation and the maintenance of adequate bone mass [9]. This is known as bone remodeling and occurs in so-called bone multicellular units (BMU), in which osteoclasts and osteoblasts renew bone at any location in the skeleton to maintain its integrity and mineral homeostasis [9].

Bone resorption is the role of osteoclasts, which in this way eliminate areas that are damaged due to repeated loading. The formed cavities are then occupied by osteoblasts, which deposit osteoid, the proteinaceous matrix that will be slowly mineralized to produce new bone. One key duty of the BMU is the complete restitution of the digested bone so that the balance is neutral and no loss of bone mass occurs [8, 9].

With a half-life of 25 years, osteocytes are the most abundant cells in bone, accounting for up to 95%. Osteocytes are derived from osteoblasts, which are buried in the mineralized bone they helped to create [10]. Osteocytes occupy a network of hollow spaces (lacuna), which are communicated by a network of canaliculi through which cytoplasmic processes interconnect other osteocytes to form a full network. Osteocytes communicate with osteoclasts and osteoblasts via different signaling molecules, including the receptor activator of NFkB ligand (RANKL)/osteoprotegerin (OPG) axis or the Sost/Dkk1/Wnt axis [11], forming a functional syncytium. Although their functions are not fully understood, osteocytes are involved in the maintenance of the bone matrix and are the main mechano-sensors of bone tissue [11]. There is growing consensus in that they constitute a finely tuned sensor system detecting the bone areas in which, because of material fatigue, damage, or other reasons, remodeling is desirable. In this sense, osteocytes may be considered as the guardians of bone quality. This function seems mediated, at least in part, by the contribution of osteocytes to the pool of one cytokine, the RANKL [12], which is crucial in the differentiation of osteoclasts from progenitor cells but also of other molecules such as OPG, DKK1, and sclerostin, among others [13, 14]. The differentiation of osteoclasts is coupled, as previously mentioned, to that of osteoblasts, which refill the resorbed cavity and keep unaltered the structure of the bone. A scheme of the bone cells is presented in Fig. 8.2.

8.2.3 Estrogen Regulation

Albright's initial observation that the loss of estrogens in women increases the risk of osteoporotic fractures was not fully understood until later years. Estrogen receptors were firstly described at the level of mRNA expression in cell cultures, experimental animals, and human tissues [15–18]. Both ER subtypes were subsequently detected in histological sections of the growth plate and in mineralized bone, and in

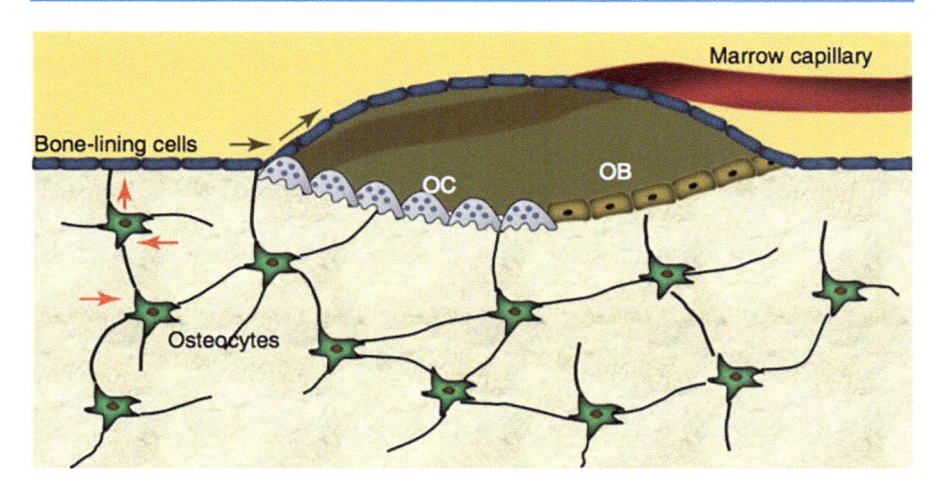

Fig. 8.2 The illustration shows a scheme of the basic multicellular unit (BMU), where the three main cellular types, osteoclasts, osteoblasts, and osteocytes, are presented. The canopy of the bone lining cells and one associated marrow capillary are also included in the figure. The network of the osteocyte canaliculi is well connected with every agent of interest, thus providing a stable structure for intercellular communication between the different cellular types in the BMU. (With permission of Elsevier from Khosla S et al. Trends Endocrinol Metab. 2012; 23:576–81. Permission conveyed through Copyright Clearance Center, Inc.)

the three basic cellular types, osteoblasts, osteoclasts, and osteocytes, although with different distribution patterns [19, 20].

In parallel, clinical observation confirmed that estrogens act as important regulators of bone metabolism not only in women but also in men [21, 22]. Moreover, pioneer data from Lindsay et al. confirmed that treatment with estrogens prevented the bone loss in ovariectomized women [23]. Details supporting the role of estrogens at different stages of bone metabolism have been confirmed by following work [24, 25].

Observational studies have described one of the primary effects of estrogen deficiency as the activation of bone remodeling, which involves both bone resorption and bone formation. However, this process is unequal, resulting in a net deficit in bone formation compared to bone resorption, ultimately leading to bone loss [25]. This is consistent with the observation of a net bone loss mainly with the decrease of estrogens and not of other hormonal candidates like follicle-stimulating hormone (FSH) [26]. The bone loss is already detected at perimenopause [27] and is maintained until late in the postmenopausal years [28]. The impact of estrogen decrease is confirmed by the clear increment of biochemical markers of bone resorption, at rates of 79%–97% [28], in both blood and urine in postmenopausal women. The biological basis of this observation is the acceleration in the activation of BMUs, in which the differentiation of both osteoclasts and osteoblasts from progenitor cells is increased, but with a deviation in favor of bone resorption in all cases. A net loss of bone, consequently, results.

One of the first effects of estrogen is on bone remodeling through direct action on osteocytes, the main regulatory bone cells [29]. Studies in humans have shown that increased osteocyte apoptosis, as demonstrated in bone biopsies, associates with depletion of estrogens by GnRH analogues administered to premenopausal women [30] and that this effect is followed by the activation of BMUs. In addition, estrogen depletion is associated with decreased expression of sclerostin and impaired integrin alpha-beta3-mediated mechano-sensation by osteocytes, altering osteoclastogenic paracrine signaling [31, 32].

Further experimental work has confirmed that there is a direct effect of estrogens on osteoclasts too. For example, the selective deletion of ERα in mice is followed by loss of bone mass and the extension of the lifespan of osteoclasts in trabecular bone [33]. Vice versa, estrogens have been demonstrated to suppress the differentiation of osteoclasts by several mechanisms, including the interference with RANKL and several miRNAs [34–36], the overexpression of OPG, the decoy receptor of RANKL, or the own reduction in the production of RANKL and other pro-resorption cytokines by different cell types [25].

Together with the activation of bone resorption, the deficiency in estrogens also determines defects in bone formation through a direct action on osteoblasts. Contrary to osteoclasts, estrogens reduce apoptosis and increases lifespan of osteoblasts. The details of the mechanisms involved in this action of estrogens are being investigated although experiences in different models suggest that estrogens might interfere with oxidative stress and reduce NF-κB, the latter being involved in impairing bone formation after bone resorption in BMUs [25]. In addition, estrogens stimulate osteoblasts to synthesize IGF1, TGF-β, and OPG. IGF1 and TGF-β promote the deposition of osteoid, while TGF-β and OPG inhibit the differentiation of osteoclasts, thereby decreasing resorption [37].

8.3 Diagnosis and Management

As other NCDs, osteoporosis has a long subclinical period that is susceptible to risk reduction strategies. Menopause defines a period of particular interest because of two main reasons, the increased deterioration of bone mass that initiates at this period and the wide receptivity of women to health promotion during this phase of their lives. It is therefore important to design a most appropriate strategy, which should include both diagnosis and management.

There are not specificities that make different diagnostic strategies for osteoporosis in the particular case of the menopausal woman. The basic principle that the primary goal of disease action should be fragility fracture reduction remains a pillar of the management plan.

8.3.1 Diagnosis

8.3.1.1 Clinical Assessment
A detailed clinical anamnesis will identify whether there are clinical risk factors. They should be preferably integrated in the context of any of the available tools for calculating absolute facture risk. The FRAX risk calculator, which provides

absolute risk at 10 years, is supported by the WHO [4] and by other scientific societies, like the National Osteoporosis Foundation (NOF) [38], International Osteoporosis Foundation [39], or others. More risk calculators have been proposed, like the Q-fracture [40], but they have not demonstrated clear advantages. Advanced age, the existence of a prior fragility fracture, or a parental history of hip fracture continue to be strong risk factors, which should receive special attention, as described in most guidelines [41].

The information obtained from this diagnostic approach should make it possible to correctly identify whether there is only menopause-related osteoporosis or, on the contrary, other underlying pathologies are determining osteoporosis secondarily.

8.3.1.2 Imaging

Additional diagnostic tools include imaging techniques, where bone densitometry is the main pillar. The status of bone tissue, not only its density, may be measured by several techniques, like quantitative computed tomography, quantitative ultrasound, etc. Densitometry based on X-ray is, nonetheless, the universal priority and, therefore, we will focus on that technique. The basis of its utility resides in that the absorption of X-ray is very sensitive to the calcium content of the tissue. Dual-energy X-ray absorptiometry (DXA) is the most widely used technique, which is taken as a reference for the diagnosis of osteoporosis according to the WHO criteria [2, 3]. Both areal and volumetric density may be measured, but areal BMD is commonly used because it accounts for approximately two-thirds of bone strength and, consequently, is considered a strong risk factor for fracture. An additional advantage of DXA resides in its capacity to visualize deformities of the vertebral bodies, thus avoiding the additional use of conventional X-ray assessment.

In addition to its value to ascertain risk for future fracture, the information obtained from DXA may be also used as a referent baseline to monitor the evolution of a particular patient. This is of interest in the case of postmenopausal women because the rate of bone loss has an individual profile, and some women, those defined as "fast losers" in some studies, show a specific sensitivity to estrogen drop. Moreover, observational studies have confirmed that the change rate of BMD in a treated patient is useful to determine the evolution of the future fracture risk [42]. The slow response of BMD to treatment represents, however, a difficulty in taking advantage of this DXA option since the lack of an increase in BMD does not necessarily imply the absence of therapeutic response.

The option of a systematic DXA assessment in women at menopause is a matter of some debate. The majority of guidelines do not recommend its practice until the age of 65 years unless there are one of the strong risk factors mentioned above [43]. This is so because, even accepting that the proportion of women with osteoporosis at 50 years that will suffer a fracture in the next 10 years is considerable, a 96% of the fractures will occur in women without densitometric osteoporosis [41]. An Australian study has added low body mass index as an independent risk factor useful in deciding whether DXA should be recommended [44].

Trabecular bone score (TBS) is a more recent method that, based upon the spine imaging provided by some specific densitometers, may give information that relates with bone texture and microarchitecture. Some studies have suggested that TBS may improve fracture risk prediction over that provided by conventional DXA, especially in some specific cases, like diabetes [45].

8.3.1.3 Biochemical Markers

Bone biochemical markers are analytes that result from the metabolic events in bone. Some of them are produced as a consequence of resorption by osteoclasts while others are released as a result of the osteoblastic activity. Since both cell types are coupled in the remodeling process because of the activation of the BMUs, both types of markers increase during raised resorption [46].

The main potential advantage of bone markers is that if they are specific enough and the analytical method is sufficiently precise, a real-time report of the status of bone metabolism may be obtained. The degree of the treatment response, for example, might be assessed without waiting for the densitometric response. Furthermore, their baseline value may be taken as an indicator of the magnitude of the resorptive process and, should this behave as a stable phenomenon, a certain prognosis of the fracture risk might be seized [47]. This is a very important feature to better detect the most abundant profile of fractured subjects, who have normal or only slightly decreased BMD for their age [48].

The choice of bone markers keeps increasing in parallel with the better knowledge of bone metabolism. Resorption markers include collagen degradation proteins, non-collagenous proteins, osteoclastic enzymes, and, more recently, osteocyte activity markers. Degradation products of type 1 collagen are produced by the activity of cathepsin K, an osteoclastic enzyme. Both the carboxy (CTX-1) and the amino-terminals (NTX-1) may be measured and are the most consolidated options. Indeed, CTX1 in serum has been recommended as reference bone resorption marker by IOF [49].

The list of formation markers includes procollagen type I propeptides, osteocalcin and alkaline phosphatase. The procollagen type I propeptides are originating mainly from activated osteoblasts and result from the posttranslational cleavage of type I procollagen molecules by proteases. Both the N- and the C-terminal, PINP or PICP, are produced, but the most reliable and preferred is PINP, which is the reference formation marker in most studies [49].

In practice, the main limitation of bone markers is their variability, mainly due to the circadian and seasonal variation of bone metabolism. Even so, they can be taken as a complement to DXA for aspects such as the aforementioned identification of rapid losers, fracture risk prediction, and monitoring of the effect of antiresorptive treatment. This latter advantage is of value only when using antiresorptives capable of achieving a substantial reduction in bone turnover, like bisphosphonates or denosumab. Their use has also been recommended as indicators to better define the selection of the type of antiresorptive in some specific clinical scenarios, such as increased bone turnover after discontinuation of denosumab [50].

8.3.2 Management

The type of patient who comes for consultation can vary. Younger women with metabolically stable healthy bones, rapid bone losers with still reasonable bone mineral density, women with no risk factors with the exception of osteoporotic densitometry in either or both the spine or hip, high-risk osteoporosis, and very high-risk osteoporosis make up different possible clinical portraits. Because of these very different potential scenarios, it is sensible to keep in mind a sequential approach, in which all possible cases are accommodated. The advantage of sequential management is that each case can be assigned to the most appropriate step in the sequence [51].

8.3.2.1 Lifestyle as a Risk Reduction Strategy

The acceleration of bone resorption initiates prior to menopause [52], and the phenomenon keeps for many years, probably up to the end of life [28, 53]. This means that considering the global life expectancy, this state will last for 30 or more years. Moreover, it is known that most fragility fractures, including hip and vertebral, attain a significant incidence at relatively advanced age, not earlier than 65 years. Also important, most antiresorptives have shown efficacy in clinical trials in which the median age of the participating women was advanced, far from the immediate postmenopausal period, and their prolonged use is not free of disadvantages [54]. Putting all these arguments together, it seems reasonable that women entering menopause should be advised on strategies to reduce the risk of osteoporosis, for which there are several options. Indeed, both the menopausal transition and early postmenopause are excellent opportunities to implement healthy lifestyle. This includes avoidance of toxics, mainly alcohol abuse and tobacco, good nutrition, and the regular practice of exercise.

Regular physical activity may reduce the progression of aging-associated sarcopenia, slow or even equilibrate the loss of bone mass, and improve neuromotor coordination to decrease the risk of falls. In addition, it has an impact on mood and well-being, which can translate into improved quality of life and functional conditions of other organs and systems. So it is a most appropriate option, which should be strongly recommended during this period in the life of women [55].

Nutrition has received attention, particularly in what refers to the adequate intake of protein, calcium, and vitamin D. The literature on the effect of calcium and vitamin D on the reduction of fracture is mixed, specifically in what refers to pharmacologic calcium. Data from Swedish women attending the mammography national program and followed for 19 years showed that women with higher calcium intakes, well above the 1 g/day, had an increased risk for hip fracture [56]. Moreover, some studies have shown that high dosages of pharmacologic calcium may be harmful in that there is an increase in kidney stones [57] and even myocardial infarction (24% increased risk in a meta-analysis pooling randomized studies) [58].

The possibility that high intakes of calcium, with or without vitamin D, may be harmful has moved scientific societies to strengthen a clear message. The recommended nutritional intake (RNI) for calcium ranges from 700 to 1000 mg/day, which should increase slightly to 1200 mg/day in higher-risk populations [59]. Dietary sources of calcium are the preferred option. The corresponding dose of vitamin D should be 800 UI/day, which may be acquired from diet and from fortified dairy products. Fortified yoghurts, for example, use to contain 200 UI vitamin D.

Some debate has also arisen about the potential of vitamin D to reduce the risk for falls. No definitive conclusion has been reached, especially since some data have been published that, paradoxically, high doses of vitamin D may even increase this risk [60].

8.3.2.2 Menopausal Hormone Therapy

The whole cascade of symptoms, quality of life deterioration, and health threats presenting in women's lives at menopause is precipitated and caused by the drastic decline in hormone output and, more specifically, the fall of estrogens. Consequently, it may be conceived that the reposition of the hormone should reinstate several, if not all, of the lost benefits.

In the case of osteoporosis, the pathophysiological features described above are clearly linked with estrogen loss. Accordingly, estrogen replacement should act to reverse every observed action, something consistently reproduced at each step. So experimental data confirm that estrogens impair osteoclast differentiation and maintain osteocyte survival and osteoblast function [25].

At the clinical level, data obtained years ago with the most primitive densitometers clearly confirmed that estrogens could prevent menopause-associated loss of bone mineral content, as described at the metacarpus in a landmark study by Lindsay et al. [23]. More than 20 years later, the same group performed a dose-dependent study showing that even low dosages of estrogens were able to maintain, and even to slightly increase, BMD at the spine [61]. Similar results have been observed with low-dose transdermal estradiol [62] and have been widely reproduced. The consistence of the findings confirms that the protective effect on the bone may be attained with dosages below those required for symptom control.

More ambitious studies have taken the reduction of fracture as an endpoint. Good quality clinical data, as derived from both randomized controlled trials (RCT) and meta-analyses, support the effect of menopause hormone therapy (MHT) against the two most relevant osteoporotic fractures, with a reduction of 35% [hazard ratio, HR, 0.65 (95% confidence intervals, CI: 0.46–0.92)] at the spine and of 33% [HR, 0.67, (95% CI: 0.47–0.96)] at the hip [63, 64]. Importantly, fracture reduction was also found at a territory considered more challenging, such as the lower arm wrist, where again data from the large US *Women's Health Initiative* (WHI) Study found a 29% reduction [HR, 071 (95% CI: 0.59–0.85)] [63].

The concurrence of both conditions, a physiopathological approach together with proven efficacy, made MHT an ideal therapeutic resource against postmenopausal osteoporosis. Moreover, data obtained from long-term follow-up of women participating in the WHI trial suggested that there was no rebound effect, so there was no increased risk of fractures in treated compared to untreated women after discontinuation of MHT [65].

The wide distribution of ER in the body means that MHT can add benefit in other therapeutic targets affected by estrogen depletion. This is the case of menopausal symptoms, a varied group of discomforts affecting the genital tract, such as the genitourinary syndrome; the central nervous system, such as vasomotor symptoms or mood swings; and other territories, which are especially bothersome in the menopausal transition or in the first years after menopause [66]. However, the prolongation of hormone action conveyed by MHT has been also associated with some risks. The increase risks of breast cancer diagnoses and, contrary to previous observational studies, of cardiovascular disease, both coronary heart disease and stroke, were most influential in reaching the preliminary conclusion that, apart from the demonstrated protection against menopausal symptoms, the balance in terms of health was negative, with more risk than benefits [67]. Subsequent reanalyses of the WHI data, along with follow-up of participants for years after study completion, in addition to the publication of new studies, have suggested that the effect of MHT is highly dependent on the components, both estrogen and progestin, as well as the timing of use in relation to age and years since menopause [68].

In that regard, an important finding has been that the increased risk of breast cancer was related to the progestogenic component and that the type of progestogen was substantially relevant with regard to that risk. Natural progesterone and dydrogesterone have been shown to have a much lower risk than medroxyprogesterone acetate, the progestogen used in the WHI study [69–71].

The timing of MHT use was also shown to matter as no increased cardiovascular risk was observed in younger women when participants were stratified by chronological or menopausal age [72]. Although the ultimate reasons for this so-called "timing hypothesis" remain elusive [73], experimental studies have shown that estrogens may protect against atherosclerosis when plaques are not yet established, such as in younger women, whereas that protective effect may turn into risk when atherosclerotic plaques are more advanced and unstable, such as in older age [74].

Therefore, the use of MHT in the treatment of osteoporosis has been very limited in the guidelines published in the years immediately following the publication of the WHI trials. Treatment of menopausal symptoms has been the only accepted indication, and only when other options could not be used, for the treatment or prevention of osteoporosis in asymptomatic women. In light of new findings, this position has been qualified in some guidelines. The use of MHT is contemplated as a first option in women younger than 60 years or less than 10 years since menopause in the recent position statement on MHT by the North American Menopause Society [75].

In the frequent event that continued anti-osteoporotic therapy is necessary, there are no established protocols to facilitate the transition between MHT and other anti-osteoporotic drugs. A progressive tapering of MHT seems a practical approach in asymptomatic women, but the evidence supporting this strategy is sparse and based only on expert opinion. The sequential use of selective estrogen receptor modulators (SERMs) has been suggested as a well-founded approach, given the more selective protection of SERMs against vertebral fractures, which are more prevalent at younger ages [76]. Alternative options exist when menopausal symptoms persist, the main ones being local preparations, including estrogens, for the genitourinary syndrome [75], nonhormonal management of hot flashes with antagonists of neurokinin-3 receptors [77], and others.

8.3.2.3 Pharmacological Compounds

Selective Estrogen Receptor Modulators (SERMs)
Advances in pharmacological chemistry together with the better knowledge of ER biochemistry have generated a number of synthetic compounds that have a molecular conformation distinct to estrogens but share their potential to interact with the ER. The structural differences with estrogens determine that their agonist/antagonist equilibrium changes as a result of the three-dimensional molecular configuration or the target tissue [78]. SERMs are grouped in families according to the root biochemical structure, and several of them have been approved for use with humans [79].

The most attractive property of SERMs is that molecules may be shaped to maintain the advantages of estrogens, for example, in osteoporosis, while eliminating as far as possible their associated risks. This search of the perfect SERM keeps being a constant in the latter years.

Two compounds, raloxifene and bazedoxifene, have been approved for treating osteoporosis in several countries. Both raloxifene and bazedoxifene have demonstrated increases in BMD and effective reduction of vertebral, but not hip fractures [80, 81]. There was a protective effect against nonvertebral fractures in corresponding post-hoc analyses [81, 82]. The size of the impact on the bone seems slightly lower than that achieved by estrogens. Interestingly, raloxifene has demonstrated reduction in the risk for breast cancer [83] although as for estrogens, an increase in deep vein thrombosis was apparent in the pivotal studies [80, 81]. Health economy analyses have shown acceptable cost-effectiveness of SERMs [84, 85].

Bazedoxifene has demonstrated a more antagonistic effect than raloxifene in endometrium, and this interesting property has been taken as the basis for development of a new formulation in which bazedoxifene is mixed with estrogens to counterbalance the oncogenic potential of estrogens on the endometrium or the breast [86].

The balance of benefits and risks of SERMs makes their use particularly appropriate in women with a more marked reduction in BMD at the spine than at the hip, without a higher risk of venous thromboembolism, and with a higher risk of breast cancer. Consequently, SERMs may fill a gap after hormone therapy to maintain BMD benefits in women who still require anti-osteoporotic treatment. Provided the response is satisfactory, their use can be maintained for up to 8 years, which is the interval at which reliable information on their effectiveness and safety is available [87, 88]. Supplements of calcium and vitamin D should be associated if diet is insufficient to provide adequate levels.

Bisphosphonates
These molecules are incorporated into the mineralized bone because of their affinity for calcium. Bisphosphonates are toxic for osteoclasts so that they condition cellular demise when ingested in the course of the osteoclast-dependent resorptive action. In

such a simple way, bisphosphonates drastically reduce bone turnover. Several compounds have been marketed and are now very good cost-effective options [89]. Alendronate, risedronate, clodronate, zoledronate, and ibandronate have been those with higher popularity. They may be administered by oral or intravenous route. Oral bisphosphonates may be used in weekly and monthly doses with similar impact on BMD and bone markers than the daily administration. Randomized controlled trials including high-risk women have shown that oral bisphosphonates reduce radiographic vertebral fractures by approximately 40%–50% and nonvertebral and hip fractures by 20–30% [51, 90, 91].

The use of bisphosphonates is appropriate after MHT when SERMs are not an option or as a first choice in women who are not candidates for MHT. An increased risk of hip fracture may also be an indication for bisphosphonates as a first choice.

Bisphosphonates are associated with frequent adverse effects, such as gastroesophageal irritation, when administered orally. The highly effective reduction of bone turnover, which drastically limits the activity of the BMUs, has favored two rare but serious adverse events, osteonecrosis, particularly at the jaw [92], and atypical femoral fractures [93]. This has popularized the new strategy of drug holiday [94], which aims at intercalating periods without treatment in the course of long-term use of bisphosphonates. Even so, guidelines continue to consider prolongation for up to 5 additional years with bisphosphonates if a sufficiently high risk of fragility fracture persists [95].

One of the main weaknesses of oral bisphosphonates is low adherence rates, with poor persistence rates ranging from 18% to 75% at 1 year [96]. This limitation seriously affects the clinical effect and impacts the cost to the healthcare system. The selection of an intravenous bisphosphonate, in particular the once-yearly zoledronic acid regimen, may ameliorate this problem.

Calcium supplementation, which along with vitamin D should be considered, as mentioned for SERMs, should receive special attention when zoledronic acid is used as the high potency of the drug may induce hypocalcemia. Supplementation or monitoring of calcium levels may be considered.

Denosumab

The first biological treatment in osteoporosis is represented by denosumab, a human (IgG2) antibody that binds to RANKL thus drastically reducing the differentiation of osteoclasts. The dose of 60 mg administered in the form of subcutaneous injection every 6 months achieved a reduction of vertebral fractures by 68%, of nonvertebral fractures by 40%, and of hip fractures by 20% as compared with placebo [97]. Unlike bisphosphonates, which persist long term in bone, the antiresorptive action of denosumab is rapidly reversible, with a rebound effect that must be taken into account when discontinuing treatment [98].

Denosumab can be used for indications similar to bisphosphonates, when there is no clear BMD response to bisphosphonates, or when adherence to bisphosphonates is poor. In fact, the use of denosumab after any other antiresorptive drug has shown superiority in increasing BMD in all bone territories without increasing serious adverse events [99].

Since denosumab is a potent antiresorptive, calcium supplementation or calcium monitoring may be considered. In addition, similar to bisphosphonates, the antibody has been associated with increased risk for osteonecrosis of the jaw and atypical femoral fractures [100].

Anabolic Agents
The recent expansion of drugs capable of stimulating the recruitment and activity of osteoblasts has opened up a new therapeutic field [101]. Their use was originally proposed as a subsequent or complementary step to antiresorptive drugs, when the blockade of bone resorption seemed insufficient to recover bone mass to the desired levels. This additional therapeutic action was usually limited to very high-risk patients. More recently, increased experience with anabolic agents has reinforced the so-called "anabolic first regimens" for women at high or very high risk of fracture. The rationale is to promote bone formation to optimize bone mass gains and then "seal" the gains with an antiresorptive [102].

Three main anabolic compounds have accumulated the most clinical evidence, teriparatide, abaloparatide, and romosozumab. Both teriparatide and abaloparatide are related to parathyroid hormone (PTH). Teriparatide is the human recombinant N-terminal 1–34 fragment of human PTH, while abaloparatide is a modification of PTH-related peptide (PTHrP) 1–34. Romosozumab is a humanized monoclonal antibody against sclerostin, an inhibitor of Wnt, a potent pathway that stimulates osteoblast activation [103].

The administration of the three anabolic molecules is subcutaneous for limited periods of time, 2 years, 18 months, and 1 year for teriparatide, abaloparatide, and romosozumab, respectively. Subsequent use of antiresorptives should be taken into account in all cases, with alendronate, denosumab, and even SERMs having been considered, although protocols vary and should be specifically addressed [51].

8.4 Conclusion

Osteoporosis is a disease with a strong gender profile. Menopause adds risk and therefore is a period of particular attention. Moreover, the age at menopause is still early enough to implement lifestyle measures that will provide benefit not only for bone but also for other systems, like the vasculature, the muscle, the central nervous system, or others.

Fractures are rare at the age of menopause unless women suffer from additional risk factors. This is why the health exams at this period of the women's life should include a review of the risk factors for osteoporosis. Most women will be free of them and, consequently, should be advised healthy lifestyle only. This will include the avoidance of toxics, tobacco, or excessive consumption of alcohol, a balanced diet in which the recommended amount of calcium (1200 mg/day) plus vitamin D (800 UI) is achieved, and regular physical activity. These measures will improve general health and quality of life and, again, should be the only recommendation to the majority of women.

Women with risk factors should be studied adequately. This adds a bone densitometry and, if risk is sufficiently high, the use of anti-osteoporotic drugs. The selection of the drug should account that women living the early stages of postmenopause, usually aged less than 60 years, have a long life expectancy in front. Since one of the main risk factors for osteoporosis is age, the indication for treatment will continue to strengthen over the years, and a lifelong strategy, with a sequential arrangement of anti-osteoporotic drugs, is mandatory (Fig. 8.3). This is why MHT needs to be considered as an initial choice when there are menopausal symptoms, and even in their absence, according to some recent guidelines. Another

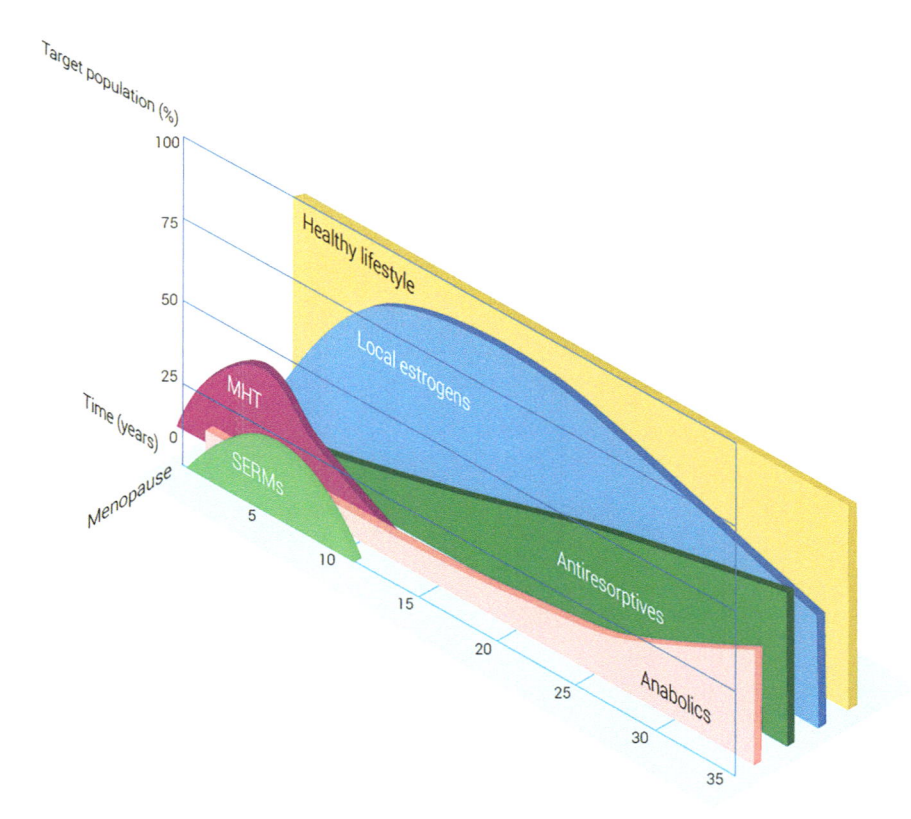

Fig. 8.3 Proposal for sequential use of anti-osteoporotic strategies based on the profile of each therapeutic group. The X axis represents the menopausal age (years since menopause) at which each therapeutic option can be placed. The Y axis represents the percentage of the population that is a candidate for each therapeutic option. The figures on each of the X and Y axes are merely an approximation based on current literature data and are subject to drastic changes depending on the variables involved. The healthy lifestyle applies to 100% of the population at all ages of menopause. MHT, menopausal hormone therapy; SERMs, selective estrogen receptor modulators. (With permission of Elsevier from Calaf-Alsina et al. Maturitas 2023; 177:107846. doi: https://doi.org/10.1016/j.maturitas.2023.107846. Permission conveyed through Copyright Clearance Center, Inc.)

important option is SERMs, which add two advantages, the reduction of the risk of breast cancer (raloxifene) and a smooth reduction of bone turnover, which discards the risks of jaw osteonecrosis or atypical femoral fracture. Also, SERMs reduce risk of vertebral fractures, which rank prior to hip fracture in the chronologic sequence of osteoporotic fractures. After a certain number of years, SERMs may be changed for bisphosphonates or denosumab [104]. This sequence, however, results from clinical judgment and has not been substantiated by any study. Therefore, initiation with bisphosphonates or denosumab, for example, may be an acceptable option under some conditions. Finally, anabolic drugs have emerged strongly and are now proposed as the first option in women at high or very high risk, always followed by an antiresorptive drug.

References

1. https://www.osteoporosis.foundation/facts-statistics/epidemiology-of-osteoporosis-and-fragility-fractures, accessed on 26 Mar 2024.
2. http://apps.who.int/iris/bitstream/10665/39142/1/WHO_TRS_843_eng.pdf, accessed on 27 Mar 2024.
3. Kanis JA, Melton LJ 3rd, Christiansen C, Johnston CC, Khaltaev N. The diagnosis of osteoporosis. J Bone Miner Res. 1994;9:1137–41.
4. https://www.shef.ac.uk/FRAX/tool.jsp?lang=en, accessed on 26 Mar 2024.
5. Curtis EM, van der Velde R, Moon RJ, van den Bergh JP, Geusens P, de Vries F, van Staa TP, Cooper C, Harvey NC. Epidemiology of fractures in the United Kingdom 1988–2012: variation with age, sex, geography, ethnicity and socioeconomic status. Bone. 2016 Jun;87:19–26. https://doi.org/10.1016/j.bone.2016.03.006.
6. Reifenstein EC Jr, Albright F. The metabolic effects of steroid hormones in osteoporosis. J Clin Invest. 1947;26:24–56.
7. Hernlund E, Svedbom A, Ivergård M, Compston J, Cooper C, Stenmark J, McCloskey EV, Jönsson B, Kanis JA. Osteoporosis in the European Union: medical management, epidemiology and economic burden. A report prepared in collaboration with the International Osteoporosis Foundation (IOF) and the European Federation of Pharmaceutical Industry Associations (EFPIA). Arch Osteoporos. 2013;8(1):136. https://doi.org/10.1007/s11657-013-0136-1.
8. Seeman E, Delmas PD. Bone quality—the material and structural basis of bone strength and fragility. N Engl J Med. 2006;354(21):2250–61. https://doi.org/10.1056/NEJMra053077.
9. Bolamperti S, Villa I, Rubinacci A. Bone remodeling: an operational process ensuring survival and bone mechanical competence. Bone Res. 2022;10:48. https://doi.org/10.1038/s41413-022-00219-8.
10. Robling AG, Bonewald LF. The osteocyte: new insights. Annu Rev Physiol. 2020;82:485–506. https://doi.org/10.1146/annurev-physiol-021119-034332.
11. Prideaux M, Findlay DM, Atkins GJ. Osteocytes: the master cells in bone remodelling. Curr Opin Pharmacol. 2016;28:24–30. https://doi.org/10.1016/j.coph.2016.02.003.
12. Nakashima T, Hayashi M, Fukunaga T, Kurata K, Oh-Hora M, Feng JQ, et al. Evidence for osteocyte regulation of bone homeostasis through RANKL expression. Nat Med. 2011;17:1231–4.
13. Boyle WJ, Simonet WS, Lacey DL. Osteoclast differentiation and activation. Nature. 2003;423:337–42. https://doi.org/10.1038/nature01658.
14. Udagawa N, Koide M, Nakamura M, Nakamichi Y, Yamashita T, Uehara S, Kobayashi Y, Furuya Y, Yasuda H, Fukuda C, Tsuda E. Osteoclast differentiation by RANKL and

OPG signaling pathways. J Bone Miner Metab. 2021;39:19–26. https://doi.org/10.1007/s00774-020-01162-6.
15. Braidman IP, Davenport LK, Carter DH, Selby PL, Mawer EB, Freemont AJ. Preliminary in situ identification of estrogen target cells in bone. J Bone Miner Res. 1995;10:74–80.
16. Arts J, Kuiper GGJM, Janssen JMMF, Gustafsson J-A, Lowik CWGM, Pols HAP, et al. Differential expression of estrogen receptors and during differentiation of human osteoblast SV-HFO cells. Endocrinology. 1997;138:5067–70.
17. Vidal O, Kindblom L-G, Ohlsson C. Expression and localization of estrogen receptor in murine and human bone. J Bone Miner Res. 1999;14:923–6.
18. Bord S, Horner A, Beavan S, Compston J. Estrogen receptors alpha and beta are differentially expressed in developing human bone. J Clin Endocrinol Metab. 2001;86:2309–14.
19. Nilsson O, Chrysis D, Pajulo O, Boman A, Holst M, Rubinstein J, et al. Localization of estrogen receptors-alpha and -beta and androgen receptor in the human growth plate at different pubertal stages. J Endocrinol. 2003;177:319–26.
20. Khalid AB, Krum SA. Estrogen receptors alpha and beta in bone. Bone. 2016;87:130–5. https://doi.org/10.1016/j.bone.2016.03.016.
21. Bilezikian JP, Morishima A, Bell J, Grumbach MM. Increased bone mass as a result of estrogen therapy in a man with aromatase deficiency. N Engl J Med. 1998;339:599–603.
22. Falahati-Nini A, Riggs BL, Atkinson EJ, O'Fallon WM, Eastell R, Khosla S. Relative contributions of testosterone and estrogen in regulating bone resorption and formation in normal elderly men. J Clin Invest. 2000;106:1553–60.
23. Lindsay R, Hart DM, Aitken JM, MacDonald EB, Anderson JB, Clarke AC. Long-term prevention of postmenopausal osteoporosis by oestrogen. Evidence for an increased bone mass after delayed onset of oestrogen treatment. Lancet. 1976;1:1038–41.
24. Almeida M, Laurent MR, Dubois V, Claessens F, O'Brien CA, Bouillon R, Vanderschueren D, Manolagas SC. Estrogens and androgens in skeletal physiology and pathophysiology. Physiol Rev. 2017;97:135–87. https://doi.org/10.1152/physrev.00033.2015.
25. Khosla S, Monroe DG. Regulation of bone metabolism by sex steroids. Cold Spring Harb Perspect Med. 2018;8(1):a031211. https://doi.org/10.1101/cshperspect.a031211.
26. Khosla S. Estrogen versus FSH effects on bone metabolism: evidence from interventional human studies. Endocrinology. 2020;161(8):bqaa111. https://doi.org/10.1210/endocr/bqaa111.
27. Karlamangla AS, Burnett-Bowie SM, Crandall CJ. Bone health during the menopause transition and beyond. Obstet Gynecol Clin N Am. 2018;45:695–708. https://doi.org/10.1016/j.ogc.2018.07.012.
28. Garnero P, Sornay-Rendu E, Chapuy MC, Delmas PD. Increased bone turnover in late postmenopausal women is a major determinant of osteoporosis. J Bone Miner Res. 1996;11:337–49.
29. McNamara LM. Osteocytes and estrogen deficiency. Curr Osteoporos Rep. 2021;19:592–603. https://doi.org/10.1007/s11914-021-00702-x.
30. Tomkinson A, Reeve J, Shaw RW, Noble BS. The death of osteocytes via apoptosis accompanies estrogen withdrawal in human bone. J Clin Endocrinol Metab. 1997;82:3128–35.
31. Fujita K, Roforth MM, Demaray S, McGregor U, Kirmani S, McCready LK, Peterson JM, Drake MT, Monroe DG, Khosla S. Effects of estrogen on bone mRNA levels of sclerostin and other genes relevant to bone metabolism in postmenopausal women. J Clin Endocrinol Metab. 2014;99:E81–8. https://doi.org/10.1210/jc.2013-3249.
32. Geoghegan IP, Hoey DA, McNamara LM. Estrogen deficiency impairs integrin $\alpha_v\beta_3$-mediated mechanosensation by osteocytes and alters osteoclastogenic paracrine signalling. Sci Rep. 2019;9:4654. https://doi.org/10.1038/s41598-019-41095-3.
33. Martin-Millan M, Almeida M, Ambrogini E, Han L, Zhao H, Weinstein RS, et al. The estrogen receptor-alpha in osteoclasts mediates the protective effects of estrogens on cancellous but not cortical bone. Mol Endocrinol. 2010;24:323–34.
34. Guo L, Chen K, Yuan J, Huang P, Xu X, Li C, Qian N, Qi J, Shao Z, Deng L, He C, Xu J. Estrogen inhibits osteoclasts formation and bone resorption via microRNA-27a targeting PPARγ and APC. J Cell Physiol. 2018;234:581–94. https://doi.org/10.1002/jcp.26788.

35. Huang Y, Yang Y, Wang J, Yao S, Yao T, Xu Y, Chen Z, Yuan P, Gao J, Shen S, Ma J. miR-21-5p targets SKP2 to reduce osteoclastogenesis in a mouse model of osteoporosis. J Biol Chem. 2021;296:100617. https://doi.org/10.1016/j.jbc.2021.100617.
36. Srivastava S, Toraldo G, Weitzmann MN, Cenci S, Ross FP, Pacifici R. Estrogen decreases osteoclast formation by down-regulating receptor activator of NF-kappa B ligand (RANKL)-induced JNK activation. J Biol Chem. 2001;276:8836–40.
37. Spelsberg TC, Subramaniam M, Riggs BL, Khosla S. The actions and interactions of sex steroids and growth factors/cytokines on the skeleton. Mol Endocrinol. 1999;13:819–28. https://doi.org/10.1210/mend.13.6.0299.
38. https://www.nof.org, accessed 27 Mar 2024.
39. https://www.osteoporosis.foundation/health-professionals/diagnosis/other-diagnostic-tools, accessed 27 Mar 2024.
40. Hippisley-Cox J, Coupland C. Derivation and validation of updated QFracture algorithm to predict risk of osteoporotic fracture in primary care in the United Kingdom: prospective open cohort study. BMJ. 2012;344:e3427.
41. Kanis JA, Cooper C, Rizzoli R, Reginster JY. Scientific Advisory Board of the European Society for Clinical and Economic Aspects of Osteoporosis (ESCEO) and the Committees of Scientific Advisors and National Societies of the International Osteoporosis Foundation (IOF). European guidance for the diagnosis and management of osteoporosis in postmenopausal women. Osteoporos Int. 2019;30:3–44. https://doi.org/10.1007/s00198-018-4704-5.
42. Leslie WD, Majumdar SR, Morin SN, Lix LM. Change in bone mineral density is an indicator of treatment-related antifracture effect in routine clinical practice: a registry-based cohort study. Ann Intern Med. 2016;165:465–72.
43. Papaioannou A, Morin S, Cheung AM, Atkinson S, Brown JP, Feldman S, et al. 2010 clinical practice guidelines for the diagnosis and management of osteoporosis in Canada: summary. CMAJ. 2010;182:1864–73.
44. Davis SR, Tan A, Bell RJ. Targeted assessment of fracture risk in women at midlife. Osteoporos Int. 2015;26:1705–12.
45. Silva BC, Leslie WD. Trabecular bone score: a new DXA-derived measurement for fracture risk assessment. Endocrinol Metab Clin N Am. 2017;46:153–80.
46. Schini M, Vilaca T, Gossiel F, Salam S, Eastell R. Bone turnover markers: basic biology to clinical applications. Endocr Rev. 2023;44:417–73. https://doi.org/10.1210/endrev/bnac031.
47. Garnero P, Sornay-Rendu E, Claustrat B, Delmas PD. Biochemical markers of bone turnover, endogenous hormones and the risk of fractures in postmenopausal women: the OFELY study. J Bone Miner Res. 2000;15:1526–36.
48. Siris ES, Miller PD, Barrett-Connor E, Faulkner KG, Wehren LE, Abbott TA, et al. Identification and fracture outcomes of undiagnosed low bone mineral density in postmenopausal women: results from the National Osteoporosis Risk Assessment. JAMA. 2001;286:2815–22.
49. Vasikaran S, Eastell R, Bruyère O, Foldes AJ, Garnero P, Griesmacher A, McClung M, Morris HA, Silverman S, Trenti T, Wahl DA, Cooper C, Kanis JA, IOF-IFCC Bone Marker Standards Working Group. Markers of bone turnover for the prediction of fracture risk and monitoring of osteoporosis treatment: a need for international reference standards. Osteoporos Int. 2011;22:391–420. https://doi.org/10.1007/s00198-010-1501-1.
50. Tsourdi E, Zillikens MC, Meier C, Body JJ, Gonzalez Rodriguez E, Anastasilakis AD, Abrahamsen B, McCloskey E, Hofbauer LC, Guañabens N, Obermayer-Pietsch B, Ralston SH, Eastell R, Pepe J, Palermo A, Langdahl B. Fracture risk and management of discontinuation of denosumab therapy: a systematic review and position statement by ECTS. J Clin Endocrinol Metab. 2021:dgaa756. https://doi.org/10.1210/clinem/dgaa756.
51. Calaf-Alsina J, Cano A, Guañabens N, Palacios S, Cancelo MJ, Castelo-Branco C, Larrainzar-Garijo R, Neyro JL, Nogues X, Diez-Perez A. Sequential management of postmenopausal health and osteoporosis: an update. Maturitas. 2023;177:107846. https://doi.org/10.1016/j.maturitas.2023.107846.
52. Sowers MR, Finkelstein JS, Ettinger B, Bondarenko I, Neer RM, Cauley JA, et al. Study of Women's Health Across the Nation. The association of endogenous hormone concentrations

and bone mineral density measures in pre- and perimenopausal women of four ethnic groups: SWAN. Osteoporos Int. 2003;14:44–52.
53. Zebaze RM, Ghasem-Zadeh A, Bohte A, Iuliano-Burns S, Mirams M, Price RI, et al. Intracortical remodelling and porosity in the distal radius and post-mortem femurs of women: a cross-sectional study. Lancet. 2010;375:1729–36.
54. Walker MD, Shane E. Postmenopausal Osteoporosis. N Engl J Med. 2023;389:1979–91. https://doi.org/10.1056/NEJMcp2307353.
55. Stojanovska L, Apostolopoulos V, Polman R, Borkoles E. To exercise, or, not to exercise, during menopause and beyond. Maturitas. 2014;77:318–23.
56. Warensjö E, Byberg L, Melhus H, Gedeborg R, Mallmin H, Wolk A, et al. Dietary calcium intake and risk of fracture and osteoporosis: prospective longitudinal cohort study. BMJ. 2011;342:d1473.
57. Wallace RB, Wactawski-Wende J, O'Sullivan MJ, Larson JC, Cochrane B, Gass M, et al. Urinary tract stone occurrence in the Women's Health Initiative (WHI) randomized clinical trial of calcium and vitamin D supplements. Am J Clin Nutr. 2011;94:270–7.
58. Bolland MJ, Grey A, Avenell A, Gamble GD, Reid IR. Calcium supplements with or without vitamin D and risk of cardiovascular events: reanalysis of the Women's Health Initiative limited access dataset and meta-analysis. BMJ. 2011;342:d2040.
59. Cano A, Chedraui P, Goulis DG, Lopes P, Mishra G, Mueck A, Senturk LM, Simoncini T, Stevenson JC, Stute P, Tuomikoski P, Rees M, Lambrinoudaki I. Calcium in the prevention of postmenopausal osteoporosis: EMAS clinical guide. Maturitas. 2018;107:7–12. https://doi.org/10.1016/j.maturitas.2017.10.004.
60. Gallagher JC. Vitamin D and falls – the dosage conundrum. Nat Rev Endocrinol. 2016;12:680–4. https://doi.org/10.1038/nrendo.2016.123.
61. Lindsay R, Gallagher JC, Kleerekoper M, Pickar JH. Effect of lower doses of conjugated equine estrogens with and without medroxyprogesterone acetate on bone in early postmenopausal women. JAMA. 2002;287:2668–76.
62. García-Pérez MA, Moreno-Mercer J, Tarín JJ, Cano A. Similar efficacy of low and standard doses of transdermal estradiol in controlling bone turnover in postmenopausal women. Gynecol Endocrinol. 2006;22:179–84.
63. Cauley JA, Robbins J, Chen Z, Cummings SR, Jackson RD, LaCroix AZ, et al. Women's Health Initiative Investigators. Effects of estrogen plus progestin on risk of fracture and bone mineral density: the Women's Health Initiative randomized trial. JAMA. 2003;290:1729–38.
64. Zhu L, Jiang X, Sun Y, Shu W. Effect of hormone therapy on the risk of bone fractures: a systematic review and meta-analysis of randomized controlled trials. Menopause. 2016;23:461–70. https://doi.org/10.1097/GME.0000000000000519.
65. Watts NB, Cauley JA, Jackson RD, LaCroix AZ, Lewis CE, Manson JE, Neuner JM, Phillips LS, Stefanick ML, Wactawski-Wende J, Crandall C, Women's Health Initiative Investigators. No increase in fractures after stopping hormone therapy: results from the women's health initiative. J Clin Endocrinol Metab. 2017;102:302–8. https://doi.org/10.1210/jc.2016-3270.
66. Gold EB, Sternfeld B, Kelsey JL, Brown C, Mouton C, Reame N, Salamone L, Stellato R. Relation of demographic and lifestyle factors to symptoms in a multi-racial/ethnic population of women 40–55 years of age. Am J Epidemiol. 2000;152:463–73. https://doi.org/10.1093/aje/152.5.463.
67. Rossouw JE, Anderson GL, Prentice RL, LaCroix AZ, Kooperberg C, Stefanick ML, Jackson RD, Beresford SA, Howard BV, Johnson KC, Kotchen JM, Ockene J, Writing Group for the Women's Health Initiative Investigators. Risks and benefits of estrogen plus progestin in healthy postmenopausal women: principal results from the Women's Health Initiative randomized controlled trial. JAMA. 2002;288:321–33. https://doi.org/10.1001/jama.288.3.321.
68. Manson JE, Kaunitz AM. Menopause management—getting clinical care back on track. N Engl J Med. 2016;374:803–6. https://doi.org/10.1056/NEJMp1514242.
69. Fournier A, Berrino F, Clavel-Chapelon F. Unequal risks for breast cancer associated with different hormone replacement therapies: results from the E3N cohort study. Breast Cancer Res Treat. 2008;107:103–11. https://doi.org/10.1007/s10549-007-9523-x.

70. Vinogradova Y, Coupland C, Hippisley-Cox J. Use of hormone replacement therapy and risk of breast cancer: nested case-control studies using the QResearch and CPRD databases. BMJ. 2020;371:m3873. https://doi.org/10.1136/bmj.m3873.
71. Saul H, Gursul D, Cassidy S, Vinogradova Y. Risk of breast cancer with HRT depends on therapy type and duration. BMJ. 2022;376:o485. https://doi.org/10.1136/bmj.o485.
72. Rossouw JE, Prentice RL, Manson JE, Wu L, Barad D, Barnabei VM, Ko M, LaCroix AZ, Margolis KL, Stefanick ML. Postmenopausal hormone therapy and risk of cardiovascular disease by age and years since menopause. JAMA. 2007;297:1465–77. https://doi.org/10.1001/jama.297.13.1465.
73. Bassuk SS, Manson JE. The timing hypothesis: do coronary risks of menopausal hormone therapy vary by age or time since menopause onset? Metabolism. 2016;65:794–803. https://doi.org/10.1016/j.metabol.2016.01.004.
74. Clarkson TB, Appt SE. Controversies about HRT—lessons from monkey models. Maturitas. 2005;51:64–74. https://doi.org/10.1016/j.maturitas.2005.02.016.
75. The 2022 Hormone Therapy Position Statement of The North American Menopause Society Advisory Panel. The 2022 hormone therapy position statement of The North American Menopause Society. Menopause. 2022;29:767–94. https://doi.org/10.1097/GME.0000000000002028.
76. Calaf J. The role of SERMs in the management of postmenopausal women. In: Cano, Calaf I Alsina, Dueñas-Díez, editors. Selective estrogen receptor modulators. Heildelberg: Springer-Verlag; 2006. p. 333–49.
77. Lederman S, Ottery FD, Cano A, Santoro N, Shapiro M, Stute P, Thurston RC, English M, Franklin C, Lee M, Neal-Perry G. Fezolinetant for treatment of moderate-to-severe vasomotor symptoms associated with menopause (SKYLIGHT 1): a phase 3 randomised controlled study. Lancet. 2023;401:1091–102. https://doi.org/10.1016/S0140-6736(23)00085-5.
78. Cano A, Hermenegildo C. Modulation of the oestrogen receptor: a process with distinct susceptible steps. Hum Reprod Update. 2000;6:207–11.
79. Riggs BL, Hartmann LC. Selective estrogen-receptor modulators—mechanisms of action and application to clinical practice. N Engl J Med. 2003;348:618–29.
80. Ettinger B, Black DM, Mitlak BH, Knickerbocker RK, Nickelsen T, Genant HK, et al. Reduction of vertebral fracture risk in postmenopausal women with osteoporosis treated with raloxifene: results from a 3-year randomized clinical trial. Multiple Outcomes of Raloxifene Evaluation (MORE) Investigators. JAMA. 1999;282:637–45.
81. Silverman SL, Christiansen C, Genant HK, Vukicevic S, Zanchetta JR, de Villiers TJ, et al. Efficacy of bazedoxifene in reducing new vertebral fracture risk in postmenopausal women with osteoporosis: results from a 3-year, randomized, placebo-, and active-controlled clinical trial. J Bone Miner Res. 2008;23:1923–34.
82. Delmas PD, Genant HK, Crans GG, Stock JL, Wong M, Siris E, et al. Severity of prevalent vertebral fractures and the risk of subsequent vertebral and nonvertebral fractures: results from the MORE trial. Bone. 2003;33:522–32.
83. Vogel VG, Costantino JP, Wickerham DL, Cronin WM, Cecchini RS, Atkins JN, et al. National Surgical Adjuvant Breast and Bowel Project (NSABP). Effects of tamoxifen vs raloxifene on the risk of developing invasive breast cancer and other disease outcomes: the NSABP Study of Tamoxifen and Raloxifene (STAR) P-2 trial. JAMA. 2006;295:2727–41.
84. Borgström F, Ström O, Kleman M, McCloskey E, Johansson H, Odén A, et al. Cost-effectiveness of bazedoxifene incorporating the FRAX® algorithm in a European perspective. Osteoporos Int. 2011;22:955–65.
85. Kim K, Svedbom A, Luo X, Sutradhar S, Kanis JA. Comparative cost-effectiveness of bazedoxifene and raloxifene in the treatment of postmenopausal osteoporosis in Europe, using the FRAX algorithm. Osteoporos Int. 2014;25:325–37.
86. Pinkerton JV, Harvey JA, Lindsay R, Pan K, Chines AA, Mirkin S, Archer DF. SMART-5 Investigators. Effects of bazedoxifene/conjugated estrogens on the endometrium and bone: a randomized trial. J Clin Endocrinol Metab. 2014;99:E189–98. https://doi.org/10.1210/jc.2013-1707.

87. Siris ES, Harris ST, Eastell R, Zanchetta JR, Goemaere S, Diez-Perez A, Stock JL, Song J, Qu Y, Kulkarni PM, Siddhanti SR, Wong M, Cummings SR. Continuing Outcomes Relevant to Evista (CORE) Investigators. Skeletal effects of raloxifene after 8 years: results from the continuing outcomes relevant to Evista (CORE) study. J Bone Miner Res. 2005;20:1514–24. https://doi.org/10.1359/JBMR.050509.
88. Yavropoulou MP, Makras P, Anastasilakis AD. Bazedoxifene for the treatment of osteoporosis. Expert Opin Pharmacother. 2019 Jul;20(10):1201–10. https://doi.org/10.1080/1465656 6.2019.1615882.
89. Khosla S, Bilezikian JP, Dempster DW, Lewiecki EM, Miller PD, Neer RM, et al. Benefits and risks of bisphosphonate therapy for osteoporosis. J Clin Endocrinol Metab. 2012;97:2272–82.
90. Black DM, Cummings SR, Karpf DB, Cauley JA, Thompson DE, Nevitt MC, et al. Randomised trial of effect of alendronate on risk of fracture in women with existing vertebral fractures. Lancet. 1996;348:1535–41.
91. McClung MR, Geusens P, Miller PD, Zippel H, Bensen WG, Roux C, et al. Effect of risedronate on the risk of hip fracture in elderly women. N Engl J Med. 2001;344:333–40.
92. Khan A, Morrison A, Cheung A, Hashem W, Compston J. Osteonecrosis of the jaw (ONJ): diagnosis and management in 2015. Osteoporos Int. 2016;27:853–9.
93. Shane E, Burr D, Abrahamsen B, Adler RA, Brown TD, Cheung AM, et al. Atypical subtrochanteric and diaphyseal femoral fractures: second report of a task force of the American Society for Bone and Mineral Research. J Bone Miner Res. 2014;29:1–23.
94. Silverman SL, Adachi JD, Dennison E, International Osteoporosis Foundation Epidemiology/Quality of Life Working Group. Bisphosphonate drug holidays: we reap what we sow. Osteoporos Int. 2016;27:849–52.
95. Camacho PM, Petak SM, Binkley N, Diab DL, Eldeiry LS, Farooki A, Harris ST, Hurley DL, Kelly J, Lewiecki EM, Pessah-Pollack R, McClung M, Wimalawansa SJ, Watts NB. American Association of Clinical Endocrinologists/American College of Endocrinology Clinical Practice Guidelines for the diagnosis and treatment of postmenopausal osteoporosis-2020 update. Endocr Pract. 2020;26(Suppl 1):1–46. https://doi.org/10.4158/GL-2020-0524SUPPL.
96. Fatoye F, Smith P, Gebrye T, Yeowell G. Real-world persistence and adherence with oral bisphosphonates for osteoporosis: a systematic review. BMJ Open. 2019;9:e027049. https://doi.org/10.1136/bmjopen-2018-027049.
97. Cummings SR, San Martin J, McClung MR, Siris ES, Eastell R, Reid IR, et al. Denosumab for prevention of fractures in postmenopausal women with osteoporosis. N Engl J Med. 2009;361:756–65.
98. Anastasilakis AD, Makras P, Yavropoulou MP, Tabacco G, Naciu AM, Palermo A. Denosumab discontinuation and the rebound phenomenon: a narrative review. J Clin Med. 2021;10:152. https://doi.org/10.3390/jcm10010152.
99. Fontalis A, Kenanidis E, Prousali E, Potoupnis M, Tsiridis E. Safety and efficacy of denosumab in osteoporotic patients previously treated with other medications: a systematic review and meta-analysis. Expert Opin Drug Saf. 2018;17:413–28. https://doi.org/10.1080/1474033 8.2018.1430764.
100. Cano A, Silvan JM, Estévez A, Baró F, Villero J, Quereda F, et al. Spanish Menopause Society position statement: use of denosumab in postmenopausal women. Maturitas. 2014;79:117–21.
101. Ruiz C, Abril N, Tarín JJ, García-Pérez MA, Cano A. The new frontier of bone formation: a breakthrough in postmenopausal osteoporosis? Climacteric. 2009;12:286–300.
102. Reid IR, Billington EO. Drug therapy for osteoporosis in older adults. Lancet. 2022;399:1080–92. https://doi.org/10.1016/S0140-6736(21)02646-5.
103. Cosman F. Anabolic therapy and optimal treatment sequences for patients with osteoporosis at high risk for fracture. Endocr Pract. 2020;26:777–86. https://doi.org/10.4158/EP-2019-0596.
104. Cano A, Mendoza N, Sánchez-Borrego R, Osteoporosis Guideline Writing Group from the Spanish Menopause Society. Sequential use of antiresorptives in younger women. Osteoporos Int. 2014;25:1191–2.

The Metabolic Syndrome During Female Midlife and Beyond

9

Peter Chedraui and Faustino R. Pérez-López

Abstract

The prevalence of the metabolic syndrome (METS) increases as women transit the menopause. Diagnostic features include obesity, hypertension, dyslipidemia, and hyperglycemia, many which are related to insulin resistance, lifestyle and excessive weight. Throughout time, definitions of the syndrome have changed, fruit of the consensus of various scientific organizations, but overall, it has helped improve the knowledge of its biology. The syndrome is accompanied by alterations of cytokines, digestive hormones, and anti-oxidative capacity. Associated comorbidities and risks mainly include insulin resistance and type 2 diabetes mellitus, cardiovascular disease, and other conditions such as sexual dysfunction, sleep disorders, gynecological pathology, urinary complaints, and osteoporosis.

9.1 Introduction

Marañon (in Spain) and Kylin (in Sweden) independently described in the first quarter of the twentieth century the metabolic disturbances associated with diabetes mellitus and hypertension [1, 2]. More than 50 years later, features composing of what now is known as the metabolic syndrome (METS) have been redefined [3, 4]. This condition has been the focus of extensive investigation since the first case of METS was described. Research has involved many areas of knowledge and the syndrome has been linked to numerous conditions or diseases; however, as a

P. Chedraui (✉)
Escuela de Postgrado en Salud, Universidad Espíritu Santo, Samborondón, Ecuador
e-mail: pchedraui@uees.edu.ec

F. R. Pérez-López
Department of Obstetrics and Gynecology, Universidad de Zaragoza Facultad de Medicina, Zaragoza, Spain
e-mail: faustino.perez@unizar.es

syndrome (not a disease), it generates overlapping and multidirectional relationships with various medical diseases or circumstances. To meet the diagnosis of METS, three of the following criteria are required: low high-density lipoprotein-cholesterol (HDL-C), high triglycerides, high glucose levels, hypertension, and/or obesity [5, 6]. The METS increases the risk of developing type 2 diabetes mellitus (T2DM), cardiovascular disease (CVD), and stroke, among other conditions. For middle-aged and older women, preventing and treating this syndrome is a health priority [7, 8]. As the prevalence of excessive weight and/or obesity increases so does that of the METS [9]. The pernicious effects of the METS over cardiovascular health are very similar to that of smoking. Fortunately, changes in health styles and diet, increase of physical activity, pharmacological treatment, and the support of qualified professionals may in fact control the syndrome.

The causes of the METS have not been clearly identified yet related to overweight and obesity, sedentary lifestyle, and insulin resistance. The latter associations are accompanied by oxidative stress, a pro-inflammatory status, and the risk of atherosclerosis that alter numerous cellular functions throughout the body. Nevertheless, other etiological possibilities have been sorted out such as alterations of the digestive microbiome, hypovitaminosis D, differences in epigenetic patterns, mitochondrial alterations, and the activation of inflammatory pathways [10–14]. The utility of performing ultrasound of the visceral and subcutaneous adipose tissue as a diagnostic for the METS is controversial. Visceral adipose tissue (VAT) is associated with the METS, hypertension, elevated alanine transaminase (>30 U/L), and uric acid [15]. The pattern of VAT differs by gender; for instance, women display higher VAT measures and lower subcutaneous adipose tissue in the waist region between the iliac crest and lower ribs.

9.2 Diagnostic Criteria for the METS

Throughout time, the definitions of the METS have changed, fruit of the consensus of various scientific organizations, but overall, it has helped improve the knowledge of its biology. While the World Health Organization focuses the definition on insulin resistance [16], the International Diabetes Federation (FID) [17, 18] and the consensus of various scientific societies consider obesity the key diagnostic element of the syndrome, even after adjusting for ethnicity and other covariates [6, 19]. As body mass index (BMI) and other indicators of obesity increase, so does the prevalence of the METS. Hence, the risk of the METS is higher among individuals with excessive weight or visceral adiposity as compared to those with normal anthropometric measures [20]. Nonetheless, even lean individuals could have the METS [21]. The conventional diagnosis of the METS should consider new diagnostic aiding options like multimodality images that allow improving diagnosis and stratification of risk and complications. Thus, computed tomography and magnetic resonance imaging can improve the assessment of excessive fat mass, subcutaneous and visceral adipose accumulation affecting cardiac, pancreatic, kidney, gastrointestinal, and liver structures [22].

The METS prevalence is generally similar even when different classifications are used within a given population. However, each diagnostic criterion determines the inclusion of different subjects; hence, prevalence may differ. For instance, diagnosis maybe centered on central obesity or abdominal obesity using various adiposity cutoff values or it may be based on insulin resistance or cardiovascular risk parameters.

9.3 The Metabolic Syndrome in Middle-Aged Women and Beyond

The exact etiology of the METS has not been established; however, there is an evident relationship with lifestyle and dietary patterns. Many features are similar to those of impaired insulin sensitivity and hyperglycemia (and other metabolic alterations). As the pancreas tries to overcome the metabolic dysfunction by producing more insulin (hyperinsulinism), the consequent impairment of insulin sensitivity produces cortisol elevations which in turn creates an inflammatory reaction with subsequent negative effects on all body tissues. Due to the ineffective metabolization of glucose in skeletal muscles, fatigue is very common. Also, gain in body weight (fat accumulation) enhances the inflammatory status, leading to a vicious circle which is difficult to close (Fig. 9.1). Additional hormonal, sociological and personal factors appearing during the menopausal transition may enhance the severity and the risk of presenting the METS. Dietary and food components, as well as reduced physical activity, may also increase the risk of the METS and hyperinsulinism. Obesity, insulin resistance, and components of the METS have been linked to precooked foods, synthetic snacks and sodas, salad dressings, and many industrial food products.

Physical activity is usually reduced in peri- and postmenopausal women that, in addition to the adjustments of ovarian steroid hormones, the final effect will be changes in body composition, fat mass infiltration in the muscle mass, and then the aggravation of insulin resistance and the pro-inflammatory status [23, 24]. The prevalence of METS differs among pre- and postmenopausal women, but in general, the increase in the prevalence is correlated to weight gain, changes in lifestyles, and endocrine adjustments, which usually change as women age. Although total testosterone levels remain constant during the menopause transition, the decline in estradiol contributes to the relative androgenic endocrine milieu while the change in fat mass and distribution increase insulin resistance and hypertension [25]. These adjustments and changes contribute to a pro-inflammatory status and the increase of free fatty acids which increase the prevalence of hypertension and insulin resistance [26] that is more common among those women from low- and middle-income countries. One study determined that 41.5% of postmenopausal women (mean age 55.9 years) living in Ecuador had the METS [27]. The menopausal transition is associated to an increase of 2–3 kg during a 3-year period with changes in body composition. In a sample of Spanish mid-aged women, with a mean age of 49.9, the prevalence of the METS was 23.1%, with 66% having natural menopause and

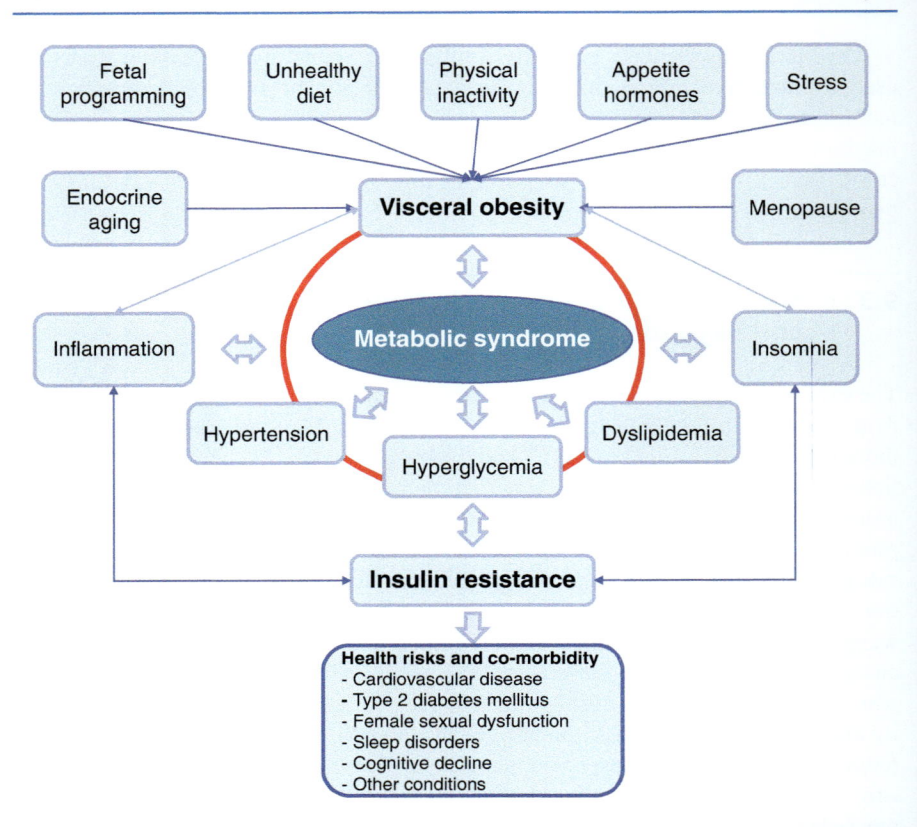

Fig. 9.1 Clinical, behavioral, and endocrine factors associated with the risk of METS. Visceral obesity and insulin resistance and their relationships with health risks and comorbid conditions. (Revised and with permission from Pérez-López FR, Chedraui P [35])

38.9% obesity. Women living in Spain with the METS were older, married at a higher rate, had altered glucose and lipid levels, and had higher Kupperman Index scores as compared to those without the syndrome [28]. On the other hand, 10 years of menopausal hormone therapy did not increase the risk of the METS in comparison to nonusers although treated women had higher baseline glucose levels as compared to untreated controls [29]. The recent meta-analysis by Chikwati [26], comparing pre- and postmenopausal women living in low- and middle-income countries, pointed out that the lack of menstrual function was associated with significantly increased risk of METS, hyperglycemia, and hypertriglyceridemia.

BMI is higher in postmenopausal women (mean age 55) with the METS as compared to those without the syndrome but had similar levels of interleukin 6 and tumor necrosis factor-alpha. Nevertheless, upon pooled analysis, those with abdominal obesity had higher interleukin 6 levels, and those with hypertension had increased levels of both cytokines. Moreover, there was a correlation between the number of positive components of the METS and levels of both cytokines [30]. In the same cohort, nitric oxide levels correlated inversely with HDL-C levels and positively with glucose and triglyceride levels and the number of positive METS items [31].

The prevalence of the METS (and its components) increases after menopause onset, consequently increasing cardiovascular risk which could be explained, at least in part, due to changes in the secretion of sex steroids and cytokines [7, 32]. Postmenopausal women with the METS display higher adipsin, leptin, resistin, and insulin levels and homeostasis model assessment-estimated insulin resistance (HOMA-IR) values, together with lower adiponectin levels. Lower adiponectin levels correlated to lower HDL-C, triglyceride, and glucose levels. In this series, women with the METS had higher interleukin 6 (inflammation marker) and lower urokinase-type plasminogen activator levels (a marker of endothelial dysfunction) [33, 34].

9.4 Female Sexual Dysfunction

Female sexual dysfunction is a multidimensional problem related to several biological, psychological, and social determinants. The METS may negatively affect sexuality of pre- and postmenopausal women, with impact on several of its domains such as satisfaction, pain, and desire as determined with the Female Sexual Function Index (FSFI) [36]. Sexual dysfunction in postmenopausal women has been related to hyperglycemia [37]. Maseroli et al. [38] have studied the pulsatility index of the clitoris using color Doppler ultrasound. Women with obesity or the METS displayed high pulsatility indices (vascular resistance), which are higher as the number of positive components of the syndrome increase. Moreover, indices correlated negatively with the arousal and satisfaction domain scores of the FSFI; hence, vascular resistance of the clitoris positively correlates with the METS, and especially with insulin resistance.

In an Italian study, premenopausal women with the METS presented a higher prevalence of sexual dysfunction compared to those metabolically healthy. The METS was associated with lower total FSFI scores and there was an inverse correlation between FSFI scores and the number of METS risk factors. In addition, high triglyceride levels and somatization were associated with female sexual dysfunction (FSD) [39]. Dutra et al. [40] reported results from a postmenopausal population living in Brazil aged 40–65, in which the prevalence of hypoactive sexual desire disorder was higher in women with METS as compared to a control group without the syndrome. Total FSFI scores, but not pain domain scores, were lower in postmenopausal women with the METS. In addition, hypoactive sexual desire disorder was significantly linked to hypertension and hypertriglyceridemia. A recent systematic review and meta-analysis provided more details regarding the relationship between METS and sexual function [41], being the prevalence of FSD among women with METS 39.3%, and in the subgroup analysis of postmenopausal women with the METS 49.8% presented FSD. In addition, the prevalence of FSD increases with the mean of age women affected with the METS.

The FSFI was also used to evaluate postmenopausal older women of the Rancho Bernardo cohort. These women had a mean age of 73 years, and 39% were sexually active and 41.5% had the METS. Total FSFI scores were similar between sexually active and inactive women although the number of METS components was significantly associated with lower sexual activity, desire, and satisfaction. Also, waist girth, diabetes, and hypertension were related to decreased sexual activity and elevated triglycerides to low desire. In addition, sexual activity was limited in women with coronary heart disease [42].

9.5 Hyperinsulinism, Type 2 Diabetes, and Cardiovascular Risk

Many symptoms and changes related to the menopause, such as weight gain, fatigue, weakness, irritability, thirst, increased appetite, sexual dysfunction, or polyuria, are in fact associated with disorders of carbohydrate metabolism and hyperinsulinism [43]. During the postmenopausal period, serum levels of sex hormone binding globulin have an inverse correlation with insulin resistance and the risk of T2DM [44]. Within this scenario, one should add increased risk of T2DM related to age. Other factors that contribute to insulin resistance include obesity, sedentary lifestyle, sleep problems, unbalanced diet, excessive consumption of tobacco and alcohol, and calcium and vitamin D deficiency. In addition, the presence of the METS increases T2DM risk and has a predictive value for insulin resistance which can be increased five-fold [45]. However, we cannot omit genetic driving factors involved in the pathophysiology of T2DM [46, 47].

After the menopause, low levels of estradiol increase the risk of CVD [32, 48, 49]. Dyslipidemia in the postmenopausal period is characterized by an increase in low-density lipoprotein cholesterol (LDL-C) and a decrease in HDL-C. After menopause, the antiatherogenic effects of HDL-C decrease, possibly in relation to the profile of subclasses of lipoproteins, that clearly has a negative impact, accelerating atherosclerosis [50]. Obesity (BMI $\geq$ 30 kg/m^2) has a negative effect on all cardiovascular risk factors. Indeed, it increases insulin resistance, blood pressure, and blood glucose, and triglycerides levels and decreases HDL-C values [51]. The digestive hormone ghrelin influences insulin sensitivity but also has negative effects on blood pressure, lipoprotein metabolism, coagulation, immunity, and inflammation [32]. The link between the METS and increased CVD risk has been reported repeatedly, regardless of the criteria used to define the syndrome. The increased risk of CVD and mortality due to coronary heart disease may range in several prospective cohorts from 1.5 to 3 times higher [52]. One meta-analysis reported that the METS increased two-fold the risk of CVD while increasing 1.5 times the mortality rate due to all causes [53]. These increased risks have been related to the criteria used to define the METS. However, a multiethnic, large-scale international research study reported that the risk of myocardial infarction is 2.5-fold higher in the presence of the METS as compared to its absence, yet similar for CVD, using WHO definition and that of the International Diabetes Federation

[54]. Guembe et al. [55] evaluated the association of cardiovascular risk and the METS and its single components by estimating their impact on the premature occurrence of cardiovascular events using rate advancement periods. For this, they analyzed data of a total of 3976 participants with an age range of 35–84 (55% were Women) of the Vascular Risk in Navarre Study. This study was a Spanish population-based cohort consuming a Mediterranean diet that used the modified criteria of the American Heart Association/National Heart, Lung, and Blood Institute and the International Diabetes Federation to define the METS. The syndrome was independently associated with CVD risk and all-cause mortality. Components of the syndrome were associated with a similar magnitude of increased CVD, suggesting that the METS was not in excess of the level explained by the presence of its single components.

Hosseinpour-Niazi et al. [56] examined the joint effect of the METS and insulin resistance with the status of ideal cardiovascular health on incident CVD. For this, a total of 6240 Iranian adults ≥30 years were included who were free of prior CVD. Ideal cardiovascular health was determined based on American Heart Association's Life Simple 7, the METS was defined according to the Joint Interim Statement Criteria, and insulin resistance was defined as a HOMA-IR value ≥1.85 in women and ≥ 2.17 in men. After a median follow-up of 14.0 years, 909 cases of CVD occurred. The METS and insulin resistance were significantly associated with incident CVD events. In the poor and intermediate status, METS increased CVD events with hazard ratios (HRs) of 1.83 and 1.57, respectively, and the corresponding values for insulin resistance in the mentioned categories were 1.91 and 1.25, respectively. In the intermediate and poor status of ideal cardiovascular health status, hypertriglyceridemia was linked to a 40% and 35% higher risk of CVD; the corresponding values for low HDL-C were 20% and 60%, respectively. The METS and the dyslipidemia component had significant improvement in the prediction of CVD among individuals with nonoptimal ideal cardiovascular health status. Chikwati et al. [26] evaluated, through a systematic review and meta-analysis, differences in cardiometabolic disease risk factors between pre- and postmenopausal midlife women living in low- and middle-income countries. They found that compared to premenopausal women, those postmenopausal were associated with the METS, high waist-to-hip ratio, hypertension, elevated triglycerides, and elevated plasma glucose levels. Thus, cardiometabolic disease risk factors are present at higher levels in postmenopausal women than premenopausal ones.

9.6   Sleep Disorders

Thus, the repeated decrease of sleep turns into a risk factor for obesity and T2DM. During sleep, growth hormone is released while cortisol secretion is inhibited. Conversely, sleep problem disturbances are associated with cortisol release that mobilizes glucose storage and stimulates insulin secretion. Therefore, the control and improvement of sleep quality are desirable interventions that aim at reducing obesity, the METS, hyperinsulinism, and T2DM. Interrupted sleep and insomnia may also alter hormonal circadian rhythms (i.e., growth hormone, cortisol) and insulin growth factors (IGFs). The relationship between the increased risk of obesity and sleep disorder is pivotal for the regulation of hormones that control appetite and energy expenditure, such as ghrelin and leptin [33]. IGF-1 has protective effects against the deleterious pro-inflammatory changes that cause the progression of insulin resistance and the METS. Inadequate nutrition may decrease insulin concentration in the portal vein system producing a reduction of hepatic IGF-1 synthesis [57]. Sleep disturbances may be accompanied by alterations in the digestive microbiota that can aggravate the METS and have negative metabolic consequences in terms of weight gain and an increase of insulin resistance [58].

In a sample of postmenopausal women, as assessed with the Athens Insomnia Scale, 33% presented insomnia, with no differences observed with the presence or not of the METS. Upon multiple regression analysis, it was found that higher total insomnia scores correlated with the use of psychotropic substances, the intensity of hot flashes and female depressive or anxiety symptoms, and partner premature ejaculation but not the METS [59]. The most frequent features of insomnia, such as difficulty in initiating and maintaining sleep, early awakenings, and excessive daytime sleepiness may be associated with the METS and CVD risk. In a cross-sectional study, Lin et al. [60] reported that the METS was related to difficulty in initiating and maintaining sleep. Also, after stratifying sleep duration as <7, 7–8, and ≥ 9 h/night, METS prevalence was associated with short sleep duration regardless of insomnia symptoms. Despite this, there was no association between METS prevalence and the combination of insomnia symptoms and sleep duration. In the three cities cross-sectional study, several symptoms of insomnia were observed in older individuals: difficulty in initiating and maintaining sleep, early awakenings, and excessive daytime sleepiness. Excessive daytime sleepiness increases METS risk and this association is independent of a previous history of CVD, insomnia symptoms, obesity, and snoring [61]. Due to the bidirectional possibilities of this relationship, prospective studies are warranted to clarify the results.

A prospective lifestyle intervention (diet and exercise), among individuals with a recent diagnosis of T2DM (with high obesity rates at baseline), found that after 6 months, insomnia was associated with obesity and insulin resistance, and after 12 months of sleep impairment, insulin metabolism was also severely impaired. It is estimated that after one year, for every 30 min lost per day of sleep, obesity and insulin resistance risk increased by 18% and 41%, respectively [62]. Poor sleep quality has been linked to insulin resistance in healthy adults although the association in adults with METS is not clear. Kline et al. [63] studied sleep quality in a population of overweight/obese postmenopausal women without T2DM using the HOMA-IR. They found that women with poor quality of sleep significantly had higher HOMA-IR values than those without the METS. In addition, women with the worst quality of sleep displayed the highest HOMA-IR values than all other women. Therefore, there is a relevant correlation between sleep quality and insulin resistance in postmenopausal women with and without METS.

The duration of sleep may also influence METS risk as determined in the Women's Health Initiative population-based arm, in which longitudinal repeated measurements of sleep duration were performed in women aged 50–79 who did not have diabetes at enrollment [64]. Women with sleep duration ≥9 h had a higher METS risk which was associated with a waist circumference >88 cm and triglycerides ≥150 mg/dL. There was no association between insomnia and the METS. This cohort study suggests that sleep duration and insomnia are associated with current and future risks of METS or some of its components. Sun et al. [65] investigated the correlation between sleep and METS in a Chinese community population of 45 years of age and older, including a total of 9096 participants. They found that long habitual daytime sleep had a positive influence on the METS. For elderly, short daytime sleep significantly increased the risk of the METS. Females with long daytime sleep was associated with an increased risk of the syndrome. The authors concluded that daytime sleep significantly increased risk of the METS for middle-aged and elderly. The hazard rate of daytime sleep on the METS varied depending on age and sex groups.

9.7 Gynecological Pathology

In postmenopausal women, the METS has been associated with endometrial, ovarian, and breast cancer, as well as non-gynecological neoplasms. Some METS components have been linked to cancer risk although this is not a universal phenomenon or relationship. The influence is not the same when it comes to insulin resistance and the risk of breast, endometrial, or ovarian cancer [66–68]. Deng et al. [69] used trajectory analyses to demonstrate the epidemiology of disease progression in different malignancies, allowing to determine the involved individual metabolic factors. This approach allows to identify the time and nature of possible interventions to reduce the cancer risk associated with the METS. The authors reported a large cohort of a Chinese population, including 20,400 women recruited in 11 hospitals that underwent periodic questionnaire assessments, clinical exams, and laboratory tests three times between 2006 and 2010. The study describes four METS trajectories: low-stable, moderate-low, moderate-high, and elevated-increasing. As compared to the low-stable METS, the elevated trajectory pattern was associated with overall cancer risk and breast, endometrial, colorectal, and kidney cancers. In addition, chronic inflammations, as evaluated with the C-reactive protein levels >3 mg/L, were significantly associated with subsequent breast, endometrial, colorectal, and liver malignancies. These results suggest that the METS, inflammation, T2DM, and excessive body weight may be involved in several relevant types of cancer [69–72].

The METS has also been associated to a higher risk of uterine fibroids which may be related to shared predisposing factors. Certain studies suggest similar risk factors for uterine fibroids and atherosclerosis such as obesity, hypertension, and metabolic derangements [73]. In a population-based long-term study (the North Finland Birth Cohort), women born in 1966 were followed up and studied again at the age of 46. It was found that the METS was associated with a hospital discharge based on the diagnosis of fibroids. Also, every one unit increase in the waist-hip ratio was related to fibroids [74]. Recent evidence demonstrates that metabolic risk factors are associated with an increased risk of uterine fibroids. A large cohort of women (≥ 18 years) with at least one consultation at the Johns Hopkins health system (n = 679,981) were more likely (i) to be obese and have the METS, essential hypertension, diabetes mellitus, and hyperlipidemia, and (ii) statin treatment was associated with lower rate of uterine fibroids [75].

In young postmenopausal women, the presence of endometrial polyps has been linked to the components of the METS. In a cross-sectional study of postmenopausal women, several variables were analyzed. Those with histologically diagnosed endometrial polyps were compared to those with controls who had no bleeding and an endometrial thickness <5 mm. A higher rate of women with polyps were obese when compared to controls (72% vs. 39%). Also, abdominal perimeter and the incidence of diabetes, hypertension, and dyslipidemias were higher in women with polyps than controls. METS prevalence was also higher in women with endometrial polyps (48.5% vs. 33.3%). The data suggest that in postmenopausal women, obesity, dyslipidemia, hyperglycemia, and the METS are predictive factors for endometrial polyps [76]. A more recent study provided information about benign endometrial pathology according to the menopausal status, METS status, and insulin resistance among women living in Turkey [77]. Benign endometrial pathology was more prevalent among women with obesity or waist circumference higher than 88 cm, and women with blood glucose higher than 110 mg/dL have a higher risk of endometrial polyps and/or hyperplasia without atypia. Therefore, it seems that some METS factors and insulin resistance may contribute to the development of benign uterine pathology.

9.8 Urinary Complaints

Both in pre- and postmenopausal women, the METS has been associated with a higher prevalence of stress urinary incontinence (SUI) when compared to those without the syndrome. Furthermore, the prevalence of SUI is higher among METS postmenopausal women as compared to METS premenopausal ones. Also, when components of the syndrome are considered separately, waist circumference and increased glucose levels were associated with SUI [78]. A systematic review found links between the overactive or neurogenic bladder and the METS and obesity as one of its components [79]. Ströher et al. [80] have reported that METS was more prevalent among women with SUI as compared to those without the syndrome (69% vs. 38%). In addition, excessive body weight-related endpoints (BMI, weight, waist) and HDL-C, triglyceride, and glucose levels were significantly higher in women with SUI as compared to controls. However, results related to excessive body weight may have some mechanic effect on SUI aside from metabolic features.

Diabetes and obesity are risk factors for urinary incontinence and chronic kidney disease. Fwu et al. [81] analyzed data from 8420 women aged 20 or more from the National Health and Nutrition Examination Survey. They found that female METS/obese participants had increased odds of any type of urinary incontinence, stress incontinence, and mixed urinary incontinence compared to non-METS/nonobese participants. The odds of co-occurring urinary incontinence and chronic kidney disease were increased relative to either condition alone in persons with diabetes. The Huang et al. [82] systematic review and meta-analysis reported that the risk of SUI is three-fold higher in women with the METS than in those without, and these results affected both pre- and postmenopausal women. Cao et al. [83] recently reported the association between the metabolic insulin resistance score for insulin resistance and urinary incontinence from the United States National Health and Nutrition Examination Survey population considering stress, urgency, and mixed urinary incontinence forms. They concluded that the metabolic score for insulin resistance was related to all forms of urinary incontinence (stress, urgency, and mixed incontinences).

Overactive bladder (OAB) is a highly prevalent condition in women, and is characterized by the sudden urge to urinate that is difficult to control and may be expressed by urgency incontinence and nocturia (waking up more than twice a night to urinate). The diagnosis of OAB is considered in the absence of urinary infection, stress incontinence, and pelvic floor disorders to withstand abdominal pressure [84]. Some women may display combined forms of OAB along with other mixed urinary symptoms. The prevalence of OAB is high in postmenopausal women with excessive body weight and may be associated with insulin resistance [85, 86]. A recent systematic review and meta-analysis reported that women with OAB have an association with METS factors: (i) low HDL-C, (ii) increased fasting glucose, triglycerides, and LDL-C levels, and (iii) increased BMI and waist circumference [87].

9.9 Osteoporosis and Fracture Risk

Bone mineral density (BMD) and fracture risk in METS individuals are determined by the balance of the dominant components of the syndrome. Hyperglycemia and diabetes tend to decrease BMD, while hypertriglyceridemia and lower HDL-C levels, related to obesity, seem to protect against fracture risk. A meta-analysis of 17 very heterogeneous studies found that the METS was associated with a nonsignificant reduction of fracture risk, and the analysis of 16 studies showed no differences in vertebral, femoral, or calcaneus BMDs compared to individuals without the syndrome [88]. The Rotterdam Study provides some information regarding the association between METS, hip bone geometry, femoral BMD, and the risk of osteoporosis and incidental fractures. After adjusting for BMI, age, and consumed drugs, METS women had a lower osteoporosis risk, and fracture risk was not increased by the METS [89]. In a meta-analysis of eight prospective epidemiological studies, the METS was not explicitly associated with prevalent or incidental fractures [90]. Moreover, no significant correlations between the METS and BMD or bone metabolic variables have been demonstrated [91]. More recently, the Babagoli et al. [92] meta-analysis of 13 cross-sectional and 7 cohort studies showed no association between the METS and fractures across the entire population. However, separate analysis of the cohort studies showed a decreased risk over the entire population and in males, but not in females, suggesting that the METS is a protective factor for bone fractures in males but has no net effect on fractures among females.

The evolution/prevalence of the METS has been studied with a focus on the menopausal transition and beyond, showing an increased prevalence of this syndrome and a reduction of BMD [93]. Among women aged 40 to 60 living in Mexico, the prevalence of the METS was 57.2%. Women with the METS, as compared to those without, had a higher prevalence of osteopenia in the lumbar spine (35.8% vs. 27.3%), with similar rates of dual femur osteopenia (14.4% vs. 18.6%, respectively). Osteoporosis in the lumbar spine and the dual femur was present in 6.8% and 1.8%, respectively, among those without the METS, whereas in women with the METS, the prevalence was 4.7% and 0.5% in the mentioned sites, respectively. There were associations between low BMD at the lumbar spine and dual femur and components of the METS in these Mexican women as follows: Waist circumference ≥ 88 cm showed an increased risk for low BMD at the femoral site in both reproductive/menopausal transition and postmenopausal women. In addition, HDL-C < 50 mg/dL was associated with low BMD in both the femur and lumbar spine. Hypertension in postmenopausal women increased the risk for low BMD in the femur. Components of the METS were associated with low BMD, thus indicating that the syndrome is associated with bone deterioration. There is evidence that the METS is associated with hypertriglyceridemia and LDL-C, and vitamin D supplementation may reduce these circumstances. In addition, there is an inverse relationship between fat mass and circulating vitamin D. The normalization of vitamin D levels may improve glucose metabolism, although there are conflictive results, and vitamin D overtreatment does not improve clinical outcomes [94, 95].

References

1. Marañon G. Über hypertonie und zuckerkrankheit. Zentralblatt für Innere Medizin. 1922;43:169–76.
2. Kylin E. Studien ueber das hypertonie-hyperglykaemie-hyperurikaemiesyndrom. Zentralblatt für Innere Medizin. 1923;44:105–27.
3. Avogadro A, Crepaldi G, Enzi G, Tiengo A, Avogardo P. Associazione di iperlipidemia, diabete mellito e obesità di medio grado. Acta Diabetol Lat. 1967;4:36–41.
4. Reaven GM. Banting lecture 1988. Role of insulin resistance in human disease. Diabetes. 1988;37(12):1595–607.
5. Cornier MA, Dabelea D, Hernandez TL, et al. The metabolic syndrome. Endocr Rev. 2008;29(7):777–822.
6. Alberti KG, Eckel RH, Grundy SM, et al. International Diabetes Federation Task Force on Epidemiology and Prevention; National Heart, Lung, and Blood Institute; American Heart Association; World Heart Federation; International Atherosclerosis Society; International Association for the Study of Obesity. Harmonizing the metabolic syndrome: a Joint Interim Statement of the International Diabetes Federation Task Force on Epidemiology and Prevention; National Heart, Lung, and Blood Institute; American Heart Association; World Heart Federation; International Atherosclerosis Society; and International Association for the Study of Obesity. Circulation. 2009;120(16):1640–5.

7. Pérez-López FR, Chedraui P, Gilbert JJ, Pérez-Roncero G. Cardiovascular risk in menopausal women and prevalent related co-morbid conditions: facing the post-Women's Health Initiative era. Fertil Steril. 2009;92(4):1171–86.
8. van Dijk GM, Kavousi M, Troup J, Franco OH. Health issues for menopausal women: the top 11 conditions have common solutions. Maturitas. 2015;80(1):24–30.
9. NCD Risk Factor Collaboration (NCD-RisC). Trends in adult body-mass index in 200 countries from 1975 to 2014: a pooled analysis of 1698 population-based measurement studies with 19·2 million participants. Lancet. 2016;387(10026):1377–96.
10. Chedraui P, Pérez-López FR. Nutrition and health during mid-life: searching for solutions and meeting challenges for the aging population. Climacteric. 2013;16(Suppl 1):85–95.
11. Ju SY, Jeong HS, Kim DH. Blood vitamin D status and metabolic syndrome in the general adult population: a dose-response meta-analysis. J Clin Endocrinol Metab. 2014;99(3):1053–63.
12. Remely M, Haslberger AG. The microbial epigenome in metabolic syndrome. Mol Asp Med. 2017;54:71–7.
13. Hand TW, Vujkovic-Cvijin I, Ridaura VK, Belkaid Y. Linking the microbiota, chronic disease, and the immune system. Trends Endocrinol Metab. 2016;27(12):831–43.
14. Dabke K, Hendrick G, Devkota S. The gut microbiome and metabolic syndrome. J Clin Invest. 2019;129(10):4050–7.
15. da Silva NF, Pinho CPS, da Silva DA. Evaluation of ultrasonographic approaches aimed at determining distinct abdominal adipose tissue depots. Arch Endocrinol Metab. 2023;67(2):162–71.
16. Alberti KG, Zimmet PZ. Definition, diagnosis and classification of diabetes mellitus and its complications. Part 1: diagnosis and classification of diabetes mellitus provisional report of a WHO consultation. Diabet Med. 1998;15(7):539–53.
17. International Diabetes Federation. The IDF consensus worldwide definition of the metabolic syndrome. Brussels: IDF Communications; 2006. Available at www.idf.org.
18. Liu J, Zhang Y, Lavie CJ, Moran AE. Trends in metabolic phenotypes according to body mass index among US adults, 1999–2018. Mayo Clin Proc. 2022;97(9):1664–79.
19. NCEP. Expert Panel on Detection, Evaluation, and Treatment of High Blood Cholesterol in Adults. Executive Summary of the Third Report of the National Cholesterol Education Program (NCEP) Expert Panel on Detection, Evaluation, and Treatment of High Blood Cholesterol in Adults (Adult Treatment Panel III). JAMA. 2001;285(19):2486–97.
20. Ervin RB. Prevalence of metabolic syndrome among adults 20 years of age and over, by sex, age, race and ethnicity, and body mass index: United States, 2003–2006. Natl Health Stat Report. 2009;13:1–7.
21. Diamanti-Kandarakis E, Papavassiliou AG, Kandarakis SA, Chrousos GP. Pathophysiology and types of dyslipidemia in PCOS. Trends Endocrinol Metab. 2007;18(7):280–5.
22. Kalisz K, Navin PJ, Itani M, Agarwal AK, Venkatesh SK, Rajiah PS. Multimodality imaging in metabolic syndrome: state-of-the-art review. Radiographics. 2024;44(3):e230083.
23. Sowers M, Zheng H, Tomey K, Karvonen-Gutierrez C, Jannausch M, Li X, Yosef M, Symons J. Changes in body composition in women over six years at midlife: ovarian and chronological aging. J Clin Endocrinol Metab. 2007;92(3):895–901.
24. Trikudanathan S, Pedley A, Massaro JM, Hoffmann U, Seely EW, Murabito JM, Fox CS. Association of female reproductive factors with body composition: the Framingham Heart Study. J Clin Endocrinol Metab. 2013;98(1):236–44.
25. Abildgaard J, Ploug T, Al-Saoudi E, Wagner T, Thomsen C, Ewertsen C, Bzorek M, Pedersen BK, Pedersen AT, Lindegaard B. Changes in abdominal subcutaneous adipose tissue phenotype following menopause is associated with increased visceral fat mass. Sci Rep. 2021;11(1):14750.
26. Chikwati RP, Chikowore T, Mahyoodeen NG, Jaff NG, George JA, Crowther NJ. The association of menopause with cardiometabolic disease risk factors in low- and middle-income countries: a systematic review and meta-analyses. Menopause. 2024;31(1):77–85.
27. Hidalgo LA, Chedraui PA, Morocho N, Alvarado M, Chavez D, Huc A. The metabolic syndrome among postmenopausal women in Ecuador. Gynecol Endocrinol. 2006;22(8):447–54.

28. Fernández-Alonso AM, Cuadros JL, Chedraui P, Mendoza M, Cuadros AM, Pérez-López FR. Obesity is related to increased menopausal symptoms among Spanish women. Menopause Int. 2010;16(3):105–10.
29. Cuadros JL, Fernández-Alonso AM, Chedraui P, Cuadros AM, Sabatel RM, Pérez-López FR. Metabolic and hormonal parameters in post-menopausal women 10 years after transdermal oestradiol treatment, alone or combined to micronized oral progesterone. Gynecol Endocrinol. 2011;27(3):156–62.
30. Chedraui P, Jaramillo W, Pérez-López FR, Escobar GS, Morocho N, Hidalgo L. Proinflammatory cytokine levels in postmenopausal women with the metabolic syndrome. Gynecol Endocrinol. 2011;27(9):685–91.
31. Chedraui P, Escobar GS, Ramírez C, Pérez-López FR, Hidalgo L, Mannella P, Genazzani A, Simoncini T. Nitric oxide and pro-inflammatory cytokine serum levels in postmenopausal women with the metabolic syndrome. Gynecol Endocrinol. 2012;28(10):787–91.
32. Pérez-López FR, Larrad-Mur L, Kallen A, Chedraui P, Taylor HS. Gender differences in cardiovascular disease: hormonal and biochemical influences. Reprod Sci. 2010;17(6):511–31.
33. Chedraui P, Pérez-López FR, Escobar GS, Palla G, Montt-Guevara M, Cecchi E, Genazzani AR, Simoncini T. Research Group for the Omega Women's Health Project. Circulating leptin, resistin, adiponectin, visfatin, adipsin and ghrelin levels and insulin resistance in postmenopausal women with and without the metabolic syndrome. Maturitas. 2014;79(1):86–90.
34. Chedraui P, Escobar GS, Pérez-López FR, Palla G, Montt-Guevara M, Cecchi E, Genazzani AR, Simoncini T. Research Group for the Omega Women's Health Project. Angiogenesis, inflammation and endothelial function in postmenopausal women screened for the metabolic syndrome. Maturitas. 2014;77(4):370–4.
35. Pérez-López FR, Chedraui P. The metabolic syndrome in mid-aged women. In: Cano A, editor. Menopause: A comprehensive Approach. 1st ed. Cham: Springer; 2017. p. 141–58.
36. Otunctemur A, Dursun M, Ozbek E, Sahin S, Besiroglu H, Koklu I, Polat EC, Erkoc M, Danis E, Bozkurt M. Effect of metabolic syndrome on sexual function in pre- and postmenopausal women. J Sex Marital Ther. 2015;41(4):440–9.
37. Chedraui P, Pérez-López FR, Blümel JE, Hidalgo L, Barriga J. Hyperglycemia in postmenopausal women screened for the metabolic syndrome is associated to increased sexual complaints. Gynecol Endocrinol. 2010;26(2):86–92.
38. Maseroli E, Fanni E, Cipriani S, Scavello I, Pampaloni F, Battaglia C, Fambrini M, Mannucci E, Jannini EA, Maggi M, Vignozzi L. Cardiometabolic risk and female sexuality: focus on clitoral vascular resistance. J Sex Med. 2016;13(11):1651–61.
39. Alvisi S, Baldassarre M, Lambertini M, et al. Sexuality and psychopathological aspects in premenopausal women with metabolic syndrome. J Sex Med. 2014;11(8):2020–8.
40. Dutra da Silva GM, Rolim Rosa Lima SM, Reis BF, Macruz CF, Postigo S. Prevalence of hypoactive sexual desire disorder among sexually active postmenopausal women with metabolic syndrome at a public Hospital Clinic in Brazil: a cross-sectional study. Sex Med. 2020;8(3):545–53.
41. Salari N, Moradi M, Hosseinian-Far A, Khodayari Y, Mohammadi M. Global prevalence of sexual dysfunction among women with metabolic syndrome: a systematic review and meta-analysis. J Diabetes Metab Disord. 2023;22(2):1011–9.
42. Trompeter SE, Bettencourt R, Barrett-Connor E. Metabolic syndrome and sexual function in postmenopausal women. Am J Med. 2016;129(12):1270–1277.e1.
43. Clark NG, Fox KM, Grandy S, SHIELD Study Group. Symptoms of diabetes and their association with the risk and presence of diabetes: findings from the Study to Help Improve Early evaluation and management of risk factors Leading to Diabetes (SHIELD). Diabetes Care. 2007;30(11):2868–73.
44. Kalyani RR, Franco M, Dobs AS, Ouyang P, Vaidya D, Bertoni A, Gapstur SM, Golden SH. The association of endogenous sex hormones, adiposity, and insulin resistance with incident diabetes in postmenopausal women. J Clin Endocrinol Metab. 2009;94(11):4127–35.

45. Ford ES, Li C, Sattar N. Metabolic syndrome and incident diabetes: current state of the evidence. Diabetes Care. 2008;31(9):1898–904.
46. DeForest N, Majithia AR. Genetics of type 2 diabetes: implications from large-scale studies. Curr Diab Rep. 2022;22(5):227–35.
47. Suzuki K, Hatzikotoulas K, Southam L, Taylor HJ, Yin X, Lorenz KM, et al. Genetic drivers of heterogeneity in type 2 diabetes pathophysiology. Nature. 2024;627(8003):347–57.
48. Matthews KA, Crawford SL, Chae CU, Everson-Rose SA, Sowers MF, Sternfeld B, Sutton-Tyrrell K. Are changes in cardiovascular disease risk factors in midlife women due to chronological aging or to the menopausal transition? J Am Coll Cardiol. 2009;54(25):2366–73.
49. Ryczkowska K, Adach W, Janikowski K, Banach M, Bielecka-Dabrowa A. Menopause and women's cardiovascular health: is it really an obvious relationship? Arch Med Sci. 2022;19(2):458–66.
50. Woodard GA, Brooks MM, Barinas-Mitchell E, Mackey RH, Matthews KA, Sutton-Tyrrell K. Lipids, menopause, and early atherosclerosis in Study of Women's Health Across the Nation Heart women. Menopause. 2011;18:376–84.
51. Bagnoli VR, Fonseca AM, Arie WM, Das Neves EM, Azevedo RS, Sorpreso IC, Soares Júnior JM, Baracat EC. Metabolic disorder and obesity in 5027 Brazilian postmenopausal women. Gynecol Endocrinol. 2014;30(10):717–20.
52. Bruno G, Merletti F, Biggeri A, Bargero G, Ferrero S, Runzo C, Prina Cerai S, Pagano G, Cavallo-Perin P, Casale Monferrato Study. Metabolic syndrome as a predictor of all-cause and cardiovascular mortality in type 2 diabetes: the Casale Monferrato Study. Diabetes Care. 2004;27(11):689–94.
53. Sattar N, McConnachie A, Shaper AG, Blauw GJ, Buckley BM, de Craen AJ, Ford I, Forouhi NG, Freeman DJ, Jukema JW, Lennon L, Macfarlane PW, Murphy MB, Packard CJ, Stott DJ, Westendorp RG, Whincup PH, Shepherd J, Wannamethee SG. Can metabolic syndrome usefully predict cardiovascular disease and diabetes? Outcome data from two prospective studies. Lancet. 2008;371(9628):1927–35.
54. Mente A, Yusuf S, Islam S, McQueen MJ, Tanomsup S, Onen CL, Rangarajan S, Gerstein HC, Anand SS, INTERHEART Investigators. Metabolic syndrome and risk of acute myocardial infarction a case-control study of 26,903 subjects from 52 countries. J Am Coll Cardiol. 2010;55(21):2390–8.
55. Guembe MJ, Fernandez-Lazaro CI, Sayon-Orea C, Toledo E, Moreno-Iribas C, RIVANA Study Investigators. Risk for cardiovascular disease associated with metabolic syndrome and its components: a 13-year prospective study in the RIVANA cohort. Cardiovasc Diabetol. 2020;19(1):195.
56. Hosseinpour-Niazi S, Afaghi S, Hadaegh P, et al. The association between metabolic syndrome and insulin resistance with risk of cardiovascular events in different states of cardiovascular health status. J Diabetes Investig. 2024;15(2):208–18.
57. Aguirre GA, De Ita JR, de la Garza RG, Castilla-Cortazar I. Insulin-like growth factor-1 deficiency and metabolic syndrome. J Transl Med. 2016;14:3.
58. Benedict C, Vogel H, Jonas W, Woting A, Blaut M, Schürmann A, Cedernaes J. Gut microbiota and glucometabolic alterations in response to recurrent partial sleep deprivation in normal-weight young individuals. Mol Metab. 2016;5(12):1175–86.
59. Chedraui P, San Miguel G, Villacreses D, Dominguez A, Jaramillo W, Escobar GS, Pérez-López FR, Genazzani AR, Simoncini T. Research Group for the Omega Women's Health Project. Assessment of insomnia and related risk factors in postmenopausal women screened for the metabolic syndrome. Maturitas. 2013;74(2):154–9.
60. Lin SC, Sun CA, You SL, Hwang LC, Liang CY, Yang T, Bai CH, Chen CH, Wei CY, Chou YC. The link of self-reported insomnia symptoms and sleep duration with metabolic syndrome: a Chinese population-based study. Sleep. 2016;39(6):1261–6.
61. Akbaraly TN, Jaussent I, Besset A, Bertrand M, Barberger-Gateau P, Ritchie K, Ferrie JE, Kivimaki M, Dauvilliers Y. Sleep complaints and metabolic syndrome in an elderly population: the Three-City Study. Am J Geriatr Psychiatry. 2015;23(8):818–28.

62. Arora T, Chen MZ, Cooper AR, Andrews RC, Taheri S. The Impact of sleep debt on excess adiposity and insulin sensitivity in patients with early type 2 diabetes mellitus. J Clin Sleep Med. 2016;12(5):673–80.
63. Kline CE, Hall MH, Buysse DJ, Earnest CP, Church TS. Poor sleep quality is associated with insulin resistance in postmenopausal women with and without metabolic syndrome. Metab Syndr Relat Disord. 2018;16(4):183–9.
64. Peila R, Xue X, Feliciano EMC, Allison M, Sturgeon S, Zaslavsky O, Stone KL, Ochs-Balcom HM, Mossavar-Rahmani Y, Crane TE, Aggarwal M, Wassertheil-Smoller S, Rohan TE. Association of sleep duration and insomnia with metabolic syndrome and its components in the Women's Health Initiative. BMC Endocr Disord. 2022;22(1):228.
65. Sun H, Zhao J, Hu X, et al. Assessing the association of self-reported sleep duration and metabolic syndrome among middle-aged and older adults in China from the China Health and Retirement Longitudinal Survey. Metab Syndr Relat Disord. 2023;21(9):509–16.
66. Esposito K, Chiodini P, Capuano A, Bellastella G, Maiorino MI, Giugliano D. Metabolic syndrome and endometrial cancer: a meta-analysis. Endocrine. 2014;45(1):28–36.
67. Hernandez AV, Pasupuleti V, Benites-Zapata VA, Thota P, Deshpande A, Perez-Lopez FR. Insulin resistance and endometrial cancer risk: a systematic review and meta-analysis. Eur J Cancer. 2015;51(18):2747–58.
68. Gianuzzi X, Palma-Ardiles G, Hernandez-Fernandez W, Pasupuleti V, Hernandez AV, Perez-Lopez FR. Insulin growth factor (IGF) 1, IGF-binding proteins and ovarian cancer risk: a systematic review and meta-analysis. Maturitas. 2016;94:22–9.
69. Deng L, Liu T, Liu CA, Zhang Q, Song MM, Lin SQ, Wang YM, Zhang QS, Shi HP. The association of metabolic syndrome scores trajectory patterns with risk of all cancer types. Cancer. 2024;130:2150. https://doi.org/10.1002/cncr.35235.
70. Esser N, Legrand-Poels S, Piette J, Scheen AJ, Paquot N. Inflammation as a link between obesity, metabolic syndrome and type 2 diabetes. Diabetes Res Clin Pract. 2014;105(2):141–50.
71. Ying M, Hu X, Li Q, Dong H, Zhou Y, Chen Z. Long-term trajectories of BMI and cumulative incident metabolic syndrome: a cohort study. Front Endocrinol. 2022;13:915394.
72. Amouzegar A, Honarvar M, Masoumi S, Khalili D, Azizi F, Mehran L. Trajectory patterns of metabolic syndrome severity score and risk of type 2 diabetes. J Transl Med. 2023;21(1):750.
73. Takeda T, Sakata M, Isobe A, Miyake A, Nishimoto F, Ota Y, Kamiura S, Kimura T. Relationship between metabolic syndrome and uterine leiomyomas: a case-control study. Gynecol Obstet Investig. 2008;66(1):14–7.
74. Uimari O, Auvinen J, Jokelainen J, Puukka K, Ruokonen A, Järvelin MR, Piltonen T, Keinänen-Kiukaanniemi S, Zondervan K, Järvelä I, Ryynänen M, Martikainen H. Uterine fibroids and cardiovascular risk. Hum Reprod. 2016;31(12):2689–703.
75. Alashqar A, El Ouweini H, Gornet M, Yenokyan G, Borahay MA. Cardiometabolic profile of women with uterine leiomyoma: a cross-sectional study. Minerva Obstet Gynecol. 2023;75(1):27–38.
76. Bueloni-Dias FN, Spadoto-Dias D, Delmanto LR, Nahas-Neto J, Nahas EA. Metabolic syndrome as a predictor of endometrial polyps in postmenopausal women. Menopause. 2016;23(7):759–64.
77. Kaya S, Kaya B, Keskin HL, Kayhan Tetik B, Yavuz FA. Is there any relationship between benign endometrial pathologies and metabolic status? J Obstet Gynaecol. 2019;39(2):176–83.
78. Otunctemur A, Dursun M, Ozbek E, Sahin S, Besiroglu H, Koklu I, Erkoc M, Danis E, Bozkurt M. Impact of metabolic syndrome on stress urinary incontinence in pre-and postmenopausal women. Int Urol Nephrol. 2014;46(8):1501–5.
79. Bunn F, Kirby M, Pinkney E, Cardozo L, Chapple C, Chester K, Cruz F, Haab F, Kelleher C, Milsom I, Sievart KD, Tubaro A, Wagg A. Is there a link between overactive bladder and the metabolic syndrome in women? A systematic review of observational studies. Int J Clin Pract. 2015;69(2):199–217.
80. Ströher RLM, Sartori MGF, Takano CC, de Araújo MP, Girão MJBC. Metabolic syndrome in women with and without stress urinary incontinence. Int Urogynecol J. 2020;31(1):173–9.

81. Fwu CW, Schulman IH, Lawrence JM, Kimmel PL, Eggers P, Norton J, Chan K, Mendley SR, Barthold JS. Association of obesity, metabolic syndrome, and diabetes with urinary incontinence and chronic kidney disease: analysis of the National Health and Nutrition Examination Survey, 2003–2020. J Urol. 2024;211(1):124–33.
82. Huang H, Han X, Liu Q, Xue J, Yu Z, Miao S. Associations between metabolic syndrome and female stress urinary incontinence: a meta-analysis. Int Urogynecol J. 2022;33(8):2073–9.
83. Cao S, Meng L, Lin L, Hu X, Li X. The association between the metabolic score for insulin resistance (METS-IR) index and urinary incontinence in the United States: results from the National Health and Nutrition Examination Survey (NHANES) 2001–2018. Diabetol Metab Syndr. 2023;15(1):248.
84. Marinkovic SP, Rovner ES, Moldwin RM, Stanton SL, Gillen LM, Marinkovic CM. The management of overactive bladder syndrome. BMJ. 2012;344:e2365.
85. Pauwaert K, Goessaert AS, Robinson D, Cardozo L, Bower W, Calders P, Mariman A, Abrams P, Tubaro A, Dmochowski R, Weiss JP, Hervé F, Depypere H, Everaert K. Nocturia in Menopausal Women: The Link Between Two Common Problems of the Middle Age. Int Urogynecol J. 2024;35(5):935–46.
86. Ng KC, Chueh JS, Chang SJ. Risk factors, urodynamic characteristics, and distress associated with nocturnal enuresis in overactive bladder-wet women. Sci Rep. 2025;15(1):235.
87. Fernández-Alonso AM, López-Baena MT, García-Alfaro P, Pérez-López FR. Systematic review and meta-analysis on the association of metabolic syndrome in women with overactive bladder. Gynecol Endocrinol. 2025;41(1):2445682.
88. Esposito K, Chiodini P, Capuano A, Colao A, Giugliano D. Fracture risk and bone mineral density in metabolic syndrome: a meta-analysis. J Clin Endocrinol Metab. 2013;98(8):3306–14.
89. Muka T, Trajanoska K, Kiefte-de Jong JC, Oei L, Uitterlinden AG, Hofman A, Dehghan A, Zillikens MC, Franco OH, Rivadeneira F. The association between metabolic syndrome, bone mineral density, hip bone geometry and fracture risk: The Rotterdam Study. PLoS One. 2015;10(6):e0129116.
90. Sun K, Liu J, Lu N, Sun H, Ning G. Association between metabolic syndrome and bone fractures: a meta-analysis of observational studies. BMC Endocr Disord. 2014;14:13.
91. Qu Y, Kang MY, Dong RP, Zhao JW. Correlations between abnormal glucose metabolism and bone mineral density or bone metabolism. Med Sci Monit. 2016;22:824–32.
92. Babagoli M, Soleimani M, Baghdadi S, Vatan MS, Shafiei SH. Does metabolic syndrome increase the risk of fracture? A systematic review and meta-analysis. Arch Osteoporos. 2022;17(1):118.
93. Salas R, Tijerina A, Cardona M, Bouzas C, Ramirez E, Martínez G, Garza A, Pastor R, Tur JA. Association between bone mineral density and metabolic syndrome among reproductive, menopausal transition, and postmenopausal women. J Clin Med. 2021;10(21):4819.
94. Pérez-López FR, Chedraui P, Pilz S. Vitamin D supplementation after the menopause. Ther Adv Endocrinol Metab. 2020;11:2042018820931291.
95. López-Baena MT, Pérez-Roncero GR, Pérez-López FR, Mezones-Holguín E, Chedraui P. Vitamin D, menopause, and aging: quo vadis? Climacteric. 2020;23(2):123–9.

The Impact of Estrogen Decline on Other Noncommunicable Diseases

10

Esperanza Navarro-Pardo, Tomi S. Mikkola, Tommaso Simoncini, Marta Millán, María Dolores Juliá, and Antonio Cano

Abstract

The widespread distribution of estrogen receptors (ER) conditions that the decline in the circulating levels of estrogens with menopause has a series of effects. Some of them may influence the risk to some noncommunicable diseases (NCD) or, if not attaining sufficient impact to modify the risk for disease, unless some level of organ dysfunctions. This chapter summarizes some remarkable changes on the

---

E. Navarro-Pardo
Department of Developmental and Educational Psychology, University of Valencia, Valencia, Spain
e-mail: esperanza.navarro@uv.es

T. S. Mikkola
Department of Obstetrics and Gynecology, Helsinki University Central Hospital, Helsinki, Finland
e-mail: tomi.mikkola@hus.fi

T. Simoncini
Division of Obstetrics and Gynecology, Department of Clinical and Experimental Medicine, University of Pisa, Pisa, Italy
e-mail: tommaso.simoncini@med.unipi.it

M. Millán
Hospital Universitario Marqués Valdecilla, University of Cantabria, Santander, Spain
e-mail: martamartinm@scsalud.es

M. D. Juliá
Department of Pediatrics, Obstetrics and Gynecology, University of Valencia, Valencia, Spain

Section of Gynecology and Reproduction, University and Polytechnic Hospital La Fe, Valencia, Spain
e-mail: M.Dolores.Julia@uv.es

A. Cano (✉)
Full Professor of Obstetrics and Gynecology, Salus Vitae Women's Health Clinical Center, Valencia, Spain
e-mail: Antonio.cano@uv.es

© The Author(s), under exclusive license to Springer Nature Switzerland AG 2025
A. Cano (ed.), *Menopause*, https://doi.org/10.1007/978-3-031-83979-5_10

central nervous system (CNS), the vasculature, and the bone joints, specifically osteoarthritis. The actions on the CNS are analyzed following a stepwise procedure so that the effect of estrogen deprivation on experimental models, from culture cells to live animals, is followed by the review of clinical studies. Both cognitive functions and mood are analyzed. The same strategy, experimental models followed by clinical data, is reproduced to revise vascular actions. The effect of estrogen deprivation on vascular physiology is reviewed along with the increased risk of diseases, such as diabetes or hyperlipidemia, which have been related to increased cardiovascular risk. The risk of atherosclerosis is therefore increased, something that is analyzed together with a concomitant clinical impact. This is more evident in the case of surgical or premature menopause. Osteoarthritis is presented, again, in a perspective in which experimental data are contrasted with clinical studies. The discrepancies between studies remain unresolved so that the loss of estrogen support, despite being frequently associated with joint pain, does not seem to be clearly related to an obvious deleterious action on cartilage function.

10.1 Introduction

The ovary is the main source of estrogens in women from menarche to menopause. Besides the key role in reproduction, estrogens have effects in several organs in the body, as confirmed by the identification of estrogen receptors (ER) in multiple tissues. This is not only a biochemical incident because there are obvious clinical manifestations, like, for example, hot flashes, which eloquently show the effect of estrogens on the central nervous system. Therefore, the key question is whether the fall in the estrogen levels in blood will have an impact on the health of women. There is the obvious case of postmenopausal osteoporosis, which is described in a separated chapter, but also important questions in relation with other chronic noncommunicable diseases. Among them, those related with the central nervous system, particularly in the area of cognition and mood, cardiovascular disease, or a highly prevalent disease as it is osteoarthritis.

10.2 Cognitive Decline and Mood

10.2.1 Menopause and Cognitive Functions

Basic neuroscience studies have provided evidence that estrogens influence aspects of brain chemistry and morphology known to be important for cognitive functions [1]. That consistency, maintained during decades, has translated with difficulty to specific neural functions because there is no unanimity on the effects of hypogonadism on measures of attention, concentration, or memory in clinical studies [2]. Thus, one issue of interest is the influence of estrogen depletion on cognition across and after menopause and, if confirmed, the mechanism through which it occurs. Moreover, brain function also includes mood states, mainly depression and anxiety. This is why, as proposed by Greendale et al. [3], the potential association of menopausal hormonal changes with brain function may be approached in two ways, directly, i.e., effects on neural cells and systems, and indirectly, i.e., effects of hormonal changes on the brain functions, mainly cognition and mood.

The interest on the action of hormones may also extend to other systems with an impact on brain functions, specifically the vascular tree, which determines the adequacy of cerebral blood perfusion [4, 5]. This area is receiving particular attention because of the changes in perfusion observed during hot flashes, a very frequent symptom of menopausal women. Indeed, recent data suggest that vasomotor symptoms might represent a female-specific risk factor for memory declines during the menopausal transition [6].

Overall, memory complaints are the most frequent claim in people older than 50 years, but the cognitive issue in menopausal women is much broader and affects cognitive functioning in general. As detailed below, not only memory (especially some subtypes as verbal recall and working memory) but also processing speed, cognitive performance, difficulty in concentrating, and, therefore, learning processes are specific functions of interest. With regard to emotional aspects, mood stability and mood disorders are the main issues (Fig. 10.1).

10.2.2 Psychobiological Feasibility

The conception that women have an increased risk of developing cognitive decline (CD) and Alzheimer's dementia (AD) compared to men is widespread in literature [7]. Moreover, it has been postulated that this higher risk may be due to a reduction

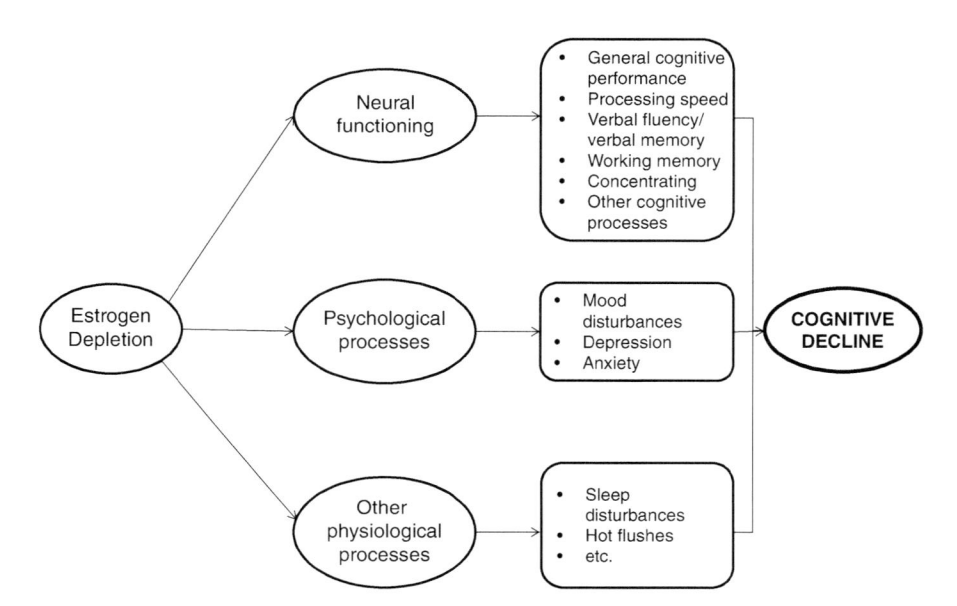

Fig. 10.1 Schematic view of ways and effects of estrogen depletion on cognition

in the neuroprotective effects of estrogen on the brain in the early postmenopausal period. This view is supported by, for example, some findings suggesting that ovariectomy in premenopausal women significantly increases the risk for the development of memory problems and AD in later life [8]. In the same way, other studies have consistently shown that induced hypogonadism is accompanied by a decline in cognitive test performance [2].

Among the biological mediators underlying the changes, a possible direct role of the raised levels of gonadotropin-releasing hormone (GnRH) on neurodegeneration has been postulated [9]. But interest has focused mainly on estrogens. There is plenty of data about a direct action of estrogens on some brain areas related with memory, mainly prefrontal cortex and hippocampus, which are rich in ER. This action may be conveyed through a modulatory effect on the levels of neurotransmitters, which may enhance neuronal growth and formation of synapses [10, 11]. The rationale, therefore, has been that if estrogens benefit the hippocampal and prefrontal cortical functions, the drop of estrogen around menopause could negatively impact on cognitive performance. In consistence with that hypothesis, data in rats show effects of estrogens on stress-induced neuroplasticity and activity changes, which has been taken to sustain the assertion that the female brain has a different innate strategy to handle stress. The pathways followed by estrogens have been described in rat models [12].

The biochemical mechanism underlying estrogen neuroprotective effect has to be elucidated considering that there are two subtypes of ER, α and β, as well as a growing number of ER splice variants. For example, mechanistic studies have described the pathways implicating ERα in the pathogenesis of AD [13]. There is also considerable information on the role of ERβ. For example, selective modulators of ERβ have been demonstrated capable of altering Alzheimer's pathology in transgenic models, and ERβ polymorphisms have been associated with risk for AD [14].

It is unclear whether the actions of ERα and ERβ are overlapping or independent of each other. There is some information obtained from immunocytochemical studies on brain from AD patients, which have suggested specific roles for each receptor subtype, but the issue is still pending clarification [15].

There is also evidence showing that insulin and insulin-like growth factor 1 (IGF1) play major roles as regulators of growth and regeneration in the central nervous system (CNS) in rodents. It has been hypothesized, for example, that exposure to estradiol may favor the action of IGF1 that, in turn, increases performance of ERα for extended periods, thus favoring protection of hippocampal functions (Fig. 10.2) [16]. Important roles for insulin, which may require the involvement of ER, have been described in spatial memory processing. Specifically, estrogen regulates different insulin-related processes with cognitive correlates (glucose transport, aerobic glycolysis, and mitochondrial function). Accordingly, decline in circulating estrogen during menopause is coincident with decrease in brain bioenergetics and shift toward a metabolically compromised phenotype [17].

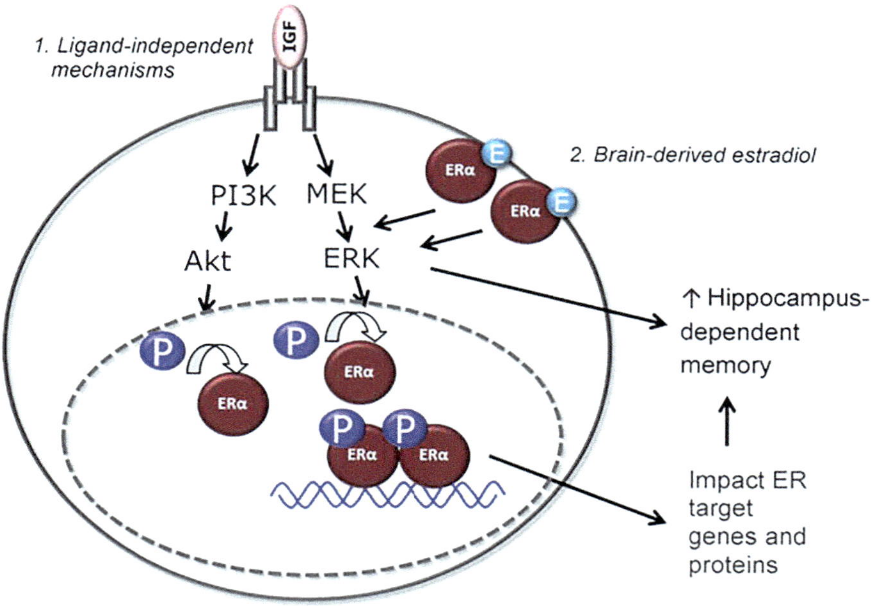

Fig. 10.2 Interactions of activated ERα with intracellular signaling cascades of IGF1 at the hippocampus. (With permission of Elsevier, Daniel, Witty, & Rodgers. Horm Behav. 2015; 74: 77–85. Permission conveyed through Copyright Clearance Center, Inc.)

10.2.3 Studies in Animals

Some studies go back to the hypothesis of effects mediated by GnRH. The point is of interest because it constitutes an alternative to the role of sex steroids. Some support is obtained from studies showing that luteinizing hormone (LH) is elevated in AD [18]. To disclose whether the elevated level on gonadotropins has an effect on the risk of AD, GnRH analogues (GnRHa) were used in an aged transgenic mouse model. GnRHa produced an acute decline in ovarian hormone output leading to a status similar to menopause. The decrease in LH by GnRHa resulted in an attenuation of amyloid-beta deposition as compared to placebo-treated animals. Also, this reduction correlated with improved cognition [19].

Despite the data in support of gonadotropins, most evidence accumulates with regard to an estrogen-mediated protective effect. So estradiol increased the synthesis of choline acetyltransferase (ChAT) in the medial septal nucleus, nucleus basalis of Meynert, and frontal cortex [20], as well as high affinity choline uptake (i.e., the rate-limiting step in acetylcholine synthesis) in the cortex and hippocampus of ovariectomized rats [21]. Also, estradiol has been shown to promote the release of acetylcholine in the cortex and hippocampus following potassium stimulation [22] and during maze learning [23].

Together with the effects on cognition, there is interest on the potential effect of estrogens on mood. Animal models are also useful to improve knowledge in emotional issues. For example, depressive-like behaviors in animals are detected by an increase in immobility time and immobile behavior and a decrease in exploratory and active behaviors. Ovarian hormone withdrawal has been associated with these features in rats [24] and macaques [25]. Thus, increased risk of affective disorders appears to be related with hormonal changes also in animal models, something that overlaps the observations in humans [26]. Other investigators have confirmed that ovariectomy influences affective and, of interest, also somatosensory processing in rats [24]. Further data in pain control are being awaited.

10.2.4 Clinical Studies

The issue of whether the menopausal transition affects cognition in women has been investigated in several trials. The Kinmen Women-Health Investigation (KIWI) [27, 28] is a longitudinal population-based study of rural women in Taiwan. During a follow-up period of 18 months, 114 out of the 495 followed women progressed to perimenopause. Interestingly, all cognitive scores slightly improved except verbal fluency, which was slightly worse. The Seattle Midlife Women's Health Study (SMWHS) explored memory functioning and, in consistence with the KIWI observations, found that perceived memory functioning was more closely related to perceived health, depressed mood, or stress than to perimenopause [29]. The positive correlation of depressed mood with nearly every indicator of memory functioning raises important questions and opens the door to indirect actions of estrogens through their well-known relationship with mood states.

The Study of Women's Health Across the Nation (SWAN) study provided a further step in terms of sophistication since investigators performed a cross-sectional analysis of a consistent cohort of 1657 women in which menopausal status was assessed together with hormonal levels, estradiol, and FSH. Again, no relationship was found between menopausal status and the cognitive performance tests when adjusting for covariates. This did not change when either estradiol or FSH levels were included in the analysis [30].

10.2.4.1 Mood and Cognition
The influence of ovarian function on mood states has been claimed in the literature for years. The issue is interesting in itself, but also in what it may affect cognition, which would then be an indirect effect. Indeed, higher levels of depressive and anxiety symptoms are directly related to slightly poorer cognitive performance because both disorders are often accompanied by attention and concentration deficit symptoms. Specifically, depression can be both a risk factor for dementia and an early indicator of incipient dementia [31]. Thus, cognitive complaints during perimenopause may result from adding perimenopausal anxiety or depressive symptoms to the brain [3].

The role of ovarian hormones on the regulation of affective disorders has been addressed in different ways. Research has demonstrated that the lifetime prevalence rate of mood disorders is significantly greater in women than in men, approximately two times more frequent [12, 32]. Data suggests that estrogens, or their absence, are strongly implicated in the regulation of mood and behavior, as well as in the pathobiology of mood disorders [33]. The interaction of estrogens with the serotonergic systems [34], has been taken to propose estradiol as a protective agent against mood changes related with serotonin withdrawal [35].

Clinical observation also confirms that estrogens play a vital role in the precipitation and course of mood disorders in women. Gender differences in mood disorders first appear after menarche and continue through reproductive age. Periods of hormonal fluctuations or estrogen instability (i.e., premenstrually, postpartum, perimenopausally) have been associated with increased vulnerability to mood disorders among susceptible women [33].

10.2.4.2 Possible Actions Through the Vascular System

There is, finally, the potential vascular deterioration as another issue that should be considered when assessing the impact of menopause on cognition. One main point relates to the vascular changes associated with vasomotor symptoms occurring across and after menopause. Again, the SWAN study evaluated whether the decrease in cognitive processing speed detected across perimenopause might have been influenced by the presence of hot flashes. Anxiety and depressive symptoms were also included in the analysis. Investigators only found a small effect associated with anxiety and depressive symptoms, but no interaction with vasomotor symptoms [30].

A possible long-term effect has been raised as well. The hypothesis that menopause might accelerate atherosclerosis and therefore future cardiovascular risk has a correlate in terms of cognitive function. Vascular factors are involved in approximately half of all dementia cases, probably because they show the cumulative impact of very different factors along lifespan [36–38].

10.3 Cardiovascular Diseases

Cardiovascular diseases (CVDs) are the number one cause of death globally, both for men and women. It is well documented that morbidity and mortality rates from CVD are higher in men than in women; however, this gender gap narrows after the menopause suggesting a role of female sex hormones and aging. In fact, the incidence of CVD in women increases substantially with aging, possibly because the menopause diminishes the gender protection contributing to an adverse impact on cardiovascular risk variables. Nevertheless, whether this higher cardiovascular risk is a function of aging or a consequence of the loss of endogenous estrogen due to the menopause, or both, has been debated in the literature for many years.

There is a wealth of data about the effect of estrogens on the vasculature or on cardiovascular risk factors, like lipids, or others. The analysis of that information will facilitate the understanding of the clinical observations.

10.3.1 Effects of Estrogen on the Cardiovascular System Physiology

Estrogens and the other sex hormones regulate some of the fundamental cardiovascular functions including blood pressure, blood flow, vasodilatation and vasoconstriction, vascular inflammation and remodeling, and atherosclerosis [39]. These actions of endogenous estrogens on the cardiovascular system can be mediated directly on the vessels or indirectly through the modulation of cardiovascular risk factors.

Estrogen exerts pleiotropic functions on the cardiovascular system through both genomic and non-genomic effects [40, 41]. Traditionally, ERs act as transcription factors regulating the expression of target genes by directly binding to specific DNA sequences, the estrogen response element (ERE). Non-genomic effects are rapid responses that occur too quickly to be mediated by gene transcription, instead involving modulation of membrane and cytoplasmic proteins, as, for example, the 7-transmembrane G protein-coupled estrogen receptor (GPER), also termed GPR30 [42].

At this level, estrogen triggers rapid vasodilatation, exerts anti-inflammatory effects, and regulates vascular cell growth and migration, leading to a protective action on vessels [43]. These rapid and non-genomic effects are reached by complex interactions with membrane-associated signaling ERs leading to the activation of downstream cascades such as mitogen-activated protein kinase (MAPK) and phosphatidylinositol 3-OH kinase (PI3K). These cascades are responsible for important cardiovascular actions of estrogens, for instance, the activation of nitric oxide (NO) synthesis or the remodeling of the endothelial actin cytoskeleton. Moreover, these cascades play crucial roles in regulating the expression of target proteins implicated in cell proliferation, apoptosis, differentiation, movement, and homeostasis [44].

Furthermore, estrogens have also systemic effects that could have influence on cardiovascular risk altering the serum lipids concentrations, the coagulation and fibrinolytic systems, and the antioxidant system. In fact, through ER, estrogens regulate hepatic expression of apoprotein genes and several coagulation and fibrinolytic protein. The net effect of these changes is to improve lipid profile and promote vasodilatation and antioxidant activities. By contrast, the menopause leads to an overturn of all these effects increasing the cardiovascular risk.

Recent advancements in the characterization of the molecular basis of estrogen's actions help us to understand the biological functions of estrogen and would be beneficial in elucidating current controversies on estrogen's clinical efficacy in the cardiovascular system.

Estrogen can regulate the level and activity of ion channels and can modulate cardiac repolarization. There are male-female differences in calcium and potassium channels and these differences are attributable, at least in part, to estrogen [45, 46].

The mRNA levels of potassium channel components, Kv4.3 and Kv1.5, are decreased with estrogen [47]. These data illustrate that estrogen can alter ion channels and transporters that can alter cardiac contractility, contractile reserve, repolarization, and susceptibility to arrhythmias. Several studies have suggested that female mitochondria generate less reactive oxygen species (ROS) when exposed to estrogens [48–50]. Female mitochondria exhibit increased phosphorylation of mitochondrial α-ketoglutarate dehydrogenase, which leads to less ROS generation by this enzyme under conditions of increased NADH. How much the effects of estrogen on mitochondrial function are mediated by nuclear ER versus acute signaling pathways versus mitochondrial localized ER will require further study. ROS at low levels is a signaling messenger, whereas at high levels, it contributes to cardiovascular disease. Estrogen-mediated differences in ROS production therefore could account for some of the male-female differences in cardiovascular function and disease.

10.3.2 Estrogen and Vascular Injury and Atherosclerosis

Endothelium represents an elective cellular target for estrogens. It is well established that estrogen improves vascular function and, that by maintaining and repairing endothelium, reduces atherosclerosis. Moreover, ERs are expressed in endothelial cells and have an athero-protective effect [51]. Through the recruitment of ERs, estradiol increases endothelial nitric oxide (NO) and prostacyclin synthesis, thus slowing early atheroma formation (Fig. 10.3). Estradiol also decreases synthesis of pro-inflammatory cytokines by circulating or resident immune cells.

The crucial role of endothelium in atherogenesis:

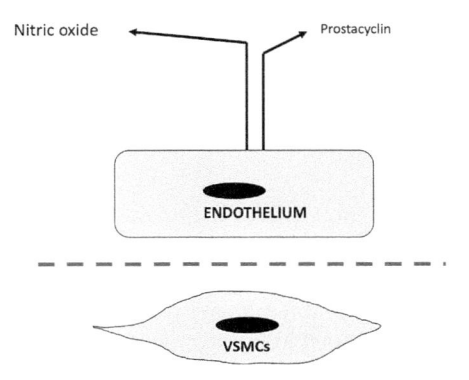

Fig. 10.3 Estrogens exert multiple effects on the cardiovascular system. Estradiol increases the synthesis of endothelial nitric oxide and prostacyclin, which, through multiple mechanisms, delay the early formation of atheroma. Among the mechanisms involved, there are anti-inflammatory actions mediated by the modulation of the tumor necrosis factor α (TNF-α) and adhesion molecules. Additional effects include the inhibition of endothelin-1 and the upregulation of the vascular endothelial growth factor (see text for further details). VSMC: vascular smooth muscle cells

In addition, estradiol facilitates endothelial vascular healing and neo-angiogenesis. While many of these effects are regulated by either ERα or ERβ, ERα is found to be dominant at vascular level. Emerging evidence suggests that estradiol also exerts vascular actions through other receptors, and particularly through the GPR30 [52]. Protective effects exerted by estrogens on endothelium include multiple cellular mechanisms, as evidenced by a number of experimental and clinical data. Estrogen has been demonstrated to activate calcium-dependent potassium channels and induce a rapid increase in NO release [53]. These non-genomic effects of estrogens on NO production are paralleled by their genomic actions exerted by activation of endothelial NO synthase (eNOS) through a receptor-mediated system [54]. Estrogens have antioxidant and anti-inflammatory properties, acting through multiple effects. Among them, estrogens may upregulate prostacyclin synthase and the expression of vascular endothelial growth factor. Conversely, they inhibit endothelin-1 release and modulate adhesion molecule and tumor necrosis factor α (TNF-α) expression and endothelial cell apoptosis [55, 56]. Moreover, estrogens can act by upregulating superoxide dismutase in the vascular district, which contributes to increased superoxide ion clearance [57]. In addition to this genomic effect, estrogens can detoxify superoxide ions through binding with the proton in the hydroxyl group of its aromatic ring. Most experimental studies suggest the protective role of estrogens in terms of oxidative stress status that can improve the oxidative balance in vascular sites, improving the local bioavailability of NO and, consequently, enhancing endothelium-dependent dilation. Estrogens may also influence the redox balance through modulation of mitochondrial enzyme activity. Thus, the antioxidant effects are regarded as one of the main mechanisms by which hormones protect women during their fertile life, when they are at lower risk of cardiovascular events with respect to men. In fact, oxidative stress is generally higher in men compared to premenopausal women. After menopause, when hormonal levels markedly fall, the risk to experience cardiovascular events rapidly rises in women, in parallel to a rapidly increase of oxidative stress biomarker levels [58].

10.3.3 Estrogen and Cardiac Hypertrophy

The details of the mechanism by which estrogen reduce cardiac hypertrophy are still undergoing investigation. One clarifying study shows that the beneficial effects of estrogens in limiting cardiac hypertrophy are attributable to estrogen-mediated degradation of calcineurin A [59]. It is likely that estrogens alter the expression of additional genes that are important in the response to cardiac hypertrophy.

10.3.4 Diabetes, Lipid Profile, and Obesity

Insulin resistance and diabetes have been associated with greater cardiovascular risk among women in different clinical trials. Moreover, data from a meta-analysis suggest that the risk for fatal coronary artery disease associated with diabetes is 50% higher in women, whereas diabetes and hypertension represent the two most important cardiovascular risk factors in women, especially when they occur in association [60]. Estrogens seem to contribute to glucose homeostasis through increased glucose transport into the cell, whereas lack of estrogens has been associated with a progressive decrease in glucose-stimulated insulin secretion and insulin sensitivity as well as insulin resistance increase [61–63]. Hormone replacement therapy has been found to exert a beneficial effect on glycated hemoglobin levels in postmenopausal women.

Early after menopause, women begin to gain weight and their body fat is redistributed from a gynecoid to an android pattern. The increase in body mass index (BMI) and proportion of visceral fat are strongly correlated with the development of hypertension, insulin resistance, and with a number of metabolic risk factors for CVD. It is otherwise known that menopause is associated with an increase in triglycerides (TGs), total cholesterol (TC), and low-density lipoprotein cholesterol (LDL-C) and lipoprotein (a) [Lp(a)]. Levels of high-density lipoprotein cholesterol (HDL-C) gradually fall after menopause, although concentration remains always significantly higher in women with respect to men. This finding is considered a protective factor for female subjects.

10.3.5 Clinical Impact of Menopause

The impact of natural menopause on CVD risk is a matter of current research. The significant fall in the circulating levels of estrogens, however, takes some years in many women. This smooth decline may perhaps obscure the cardiovascular impact of natural menopause. So it has been considered that artificial menopause is a good model for showing the clinical impact of hormonal deprivation because the fall in the levels of estrogens is both rapid and acute. Primary ovarian insufficiency, in which women are exposed to longer hypoestrogenic periods in their lives, may be also illustrative.

The data are not uniform since some studies focusing on cardiovascular risk factors have found unfavorable changes in women with surgical menopause [64–66] while others have not [67]. Of interest, the incidence of cardiovascular events, coronary heart disease and stroke, seems to be increased by early menopause [68–70]. Reviews about the topic also conclude accordingly [71, 72].

The impact of natural menopause has been thoroughly investigated too, and interest has focused in the menopausal transition.

10.3.5.1 The Menopausal Transition and Cardiovascular Risk
With regard to this, it is worth mentioning the results of the SWAN. SWAN is a multicenter, multiethnic longitudinal study designed to characterize the physiological and psychosocial changes that occur during the menopausal transition and to observe their effects on subsequent health and risk factors for age-related diseases. A total of 3302 women were enrolled at seven clinical sites between 1996

and 1997. At the time of enrollment, women were premenopausal, not taking hormones, and between 42 and 52 years of age. Participants self-identified as African American (28%), Caucasian (47%), Chinese (8%), Hispanic (8%), or Japanese (9%). SWAN has a multidisciplinary focus and thus has repeated measures of bone health, cardiovascular risk factors, psychosocial factors, and ovarian hormones [73].

In this set, Matthews et al. [74] evaluated the change in CHD risk factors in relation to a very particular and critical period of women's life that is the final menstrual period (FMP). Women who experienced a natural menopause (1054 out of the total) were analyzed independent of age and other confounders. The results showed significant increases in total cholesterol, LDL-C, and Apo B within a year of the FMP; importantly, the rate of change relative to FMP did not vary by ethnicity, suggesting that menopause had a uniform influence on lipids. The other risk factors changed in a linear pattern consistent with chronologic aging: Triglycerides, lipoprotein (a), insulin, factor VIIc, and systolic blood pressure increased; diastolic blood pressure, tissue plasminogen activator antigen, fibrinogen, and high-sensitivity C-reactive protein did not change.

10.4 Osteoarthritis

10.4.1 Introduction

Osteoarthritis (OA) is the most common degenerative joint disease. Approximately one-third of 65-year-old people suffer from OA, and the incidence is higher in women than in men. The process consists of breakdown of cartilage that affects the surfaces within the joints (Fig. 10.4). The cartilage covering the ends of the bones gradually roughens and becomes thin while the underlying bone surface becomes thicker. A reparation process initiates at the joint so that the bone edges grow outward, forming bony spurs called osteophytes, the synovium becomes thick and produces extra fluid, and both capsule and ligaments slowly thicken and contract. The consequence is that a joint affected by OA does not move as smoothly as it should. The most common symptoms are stiffness, particularly first thing in the morning or after resting, and pain. Moreover, affected joints may get swollen after extended activity. The whole picture may severely impair quality of life. Unfortunately, current treatment provided by physicians is still limited to anti-inflammatories to control pain. The pathogenesis of OA is complex because its development involves the interaction of multiple factors, and estrogens have been claimed to be one of them. The association with menopause derives from direct epidemiological observation [75], together with a higher prevalence among women and the expression of ER in joint tissues [76, 77].

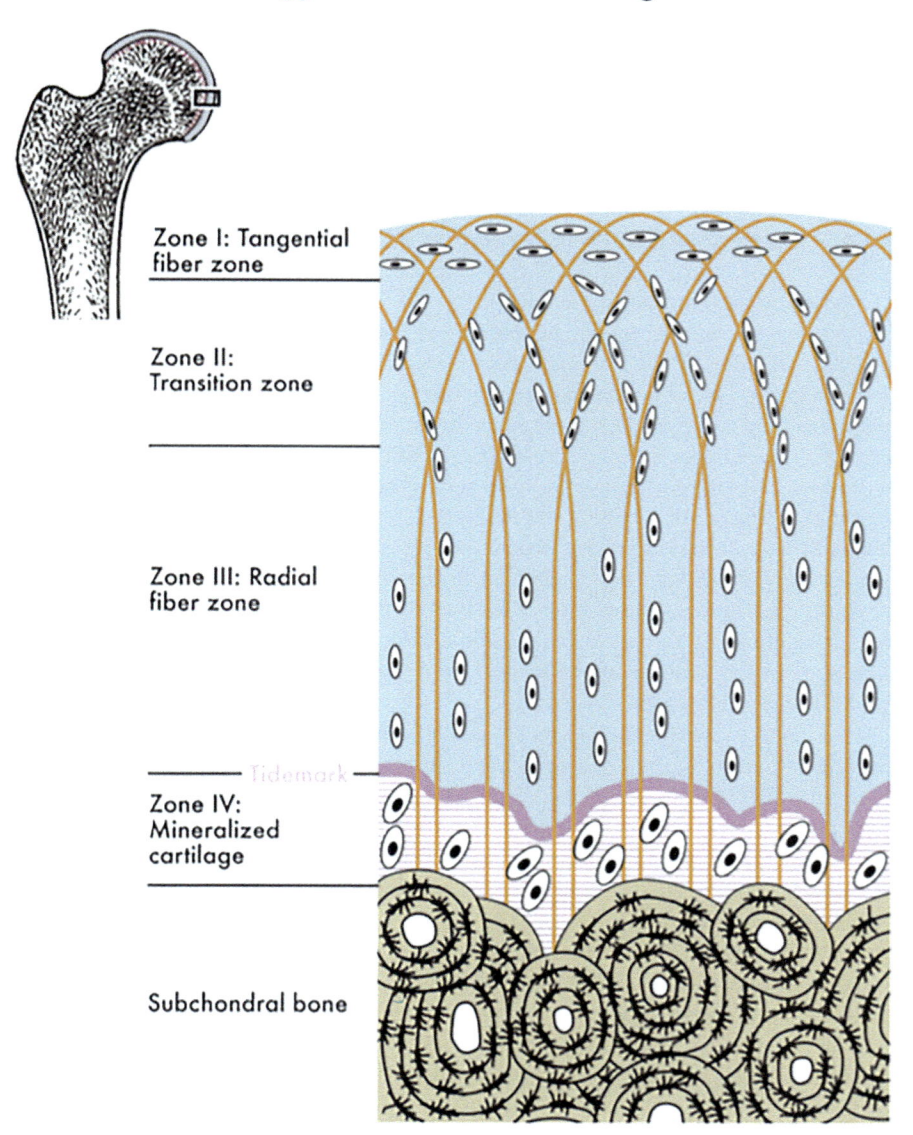

Fig. 10.4 The articular cartilage is composed of different histological layers, as shown in the figure. The mineralized cartilage (Zone IV) constitutes the transition to the subchondral bone. (With permission of Elsevier from Prog Histochem Cytochem. 2011; 45:239–93. Permission obtained through Copyright Clearance Center, Inc.)

Estrogens are involved in several biological processes through both direct and indirect molecular mechanisms. In general, acute estrogen deficiency increases the production of both pro-inflammatory cytokine and ROS and activates nuclear factor-κB. Pro-inflammatory cytokine expression, in turn, attenuates with estrogen replacement [78], an important observation because together with metalloproteinases, cellular senescence and inflammatory cytokines play an important role in the progression of OA [79, 80].

10.4.2 Evidences from In Vivo and In Vitro Experiments

The proposal that estrogen deficiency is involved in the onset and progression of OA is limited by the incomplete understanding of the underlying molecular mechanism [81, 82]. Deletion of ER in female mice results in cartilage damage, osteophytosis, and changes in the subchondral bone of the joints, supporting the hypothesis that estrogens play a role in the maintenance of the structural integrity of articular cartilage [83]. Experiments performed in ovariectomized (OVX) mice have shown that acute loss of estrogens induces similar joint damage [84]. These observations suggest that the presence of ER in the cartilage is important for joint cartilage homeostasis. Moreover, the fact that estrogen deficiency also increases subchondral bone remodeling, which has been suggested to promote osteoarthritis changes [85], has brought some concern about whether the phenotypes obtained from the models described above are either only due to the effects of estrogen deprivation on joint cartilage or to an indirect effect derived from the subchondral bone loss induced by the hormone decline [86].

In order to overcome the indirect effects of the lack of estrogen signal on the joint cartilage through the subchondral bone, different experimental approaches have been proposed. OVX rabbits, which do not suffer bone loss as much as mice, have been proposed as a model [87]. Mild abnormalities in the joint structure have been reported in 22-week-old OVX rabbits, as well as higher Mankin scores, while no significant changes in subchondral bone mineral density were developed as compared to their controls, suggesting that estrogens have a protective effect on joint cartilage through a direct mechanism [86].

Another approach used to provide evidence about the action of estrogen on joint cartilage has consisted of experiments performed in OVX rats. Ovariectomy induced a rapid increase in serum type II collagen (CII), indicating cartilage degradation, which correlated with microstructural cartilage damage [88]. The effect of estrogen deficiency on the synthesis of glycosaminoglycans (GAG), which are an important component of the connective tissue, was investigated in pigs by other researchers. A significant decrease in GAG from knee joints was found in both cryo- and paraffin sections of OVX animals compared with sham controls, indicating that loss of estrogens has detrimental effect on cartilage tissue [89].

Therefore, evidence obtained from animal models with either estrogen depletion or lack of ER supports the hypothesis that estrogens have a chondroprotective role.

10.4.3 Clinical Evidence

In line with the data observed in the experiments performed in animals, there are also clinical observations, which have contributed to gain knowledge on this potential action of estrogens.

The possible relationship between the hormonal changes of menopause and OA was already proposed in 1925, when Cecil and Archer described the *"arthritis of the menopause,"* which affects the hands of women around the time of menopause [90]. Sometimes, the process occurs in a more generalized form, as reported by Kellgren and Moore, who were first in describing a form of *"menopausal arthritis"* of rapid onset, with Heberden nodes [88]. This form, which they called "generalized primary osteoarthritis," was characterized by a rapid onset of symptoms and multiple affected joints (hands, spine, and knees). Although there is controversy on the existence of this syndrome, the increase in the prevalence of OA in the perimenopausal woman, particularly hand OA, is acknowledged [91, 92]. The progression of OA involves not only numerous risk factors and multiple joint sites but also multiple complex pathways, which directly or indirectly appear to be related to the fluctuations in hormonal levels that occur around menopause [93].

10.4.3.1 Epidemiological Studies

The prevalence of OA increases with age in men and women, but there appears to be an increase in incidence and severity with menopause [94]. Moreover, OA changes are more pronounced in the hand than in the hip or in the knee, and this pattern reproduces, although maintaining prevalence differences, between women and men [95]. So symptomatic OA affected the hands of 26% of women and of 13% of men and the knees of 11.4% of women and 6.8% of men in the Framingham cohort [96]. Also, more than 40% of women reported to have received the diagnosis of OA in the Women's Health Initiative (WHI) Study, which included postmenopausal women from the general population. As in other studies, women who were older or overweight had a higher risk indicating that there are other factors, apart from low levels of estrogens, which induce OA development [97].

The increase in the population of middle-aged women with polyarticular symptoms has further nourished the hypothesis that a relationship exists between the onset of OA and menopause [98]. In support of a role for hormones, some studies have found that hysterectomized women, who have been linked to earlier physiological menopause in several studies, suffer higher rates of OA at the knee or at the first carpometacarpal joint [99]. Additionally, a population-based nested case-control study using the National Health Insurance program database from 2000 to 2016 in Taiwan found that hysterectomy had a significant association with OA (aOR = 1.19, 95% CI = 1.09–1.30), especially knee OA (aOR = 1.25, 95% CI = 1.13–1.38) [100]. Also, an inverse association has been observed between premenopausal status and patellofemoral OA [101]. The same authors also reported that women with artificial menopause, who undergo a more drastic reduction of circulating estrogens, suffer a significantly higher rate of OA in hands and knees [99]. Moreover, a study in a population of women aged 25–45 years found that, even after adjusting for age, hand OA was more frequent in those who had already passed menopause [102]. A similar observation reproduced in the case of users of aromatase inhibitors, since younger women, with the FMP within the latter 5 years, report a higher rate of arthralgia than women in whom the FMP occurred more than 10 years ago [98].

The association of OA with estrogen, however, has not been unanimous in the literature. For example, one study could not confirm an effect of the duration of the exposure to estrogens, as measured by the age at menarche or menopause, rate of hysterectomy, parity, or use of oral contraceptives, with the onset of OA [103]. The issue, therefore, is controversial as it is whether the potential relationship applies to all forms of OA in women or only to any of the two subsets, generalized OA or OA of the menopause [104].

In summary, despite the very suggestive data in the literature, the effect of menopause on OA still requires further investigation [82].

10.4.3.2 Endogenous Sex Steroids in Women with Generalized Osteoarthritis

The studies investigating the relationship of endogenous sexual hormones and risk for OA are inconclusive. Low levels of testosterone were described in women with hand OA [102] and low levels of serum estradiol and urine 2-hydroxy-estrone were predictive of radiographic signs of knee OA [105]. However, no trend in the sex hormone concentrations was found when contrasted with the severity or radiographic hand OA in a study on 229 Caucasian women [106]. The comparison of the age and obesity adjusted sex hormone concentrations by the worst Kellgren-Lawrence score revealed little difference in the same study. Moreover, a systematic review of 16 studies examining the association between OA and hormonal exposure, including the fertile period (duration, hormone levels, age at menopause, and menarche) and the postmenopause (years since menopause, surgical menopause), concluded that the assumed relationship between the female hormonal aspects and OA could not be clearly observed [107]. There may already be a possible gender difference present throughout the reproductive lifespan so the effect of menopause could be partially attenuated and undetected in some studies [108].

10.4.3.3 Radiological Imaging Studies of the Articular Cartilage

The loss of the articular cartilage is a significant feature of OA progression. There is therefore interest in using the level of damage of articular cartilage, as measured by radiological imaging, as an indicator of either the progression of OA or the impact of therapeutic interventions [109].

There are data from both experimental and clinical studies. Wu et al. by using 3D visualization with propagation-based phase-contrast computed tomography imaging observed a decrease in cartilage volume, surface area, and thickness as well as capture subchondral bone surface and trabecular bone loss among OVX mice compared with controls, which again suggests that low levels of estrogens induce cartilage deterioration [110].

Among the clinical studies, data from the longitudinal Southeast Michigan Arthritis Cohort found that pre- and perimenopausal women who had the lowest tertile of circulating serum estradiol (<47 pg/mL) suffered a 2-fold increased risk for developing incident radiographic OA compared with those from the middle tertile (47–77 pg/mL) over a 3-year period (OR: 1.88, 95% CI: 1.07–3.51). Women in the highest tertile (>78 pg/mL) showed no increased risk of developing incident OA (OR: 1.04, 95% CI: 0.52–2.09) [105]. However, using data from almost the same cohort [102], the same investigators found that HRT was associated with a nonsignificant 2-fold increase in radiographically detected OA (OR: 2.56, 95% CI: 0.68–9.5).

There is still sparse evidence on the relationship of sex hormones and the structural damage of the articular cartilage, as measured by fine radiological methods, as for example, magnetic resonance imaging (MRI) [111]. A study on 325 subjects showed that the rate of the articular cartilage loss was higher in women than in men and that the difference started to become evident from the age of 50 years [112]. Moreover, differences between men and women were also observed between sex hormones and MRI structural changes in a group of individuals with symptomatic OA. In women but not in men, low levels of estradiol, progesterone, and testosterone were associated with MRI-detected structural changes related with OA [113].

10.5 Conclusion

OA is more prevalent in women, and the difference increases after menopause. The molecular mechanisms determining the effect of menopause are still unknown. However, both experimental data in transgenic animals devoid of estrogenic signals and observations in the human suggest that hormonal deficiency may be a determining factor in the process. Despite the progression in the knowledge of the disease, details of the interaction of estrogen deficiency with other factors to induce or influence the progression of OA remain to be clarified.

References

1. Sherwin B. Estrogen effects on cognition in menopausal women. Neurology. 1997;48:21S–6S.
2. Schmidt P, Keenan P, Schenkel L, Berlin K, Gibson C, Rubinow D. Cognitive performance in healthy women during induced hypogonadism and ovarian steroid addback. Arch Womens Ment Health. 2013;16:47–58.
3. Greendale G, Derby C, Maki P. Perimenopause & Cognition. Obstet Gynecol Clin Nort Am. 2011;38:519–35.
4. Abe T, Bereczki D, Takahashi Y, Tashiro M, Iwata R, Itoh M. Medial frontal cortex perfusion abnormalities as evaluated by positron emission tomography in women with climacteric symptoms. Menopause. 2006;13:891–901.
5. Izumi S, Muano T, Mori A, Kika G, Okuwaki S. Common carotid artery stiffness, cardiovascular function and lipid metabolism after menopause. Life Sci. 2006;78:1696–701.
6. Maki P. Verbal memory and menopause. Maturitas. 2015;82:288–90.

7. Craig M, Brammer M, Maki P, Fletcher P, Daly C, Rymer J, et al. The interactive effect of acute ovarian suppression and the cholinergic system on visuospatial working memory in young women. Psychoneuroendocrinology. 2010;35:987–1000.
8. Ryan J, Scali J, Carriere I, Amieva H, Rouaud O, Berr C, et al. Impact of a premature menopause on cognitive function in later life. BJOG. 2014;121:1729–39.
9. Skinner D, Albertson A, Navratil A, Smith A, Mignot M, et al. Effects of gonadotrophin-releasing hormone outside the hypothalamic-pituitary-reproductive axis. J Neuroendocrinol. 2009;21:282–92.
10. McEwen B. Estrogens effects on the brain: multiple sites and molecular mechanisms. J Appl Physiol. 2001;91:2785–801.
11. Hesson J. Cumulative estrogen exposure and prospective memory in older women. Brain Cogn. 2012;80:89–95.
12. Ter-Horst G, Wichmann R, Gerrits M, Westenbroek C, Lin Y. Sex differences in stress responses: focus on ovarian hormones. Physiol Behav. 2009;97:239–49.
13. Lan Y, Zhaoa J, Li S. Update on the neuroprotective effect of estrogen receptor Alpha against Alzheimer's Disease. J Alzheimers Dis. 2015;43:1137–48.
14. Zhao L, Woody S, Chhibber A. Estrogen receptor β in Alzheimer's disease: from mechanism to therapeutics. Ageing Res Rev. 2015;24:178–90.
15. Hestiantoro A, Swaab D. Changes in estrogen receptor-alpha and -beta in the infundibular nucleus of the human hypothalamus are related to the occurrence of Alzheimer's disease neuropathology. J Clin Endocrinol Metab. 2004;89:1912–25.
16. Daniel J, Witty C, Rodgers S. Long-term consequences of estrogens administered in midlife on female cognitive aging. Horm Behav. 2015;74:77–85.
17. Rettberg J, Yao J, Brinton R. Estrogen: a master regulator of bioenergetic systems in the brain and body. Front Neuroendocrinol. 2014;35:8–30.
18. Bowen R, Isley J, Atkinson R. An association of elevated serum gonadotropin concentrations and Alzheimer disease? J Neuroendocrinol. 2000;12:351–4.
19. Casadesus G, Webber K, Atwood C, Pappolla M, Perry G, Bowen R, et al. Luteinizing hormone modulates cognition and amyloid-β deposition in Alzheimer APP transgenic mice. Biochim Biophys Acta. 2006;1762:447–52.
20. Luine V. Estradiol increases choline acetyltransferase activity in specific basal forebrain nuclei and projection areas of female rats. Exp Neurol. 1985;89:484–90.
21. O'Malley C, Hautamaki R, Kelley M, Meyer E. Effects of ovariectomy and oestradiol benzoate on high-affinity choline uptake, ACh synthesis, and release from rat cerebral cortical synaptosomes. Brain Res. 1987;403:389–92.
22. Gibbs R, Hashash A, Johnson D. Effects of oestrogen on potassium-stimulated acetylcholine release in the hippocampus and overlying cortex of adult rats. Brain Res. 1997;749:143–6.
23. Marriott L, Korol D. Short-term estrogen treatment in ovariectomized rats augments hippocampal acetylcholine release during place learning. Neurobiol Learn Memory. 2003;80:315–22.
24. Li L, Wang Z, Yu J, Zhang Y. Ovariectomy results in variable changes in nociception, mood and depression in adult female rats. PLoS One. 2014;9:e94312.
25. Shively C, Bethea C. Cognition, mood disorders, and sex hormones. ILAR J. 2004;45:189–99.
26. Hall E, Steiner M. Serotonin and female psychopathology. Womens Health. 2013;9:85–97.
27. Fuh J, Wang S, Lu S, Juang K, Chiu L. The Kinmen women-health investigation (KIWI): a menopausal study of a population aged 40–54. Maturitas. 2001;39:117–24.
28. Fuh J, Wang S, Lee S, Lu S, Juang K. A longitudinal study of cognition change during early menopausal transition in a rural community. Maturitas. 2006;53:447–53.
29. Woods N, Mitchel E, Adams C. Memory functioning among midlife women: observations from the Seattle Midlife Women's Health Study. Menopause. 2000;7:257–65.
30. Luetters C, Huang M, Seeman T, Buckwalter G, Meyer P, Avis N, et al. Menopause transition stage and endogenous estradiol and follicle-stimulating hormone levels are not related to cognitive performance: cross-sectional results from the study of women's health across the nation (SWAN). J Women's Health. 2007;16:331–44.

31. Fiske A, Wetherel J, Gatz M. Depression in older adults. Annu Rev Clin Psychol. 2009;5:363–89.
32. Walf A, Frye C. A review and update of mechanisms of estrogen in the hippocampus and amygdala for anxiety and depression behavior. Neuropsychopharmacology. 2006;31:1097–111.
33. Halbreich U, Kahn L. Role of estrogen in the aetiology and treatment of mood disorders. CNS Drugs. 2001;15:797–817.
34. Amin Z, Gueorguieva R, Cappiello A, Czarkowsk K, Stiklus S, Anderson G, et al. Estradiol and tryptophan depletion interact to modulate cognition in menopausal women. Neuropsychopharmacology. 2006;31:2489–97.
35. Wharton W, Gleason C, Olson S, Carlsson C, Asthana S. Neurobiological underpinnings of the estrogen – mood relationship. Curr Psychiatr Rev. 2012;8:247–56.
36. Sonnen J, Larson E, Crane P, Haneuse S, Li G, Schellenberg G, et al. Pathological correlates of dementia in a longitudinal, population-based sample of aging. Ann Neurol. 2007;62:406–13.
37. Bowler J. Vascular cognitive impairment. J Neurol Neurosurg Psychiatry. 2005;76:35–44.
38. Gorelick P, Scuteri A, Black S, Decarli C, Greenberg S, Iadecola C, et al. Vascular contributions to cognitive impairment and dementia: a statement for healthcare professionals from the American Heart Association/American Stroke Association. Stroke. 2011;42:2672–713.
39. Mendelsohn M, Karas R. The protective effects of estrogen on the cardiovascular system. N Engl J Med. 1999;340:1801–11.
40. Fu X, Simoncini T. Non-genomic sex steroid actions in the vascular system. Semin Reprod Med. 2007;25:178–86.
41. Simoncini T, Genazzani A. Non-genomic actions of sex steroid hormones. Eur J Endocrinol. 2003;148:281–92.
42. Prossnitz ER, Barton M. The G protein-coupled oestrogen receptor GPER in health and disease: an update. Nat Rev Endocrinol. 2023;19:407–24.
43. Simoncini T, Mannella P, Fornari L, Caruso A, Varone G, Genazzani A. Genomic and non-genomic effects of estrogens on endothelial cells. Steroids. 2004;69:537–42.
44. Simoncini T. Mechanisms of action of estrogen receptors in vascular cells: relevance for menopause and aging. Climacteric. 2009;12:S6–11.
45. Jiao L, Machuki JO, Wu Q, Shi M, Fu L, Adekunle AO, et al. Estrogen and calcium handling proteins: new discoveries and mechanisms in cardiovascular diseases. Am J Physiol Heart Circ Physiol. 2020;318:H820–9.
46. Baldwin SN, Jepps TA, Greenwood IA. Cycling matters: sex hormone regulation of vascular potassium channels. Channels (Austin). 2023;17:2217637.
47. Saito T, Ciobotaru A, Bopassa J, Toro L, Stefani E, Eghbali M. Estrogen contributes to gender differences in mouse ventricular repolarization. Circ Res. 2009;105:343–52.
48. Lagranha C, Deschamps A, Aponte A, Steenbergen C, Murphy E. Sex differences in the phosphorylation of mitochondrial proteins result in reduced production of reactive oxygen species and cardioprotection in females. Circ Res. 2010;106:1681–91.
49. Razmara A, Duckles S, Krause D, Procaccio V. Estrogen suppresses brain mitochondrial oxidative stress in female and male rats. Brain Res. 2007;1176:71–81.
50. Scholtes C, Giguère V. Transcriptional regulation of ROS homeostasis by the ERR subfamily of nuclear receptors. Antioxidants (Basel). 2021;10:437.
51. Davezac M, Buscato M, Zahreddine R, Lacolley P, Henrion D, Lenfant F, et al. Estrogen receptor and vascular aging. Front Aging. 2021;2:727380.
52. Fredette NC, Meyer MR, Prossnitz ER. Role of GPER in estrogen-dependent nitric oxide formation and vasodilation. J Steroid Biochem Mol Biol. 2018;176:65–72.
53. Sader M, Celermajer D. Endothelial function, vascular reactivity and gender differences in the cardiovascular system. Cardiovasc Res. 2002;53:597–604.
54. Simoncini T. Interaction of oestrogen receptor with the regulatory subunit of phosphatidylinositol-3-OH kinase. Nature. 2000;407:538–41.
55. Nathan L, Pervin S, Singh R, Rosenfeld M, Chaudhuri G. Estradiol inhibits leukocyte adhesion and transendothelial migration in rabbits in vivo: possible mechanisms for gender differences in atherosclerosis. Circ Res. 1999;85:377–85.

56. Simoncini T. Effects of phytoestrogens derived from red clover on atherogenic adhesion molecules in human endothelial cells. Menopause. 2008;15:542–50.
57. Strehlow K. Modulation of antioxidant enzyme expression and function by estrogen. Circ Res. 2003;93:170–7.
58. Signorelli S. Duration of menopause and behavior of malondialdehyde, lipids, lipoproteins and carotid wall artery intima-media thickness. Maturitas. 2001;39:39–42.
59. Donaldson C, Eder S, Baker C, Aronovitz M, Weiss A, Hall-Porter M, et al. Estrogen attenuates left ventricular and cardiomyocyte hypertrophy by an estrogen receptor-dependent pathway that increases calcineurin degradation. Circ Res. 2009;104:265–75.
60. Hu G, Tuomilehto J, Silventoinen K, Barengo N, Jousilahti P. Joint effects of physical activity, body mass index, waist circumference and waist-to-hip ratio with the risk of cardiovascular disease among middle-aged Finnish men and women. Eur Heart J. 2004;25:2212–9.
61. Steinberg H, Paradisi G, Cronin J, Crowde K, Hempfling A, Hook G, et al. Type II diabetes abrogates sex differences in endothelial function in premenopausal women. Circulation. 2000;101:2040–6.
62. De Paoli M, Zakharia A, Werstuck GH. The role of estrogen in insulin resistance: a review of clinical and preclinical data. Am J Pathol. 2021;191:1490–8.
63. Zhu J, Zhou Y, Jin B, Shu J. Role of estrogen in the regulation of central and peripheral energy homeostasis: from a menopausal perspective. Ther Adv Endocrinol Metab. 2023;14:20420188231199359.
64. Özkaya E, Cakir E, Okuyan E, Cakir C, Ustün G, et al. Comparison of the effects of surgical and natural menopause on carotid intima media thickness, osteoporosis, and homocysteine levels. Menopause. 2011;18:73–6.
65. Farahmand M, Ramezani Tehrani F, Bahri Khomami M, Noroozzadeh M, Azizi F. Surgical menopause versus natural menopause and cardio-metabolic disturbances: a 12-year population-based cohort study. J Endocrinol Investig. 2015;38:761–7.
66. Fukuda K, Takashima Y, Hashimoto M, Uchino A, Yuzuriha T, Yao H. Early menopause and the risk of silent brain infarction in community-dwelling elderly subjects: the Sefuri brain MRI study. J Stroke Cerebrovasc Dis. 2014;23:817–22.
67. Appiah D, Schreiner P, Bower J, Sternfeld B, Lewis C, Wellons M. Is surgical menopause associated with future levels of cardiovascular risk factor independent of antecedent levels? The CARDIA Study. Am J Epidemiol. 2015;182:991–9.
68. Wellons M, Ouyang P, Schreiner P, Herrington D, Vaidya D. Early menopause predicts future coronary heart disease and stroke: the Multi-Ethnic Study of Atherosclerosis. Menopause. 2012;19:1081–7.
69. Lubiszewska B, Kruk M, Broda G, Ksiezycka E, Piotrowski W, Kurjata P, et al. The impact of early menopause on risk of coronary artery disease (PREmature Coronary Artery Disease in Women-PRECADIW case-control study). Eur J Prev Cardiol. 2012;19:95–101.
70. Honigberg MC, Zekavat SM, Aragam K, Finneran P, Klarin D, Bhatt DL, et al. Association of Premature Natural and Surgical Menopause with Incident Cardiovascular Disease. JAMA. 2019;322:2411–21.
71. Faubion S, Kuhle C, Shuster L, Rocca W. Long-term health consequences of premature or early menopause and considerations for management. Climacteric. 2015;18:483–91.
72. Shuster L, Rhodes D, Gostout B, Grossardt B, Rocca W. Premature menopause or early menopause: long-term health consequences. Maturitas. 2010;65:161–6.
73. Santoro N, Sutton-Tyrrell K. The SWAN song: Study of Women's Health Across the Nation's recurring themes. Obstet Gynecol Clin N Am. 2011;38:417–23.
74. Matthews K, Crawford S, Chae C, Everson-Rose S, Sowers M, Sternfeld B, et al. Are changes in cardiovascular disease risk factors in midlife women due to chronological aging or to the menopausal transition? J Am Coll Cardiol. 2009;54:2366–73.
75. Pang H, Chen S, Klyne DM, Harrich D, Ding W, Yang S, et al. Low back pain and osteoarthritis pain: a perspective of estrogen. Bone Res. 2023;11:42.
76. Ushiyama T, Ueyama H, Inoue K, Ohkubo I, Hukuda S. Expression of genes for estrogen receptors alpha and beta in human articular chondrocytes. Osteoarthr Cartil. 1999;7:560–6.

77. Sciore P, Frank C, Hart D. Identification of sex hormone receptors in human and rabbit ligaments of the knee by reverse transcription-polymerase chain reaction: evidence that receptors are present in tissue from both male and female subjects. J Orthop Res. 1998;16:604–10.
78. Srikanth V, Fryer J, Zhai G, Winzenberg T, Hosmer D, Jones G. A meta-analysis of sex differences prevalence, incidence and severity of osteoarthritis. Osteoarthr Cartil. 2005;13:769–81.
79. McCulloch K, Litherland GJ, Rai TS. Cellular senescence in osteoarthritis pathology. Aging Cell. 2017;16:210–8.
80. Mehana EE, Khafaga AF, El-Blehi SS. The role of matrix metalloproteinases in osteoarthritis pathogenesis: an updated review. Life Sci. 2019;234:116786.
81. Dennison EM. Osteoarthritis: the importance of hormonal status in midlife women. Maturitas. 2022;165:8–11.
82. Gulati M, Dursun E, Vincent K, Watt FE. The influence of sex hormones on musculoskeletal pain and osteoarthritis. Lancet Rheumatol. 2023;5:e225–38.
83. Sniekers Y, van Osch G, Ederveen A, Inzunza J, Gustafsson J, van Leeuwen J, et al. Development of osteoarthritic features in estrogen receptor knockout mice. Osteoarthr Cartil. 2009;17:1356–61.
84. Ma H, Blanchet T, Peluso D, Hopkins B, Morris E, Glasson S. Osteoarthritis severity is sex dependent in a surgical mouse model. Osteoarthr Cartil. 2007;15:695–700.
85. Bellido M, Lugo L, Roman-Blas J, Castañeda S, Caeiro J, Sonia Dapia S, et al. Subchondral bone microstructural damage by increased remodelling aggravates experimental osteoarthritis preceded by osteoporosis. Arthritis Res Ther. 2010;12:R152.
86. Castañeda S, Largo R, Calvo E, Bellido M, Gómez-Vaquero C, Herrero-Beaumont G. Effects of estrogen deficiency and low bone mineral density on healthy knee cartilage in rabbits. J Orthop Res. 2010;28:812–8.
87. Castañeda S, Calvo E, Largo R, González-González R, de la Piedra C, Díaz-Curiel M. Characterization of a new experimental model of osteoporosis in rabbits. J Bone Miner Metab. 2008;26:53–9.
88. Oestergaard S, Sondergaard B, Hoegh-Andersen P, Henriksen K, Qvist P, et al. Effects of ovariectomy and estrogen therapy on type II collagen degradation and structural integrity of articular cartilage in rats: implications of the time of initiation. Arthritis Rheum. 2006;54:2441–51.
89. Claassen H, Cellarius C, Scholz-Ahrens K, Schrezenmeir J, Glüer C, Schünke M, et al. Extracellular matrix changes in knee joint cartilage following bone-active drug treatment. Cell Tissue Res. 2006;324:279–89.
90. Cecil R, Archer B. Arthritis of the menopause. JAMA. 1925;84:75–9.
91. Cooper C, Egger P, Coggon D, Hart D, Masud T, Cicuttini F, et al. Generalized osteoarthritis in women: pattern of joint involvement and approaches to definition for epidemiological studies. J Rheumatol. 1996;23:1938–42.
92. Prieto-Alhambra D, Judge A, Javaid MK, Cooper C, Diez-Perez A, Arden NK. Incidence and risk factors for clinically diagnosed knee, hip and hand osteoarthritis: influences of age, gender and osteoarthritis affecting other joints. Ann Rheum Dis. 2014;73:1659–64.
93. Hussain SM, Cicuttini FM, Alyousef B, Wang Y. Female hormonal factors and osteoarthritis of the knee, hip and hand: a narrative review. Climacteric. 2018;21:132–9.
94. Eun Y, Yoo JE, Han K, Kim D, Lee KN, Lee J, et al. Female reproductive factors and risk of joint replacement arthroplasty of the knee and hip due to osteoarthritis in postmenopausal women: a nationwide cohort study of 1.13 million women. Osteoarthr Cartil. 2022;30:69–80.
95. Katz JN, Arant KR, Loeser RF. Diagnosis and treatment of hip and knee osteoarthritis: a review. JAMA. 2021;325:568–78.
96. Felson D, Naimark A, Anderson J, Kazis L, Castelli W, Meenan R. The prevalence of knee osteoarthritis in the elderly. The Framingham Osteoarthritis Study. Arthritis Rheum. 1987;30:914–8.
97. Wright N, Riggs G, Lisse J, Chen Z. Women's Health Initiative. Self-reported osteoarthritis, ethnicity, body mass index, and other associated risk factors in postmenopausal women-results from the Women's Health Initiative. J Am Geriatr Soc. 2008;56:1.

98. Magliano M. Menopausal arthralgia: fact or fiction. Maturitas. 2010;67:29–33.
99. Spector T, Hart D, Brown P, Almeyda J, Dacre J, Doyle D, et al. Frequency of osteoarthritis in hysterectomized women. J Rheumatol. 1991;18:1877–83.
100. Lin SJ, Wu CY, Tsau CF, Yang HY. Hysterectomy and risk of osteoarthritis in women: a nationwide nested case–control study. Scand J Rheumatol. 2023;52:556–63.
101. Cicuttini F, Spector T, Baker J. Risk factors for osteoarthritis in the tibiofemoral and patellofemoral joints of the knee. J Rheumatol. 1997;24:1164–7.
102. Sowers M, Hochberg M, Crabbe J, Muhich A, Crutchfield M, Updike S. Association of bone mineral density and sex hormone levels with osteoarthritis of the hand and knee in premenopausal women. Am J Epidemiol. 1996;143:38–47.
103. Samanta A, Jones A, Regan M, Wilson S, Doherty M. Is osteoarthritis in women affected by hormonal changes or smoking? Br J Rheumatol. 1993;32:366–70.
104. Wluka A, Cicuttini F, Spector T. Menopause, oestrogens and arthritis. Maturitas. 2000;35:183–99.
105. Sowers M, McConnell D, Jannausch M, Buyuktur A, Hochberg M, al. e. Estradiol and its metabolites and their association with knee osteoarthritis. Arthritis Rheum. 2006;54:2481–7.
106. Cauley J, Kwoh C, Egeland G, Nevitt M, Cooperstein L, Rohay J, et al. Serum sex hormones and severity of osteoarthritis of the hand. J Rheumatol. 1993;20:1170–5.
107. De Klerk B, Schiphof D, Groeneveld F, Koes B, van Osch G, van Meurs J, et al. No clear association between female hormonal aspects and osteoarthritis of the hand, hip, and knee: a systematic review. Rheumatology. 2009;48:1160–5.
108. Di Martino A, Barile F, D'Agostino C, Castafaro V, Cerasoli T, Mora P, et al. Are there gender-specific differences in hip and knee cartilage composition and degeneration? A systematic literature review. Eur J Orthop Surg Traumatol. 2024;34:1901–10.
109. Raynauld J. Magnetic resonance imaging of articular cartilage: toward a redefinition of "primary" knee osteoarthritis and its progression. J Rheumatol. 2002;29:1809–10.
110. Wu T, Ni S, Cao Y, Liao S, Hu J, Duan C. Threedimensional visualization and pathologic characteristics of cartilage and subchondral bone changes in the lumbar facet joint of an ovariectomized mouse model. Spine J. 2018;18:663–73.
111. Linn S, Murtaugh B, Casey E. Role of sex hormones in the development of osteoarthritis. PM R. 2012;4:S169–73.
112. Ding C, Cicuttini F, Blizzard L, Scott F, Jones G. A longitudinal study of the effect of sex and age on rate of change in knee cartilage volume in adults. Rheumatology (Oxford). 2007;46:273–9.
113. Jin X, Wang BH, Wang X, Antony B, Zhu Z, Han W, et al. Associations between endogenous sex hormones and MRI structural changes in patients with symptomatic knee osteoarthritis. Osteoarthr Cartil. 2017;25:1100–6.

Part IV
Management of Menopause

11. Hormone Therapy (I): Estrogens, Progestogens, and Androgens

Francisco Quereda

Abstract

Most important ovarian hormones are estrogens, progestins, and androgens. Menopausal ovarian failure leads to hormonal deprivation with variable repercussions among women, such as symptoms with negative effects on quality of life, and changes in future risks of some important and prevalent pathologies. Hormone replacement therapy is the etiologic treatment to avoid all that, but it introduces modifications to these risks, in addition to some side effects. However, many types of composition, formulations, doses, pathways, and schemes are available for hormone therapy, with relevant differences in terms of pharmacokinetics, efficacy, or side effects, that may be even targets for selection, such as the bleeding pattern or lipid profile effects. Therefore, issues like information, indication, therapy selection, acceptance, and compliance are difficult or laborious in many cases and require knowledge and experience from the healthcare professional. In this chapter, we will review and discuss all these topics, the therapeutic plan approach, and follow-up management.

11.1 Introduction

Hormone deprivation is linked to a variety of symptoms and to negative changes in the risk profile of some chronic diseases in women. Although there is a great variability in severity, this deprivation implies a negative impact for many women on her present or future health and/or quality of life. Therefore, perimenopause is an important period in women's life to evaluate the following aspects:

F. Quereda (✉)
Hospital Universitario de San Juan de Alicante, Miguel Hernández University, Alicante, Spain
e-mail: fj.quereda@umh.es

- Identification of climacteric symptoms and alterations in quality of life related to hormone deprivation.
- Estimation of the level of risk of pathologies that may arise in the future, such as osteoporosis or cardiovascular diseases.
- Evaluation and discussion with the woman about whether or not the use of hormone therapy (HT) is appropriate for her.

These topics have been extensively reviewed in other chapters, so, if the decision to start HT is made, the next step is to choose which type of HT might be the most suitable. This is not always an easy decision, given the large number of different alternatives and their implication in compliance, undesirable effects, and efficiency.

In HT prescribing, formulation selection, timing, schedule, dosage, and route of administration are important issues because different alternatives have different effects and perhaps different benefit/risk profiles [1]. In addition, there are a large number of options, so the prescription can be made in a suit-tailored way, looking for the best formulation for the specific woman to be treated [2–4].

Indeed, after the assessment of menopause-related quality of life, health status and health risks in the perimenopausal period of a particular woman, and once the suitability and acceptance for HT use is agreed, it is important to identify the best HT alternative. For that, this chapter will review the role of the different hormones in HT, the alternatives in each group, the treatment schemes, the doses, and their differences. Taken together, this constitutes an important background that menopause healthcare providers must take into account in order to obtain the best final impact on their patients.

So, the final selection of HT for a woman will depend on her context and preferences, as well as on the targets to cover [5, 6]. Besides, reasons to treat or scenarios may change with time, leading to adjustments of treatment. So, a good knowledge of alternatives in the HT components is of great value for prescription, appropriate adherence, and a good effectiveness/risk ratio [7].

11.2 HT Composition and Objectives: Role of Estrogens, Progestogens, and Androgens

The purpose of HT prescription is never to achieve premenopausal hormonal levels. Instead, the objective is to suppress or alleviate the clinical symptoms of hormonal deprivation [8], and this is achieved with doses and schemes that simulate ovarian function, but also with lower doses and even with non-physiologic treatment schemes.

Therefore, once the preferences of a woman have been identified, the target of treatment should be defined, and then, the best suited compound, dose, route, and scheme for this woman should be chosen. In addition, possible collateral effects of a particular form of HT can lead the selection, in order to get or to avoid them, because in some cases they could be pursued while in others avoided [9, 10]. Table 11.1 shows the variables to keep in mind for HT prescription. They should be considered under the perspective of some **general guidelines**:

Table 11.1 Variables to consider about prescription of hormonal treatment

Composition
- Estrogens
- Estrogens and progestins
- Androgens
- Estrogens and androgens
- Estrogens, progestins, and androgens
- Tibolone
- T-SEC compounds or other combinations

Scheme of treatment
- Cyclic or continuous
- Sequential or combined
- Cycle-sequential

Route of administration
- Oral
- Transdermal
- Subcutaneous implants
- Vaginal
- Intramuscular
- Combination of routes

Dosage of treatment
- High
- Standard
- Medium
- Low
- Ultra-low

- Most objectives of HT are achieved by estrogens.
- The inclusion of progestogens in HT is lead to protect endometrium against the risk induced by estrogens use. Therefore, they should not be used when treating women without uterus, unless there is a specific reason to do so.
- In general, progestogens partially reduce some of the beneficial effects of estrogens, like the impact on cardiovascular risk profile, and perhaps introduce a little increase of breast cancer risk depending on the progestogen.
- Progestogens have remarkable differences from each other, which generate a variety of effects that can be desirable for some women, but undesirable for others.
- The inclusion of androgens adds a specific profile of effects, such as improved sexual function and mood, or self-perception of well-being.
- The overall risks profile of androgens is not well defined, but it is known that, for example, they worsen the lipid profile.

11.2.1 Estrogens: Objectives and Alternatives

Estrogens constitute the etiological treatment for climacteric syndrome. Several randomized clinical trials have demonstrated that estrogens are effective in the reduction or suppression of hot flushes and most of the other symptoms related to menopause [8]. Thus, they are the main component of HT.

At present, the evidence-based objectives for estrogens in HT are as follows:

- To avoid, suppress, or alleviate vasomotor, urogenital, and other symptoms related to hormonal deprivation, especially when they affect quality of life. This includes psychological alterations, sexual dysfunction, well-being perception, sleep disturbances, etc.
- To maintain or recover the beneficial effects on multiple targets, among them bone, endothelium, lipid profile, or skin.

Because high estrogenic potency is not required to achieve those objectives, natural estrogens are preferred to synthetic estrogens in HT.

Table 11.2 shows the molecular types of estrogens more frequently used in HT. Among them, estradiol is the most commonly used estrogen in Europe while conjugated equine estrogens (CEE) are so in the United States. In some countries, weaker estrogens like estriol have been frequently used, but it seems that the molecule is advantageous mainly when used for local vaginal treatment. Promestriene is another weak estrogen used for topical vaginal treatment in some countries.

And more recently, estetrol (a native fetal estrogen) is being tested for development as a possible menopause hormone therapy, after its approval for use in contraception [11].

At the beginning of HT treatment, it was thought that the estrogen dose should reproduce, or even exceed, the usual physiological levels of estradiol during the reproductive age. However, it soon became clear that much lower doses reached the goal [12, 13]. A standard dose was then defined (see Table 11.3), which in general afforded the estrogenic blood levels of a sixth to eighth day of the physiological menstrual cycle. The Health, Osteoporosis, Progestin, Estrogen (HOPE) trial

Table 11.2 Alternatives for hormonal treatment composition

Estrogens
– 17-beta-estradiol
– Estradiol valerianate
– Micronized estradiol
– Conjugated equine estrogens
– Estriol
– Promestriene
– Others

Gestagens
– Micronized natural progesterone
– Dydrogesterone
– Medrogestone
– Medroxyprogesterone acetate
– Levonorgestrel
– Norgestrel
– Norethisterone acetate
– Drospirenone

Androgens
– Testosterone
– Methyl-testosterone
– Others

Tibolone
– T-SEC combinations

Table 11.3 Doses of estrogens used for HT

	High dose	Standard dose	Intermediate dose	Low dose	Ultralow dose
Oral estradiol (milligrams)	4 or 3	2	–	1	0.5
Transdermal estradiol (micrograms)	100 or 75	50	37.5	25	–
Conjugated equine estrogens (milligrams)	1.25	0.625	0.45	0.3	–

showed that lower dosages are effective for many targets in women, so that HT might become a woman-tailored selection among different therapeutic possibilities and goal-adjusted [14, 15]. The higher chance for non-desirable effects with higher hormone doses was another reason to search for the lower dose able to achieve the wanted effect [16]. Of interest, the accomplishment of the target does not always correlate with the blood levels of estrogens. Therefore, against the case, of thyroid hormones, the achievement of a concrete level of serum estrogens should never be the goal of HT, nor should be taken as the way to control the treatment effect.

11.2.2 Progestogens: Objectives and Alternatives

It is now well recognized that the use of estrogens without progestogens induces endometrial proliferation, hyperplasia, and even carcinoma. And there is also good evidence about the efficacy of progestogens in the prevention of that adverse effect. So, at present, the main target for using progestogens in HT is the induction of endometrial secretory changes, even atrophy, to counteract the estrogen-induced proliferative effects [2, 3].

Because progestogens reduce the beneficial effects of estrogens on the lipid profile and other targets, they are only recommended for HT in women with uterus; thus, estrogen-only is the appropriate therapy for hysterectomized women. However, when there is risk of recurrence or reactivation of any estrogen-dependent disease, like endometriosis or early-stage endometrial cancer, progestogens are recommended despite the user being previously hysterectomized.

It is remarkable that within the progestogens are included different molecular forms that group them into families with relevant pharmacologic differences among them, with subsequent physiological impact or clinical effects. Therefore, the selection of a progestogen always results from an array of possibilities. Figure 11.1 shows that there is a variety of synthetic progestogens besides natural progesterone and derivatives. All of them protect the endometrium against the proliferative effect of estrogens [17], but their different potency and other effects, metabolic or of other nature, should be considered in the choice. Those alternative effects sometimes are not desired, but other times could be secondary objectives for treatment (androgenic effect for example), and all of that may influence the selection.

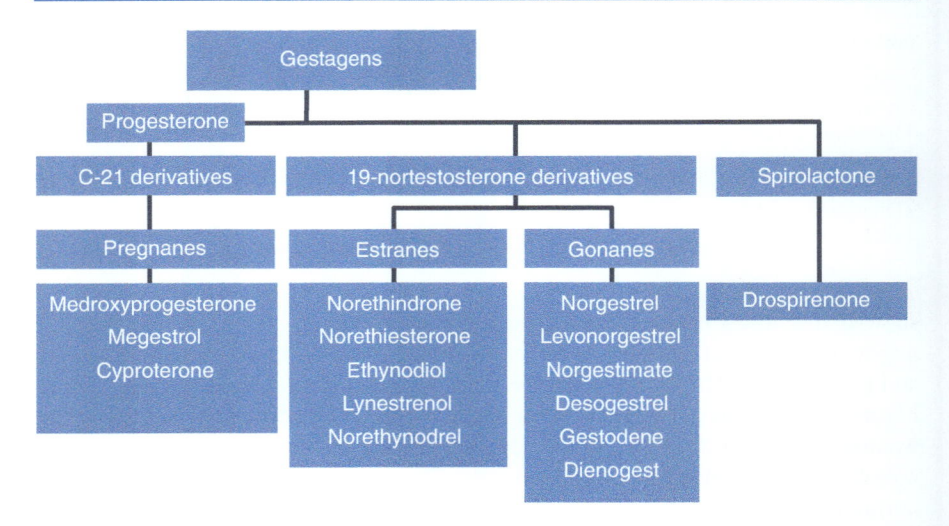

```
                        Gestagens
                            │
   ┌────────────────────────┼────────────────────────┐
Progesterone                │                        │
   │                        │                        │
C-21 derivatives   19-nortestosterone derivatives   Spirolactone
   │                        │                        │
   │               ┌────────┴────────┐               │
Pregnanes        Estranes         Gonanes         Drospirenone
Medroxyprogesterone Norethindrone  Norgestrel
Megestrol        Norethiesterone  Levonorgestrel
Cyproterone      Ethynodiol       Norgestimate
                 Lynestrenol      Desogestrel
                 Norethynodrel    Gestodene
                                  Dienogest
```

Fig. 11.1 Classification of gestagens used for HT between chemical structure

The diversity of progestogens is in part the result of the translation to HT from years of research in the field of contraception, which has searched for a lower neutralizing impact on the beneficial effects of estrogens. Progestogens from the same family share some characteristics, but some differences exist even inside each group, and those specificities should be known.

Some general guidelines and considerations are as follows [2, 3]:

- Natural progesterone has lower potency and more mineral-corticoid blocking effect. A certain diuretic effect has been shown for progesterone, although this is not necessarily reproduced with all of its derivatives, for example, medroxyprogesterone acetate.
- Norderivative progestogens, which could exert some positive effect on sexuality throughout a certain androgenic effect. They also show higher capacity of endometrial protection, although less favorable lipid profile impact than estrogen-only HT.
- Cyproterone acetate, and in a lesser extent drospirenone, has antiandrogenic effect which may be especially desirable for some women. However, drospirenone characteristically adds a weak diuretic effect that contributes to a slight decrease in weight, very much valued by some women.

11.2.3 Androgens: Objectives and Alternatives

Androgen production basically takes place in adrenal glands, ovaries, and testicles and decreases along the life in men and women after 30s. However, in women, ovarian failure determines an accelerated decrease throughout the perimenopausal and postmenopausal periods, although postmenopausal ovaries maintain some androgen production many years afterwards. In fact, when ovaries are removed, the decline in androgen levels is greater than after natural menopause.

Androgens have been related to energy, mood, well-being self-perception, and some parameters of sexuality (libido, activity, arousal, excitability, and satisfaction) [18]. Androgen deficiency has been related to adynamia, sexual dysfunction, and minor depressive states, altogether included in the so named "androgenic deficiency syndrome" [19, 20]. It is remarkable that this is a clinical diagnosis and cannot be defined by serum androgenic levels, although it is more frequent after surgical menopause (among women with the lowest serum levels).

In consistence with the above, the main potential goal for the inclusion of androgens in HT is the improvement of libido, especially when sexual desire is hypoactive and mood and well-being perception are altered. In addition, androgens may help estrogens to reduce vasomotor symptoms, increase the anabolic effect on bone, and, overall, increase sexual activity and satisfaction [21, 22].

However, androgens may induce some adverse effects—like hirsutism, acne, or virilization—particularly when used in doses over physiological threshold. For example, methyl-testosterone (5 mg/day) was satisfactorily used to improve sexuality in women, but the mentioned adverse effects and potential risks discouraged its use at those dosages.

Other concerns about androgens include a negative impact on lipid profile added to a possible increase in cardiovascular and breast cancer risk [23]. Androgens are metabolized to estrogens in a variable degree, so they may contribute to cancer risks by themselves or mediated by induced increases of estrogens. In any case, evidences for impact of androgens on breast cancer risk are scarce, controversial, and inconclusive [3].

In summary, the field in which androgens are specifically appropriate is for women with androgen deficiency syndrome and/or hypoactive sexual desire, in whom low doses have shown a significantly improvement in these aspects, clearly related to quality of life. And effectively, two decades ago, randomized clinical trials demonstrated that the use of transdermal testosterone, at doses inside the physiological premenopausal range, improved sexuality of women with that profile [24]. Testosterone patches afford transdermal administration achieving serum levels within the physiological premenopausal range and being clinically effective for these women.

The lack of commercial availability of transdermal testosterone in some countries has increased the interest on norderivative progestogens, which may be an alternative option providing some of the mentioned effects for androgens. And tibolone brings some of these androgenic effects when used for HT [25], but in many countries is not available.

11.3 HT Tailoring: Dose, Route, and Schemes of Administration

After we have reviewed the different alternatives and objectives for HT, it is necessary to analyze other aspects that contribute to individualize the selection and make it target-directed. Once composition is decided, dose, route, and scheme of treatment should be selected from a diversity of possibilities. Some general guidelines for this purpose are as follows:

- The dose of estrogen should be chosen firstly.
- The lower possible dose of progestogen is preferred, and for that, both dose and duration of treatment are main issues. This selection will depend on estrogenic dose, so that the higher the estrogen, the higher the progestogen dose and/or duration.
- There is an individual variability, and some women get a good control with lower doses than others, and, for example, smokers may need higher doses because they have an accelerated hepatic metabolism of estrogens.

11.3.1 Dose

The goals for HT are achieved in most women with doses that lead to serum estrogenic levels similar to a fifth to eighth day of a normal ovarian cycle. These are considered "standard doses" (Table 11.3). However, some randomized clinical trials showed that lower doses get the goals for many women. These findings reinforced the potential of "low-dose" HT, which is roughly understood as half the standard dose. Even more, it has been shown that even lower doses (ultralow dose of HT) have positive effects, for example, on bone metabolism in older women [26]. These doses are so low that do not induce endometrial proliferation in most cases, although the addition of a progestogen is recommended in some countries.

11.3.1.1 Selection of the Dose of Estrogen

Different approaches can be used to select the appropriate dose of HT. In general, the tendency is to use standard dose of estrogens for younger women, and low-dose HT is more often used for women between 50 and 55, and especially over 55 years of age. Actually, the dose to be used should always be adjusted in order to get the pursued objectives, at the beginning, but also later during the follow-up.

Nowadays, the rule is to give the minimal dose to get the goal [27]. The strategy to reach that stage may be starting with a low dose and then increase step by step when necessary, or either begin with standard dose and introduce changes afterwards if required, trying to reduce the dose some years later if the woman does not worsen with that.

Ultralow-dose HT is an opportunity for older symptomatic women or long-term HT users. Perhaps in the future it could be a useful strategy for some women, like older ones, or with comorbidities, in the case of potential benefits from HT [26]. For example, bone metabolism has shown sensitivity to ultralow dose of estrogens, and patients' acceptance to such a low dose may be better as well.

11.3.1.2 Selection of the Dose of Progestogen

The endometrial protection of progestogens against the proliferative estrogenic stimulus depends on total dose and duration of progestogen per cycle, although the potency of the molecule also has an effect [28]. For example, natural progesterone at a dose of 200 mg/day is needed for at least 10–12 days each cycle for a standard dose of estrogen. Lower doses of estrogen require half dose (100 mg) progesterone.

Some combinations have tried to reduce the dose of progestogen, as shown later in another section.

It is also of interest that commercial preparations of progesterone may be used by oral or vaginal route. The vaginal route avoids first liver pass, and so some secondary effects are reduced or avoided. However, this vaginal route is not well accepted by some women, and compliance may be worse.

11.3.1.3 Selection of the Dose of Androgens

The dose of testosterone approved for HT in Europe is 300 μg/day delivered by a twice-a-week transdermal patch. Randomized clinical trials demonstrated that these patches lead to serum concentrations of testosterone within physiological range and were effective with a good benefit-risk balance. The main indication for this treatment is androgen deficiency and related symptoms (hypoactive sexual disorder or complete androgen deficiency syndrome with adynamia, low well-being status, etc.).

Testosterone may be used in combination with estrogens, because so was done in the trials and especially when symptoms persist in spite of estrogenic treatment. However, testosterone is not available in some countries, and similar effects can be partially obtained with the use of norderivatives progestogens, tibolone, or androgen gel formulations. However, these last gels were designed for men and therefore require dose correction and have lower reliability and blood levels stability than patches.

11.4 Routes of Administration for HT

HT may be administered by different routes (Table 11.1). This broad variety probably means that a perfect route for all women does not exist. The available alternatives have differences in comfort, posology, acceptance, and, consequently, compliance. However, besides, there are pharmacokinetic differences that are clinically relevant when considering side effects, either beneficial or adverse. And those different characteristics may be used to select one or the other while considering women's desire, potential risks, and/or secondary goals of treatment.

11.4.1 Oral HT

This route of administration has the first-pass through the liver as a characteristic. Therefore, there is partial steroid metabolism before systemic bioavailability, which requires a higher daily dose and induces some metabolic hepatic changes. The result is a specific serum estrogenic profile, which differs from the physiological pattern in that there are higher estrone levels and proportions, even when the administered steroid is oral estradiol [4].

The disadvantage of the estrogenic induction of liver enzymes is that the thrombotic and/or hypertensive risk may increase in some women. However, in the other side, oral estrogens favorably change the lipid cardiovascular risk profile, promoting a decrease in total and LDL-cholesterol, as well as in lipoprotein (a). In contrast, HDL-cholesterol and triglycerides increase [4].

This route affords simplicity but also an increase in missing doses and requires consistency.

11.4.2 Transdermal Route

This is a route broadly used in Europe and overall in South European countries. The following aspects characterize this route of administration [29, 30]:

- Estrogenic serum levels are quite uniform and sustained.
- The first-pass through the liver is avoided and logically its related effects. Consequently a very lower dose is required and the serum estrogenic profile is dominated by estradiol, more similar to the premenopausal profile.
- Some evidences suggest a lower risk for this route of estrogenic-associated venous thrombosis and/or hypertension.
- Cholesterol levels are less reduced than with oral route, but triglycerides do not change.
- In the case of patches, some women show a variable local intolerance with erythema, eczema, and/or pruritus.
- Detachment of the patches in some women leads to variable estrogenic levels.
- The use of gel is associated with lower adherence, lower reliability of dose, and daily variability of estrogenic levels (pulse therapy depending on applied dose). Together with efficacy, gels share the characteristics of the transdermal route.

11.4.3 Transvaginal Route for HT

This route can be used for systemic treatment, but this requires higher doses than used for local treatment. In this case, vaginal route shares with transdermal systems the avoidance of the first-pass hepatic effect.

Transvaginal route for systemic HT is restricted to few countries, but vaginal formulations are broadly prescribed for local vaginal treatment using weak estrogens or very low doses of estradiol. The main indication is maintenance or recovery of trophism and improvement of vulvovaginal properties to limit symptoms like dyspareunia and dryness. In fact, vaginal HT is sometimes used associated to systemic HT when the latter is not enough to solve these problems. And of course, the vaginal route is indicated for women who do not desire or do not need systemic HT but suffer local problems.

The transvaginal route with these formulations has reduced systemic absorption and shows no evidence of endometrial proliferation. So, it is considered local HT and is available in the form of pills, ovules, creams, and gel (daily or twice a week), which in general suffer of low compliance as main difficulty and pruritus as main adverse effect.

11.4.4 Other Routes of Administration of HT

Other routes of administration have been used and deserve some comments.

- Intrauterine device (IUD) for delivery of HT only exists for progestogen administration. The doses used for contraception are effective but so high for HT and in some countries are available in different doses.
- Intramuscular depot formulations were broadly used for HT in the past, but nowadays this route is only used for very specific patients, like those with poor compliance with other routes.
- Transrectal route does not seem to add advantages versus vaginal and is not available in most countries.
- Nasal and sublingual are singular routes that contributed to develop the concept of pulse therapy, but are only available in some countries [31]. They have some pharmacokinetics differences and lower general bioavailability of hormones. Briefly, the "pulse-therapy" concept is based on a quite specific genomic effect induced throughout a quick and short peak of estrogenic serum concentration. A low dose is absorbed but is enough to induce nuclear intracellular estrogenic effects, which are sustained for some time while the concentration in serum declines quickly. It has been presumed that the adverse effects might not be induced so rapidly and therefore might be of lower importance, but evidence for that is limited.

11.5 Schemes of Treatment for HT

HT is administered following some specific treatment regimes. Although there is some confusion and controversy, perhaps the clearest terminology to denominate the more usual schemes of treatment is the following:

- Cyclic or continuous HT, based on whether there are, or there are not, periods without treatment.
- Combined or estrogen-only HT, based on whether progestogens are, or are not, associated to estrogen.
- Sequential HT, when a combined HT includes periods of changing doses of progestogen, or without progestogen. And because there is a very low use of cyclic HT nowadays, the frequently used "continuous combined HT" nomenclature denotes a regime in which both estrogen and progestogen are used without

changes in dose and without interruption. In contrast, triphasic formulations are those in which the doses of one or both estrogen and progestogen are changing during the cycle introducing at least three phases [32].
- The cyclo-sequential regime aims at reducing the total progestogen dose while maintaining amenorrhea. Estrogens are administered daily while progestogens are given in alternating phases of 1–3 days separated by 3–4 days without progestogen [33, 34].

These schemes differ sufficiently to justify the selection or one or another in order to get some goals. Concerning the endometrial protection, 12 days of progestogen and an adequate dose related to estrogenic dose are needed in cyclic regimes.

Figures 11.2 and 11.3 graphically show different schemes of associations for HT. Finally, looking for a decrease in total progestin dose and long periods of amenorrhea but accepting a pre-planned bleeding, the long cyclo-sequential schemes are used, when progestin is associated for 12–14 days at higher doses every 2 or 3 months with estrogen-only HT. This last regime requires more strict endometrial surveillance because a small increase in endometrial hyperplasia rate has been found with these regimes.

Table 11.4 summarizes the main characteristics and goals for the different schedules for HT. For example, it can be noticed how in some cases the induction of a deprivation bleeding may be an objective (especially in perimenopausal period); however, avoiding it may be the goal in other cases. Sometimes, it might be helpful to maintain some hormonal variation throughout the treatment cycle (in case of

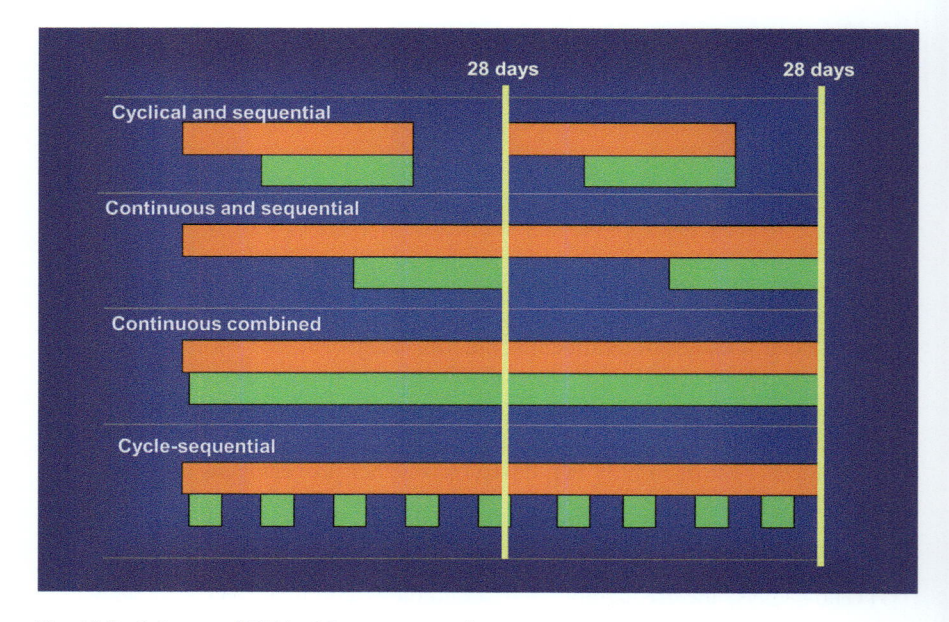

Fig. 11.2 Schemes of HT (red for estrogen and green for progestin administration)

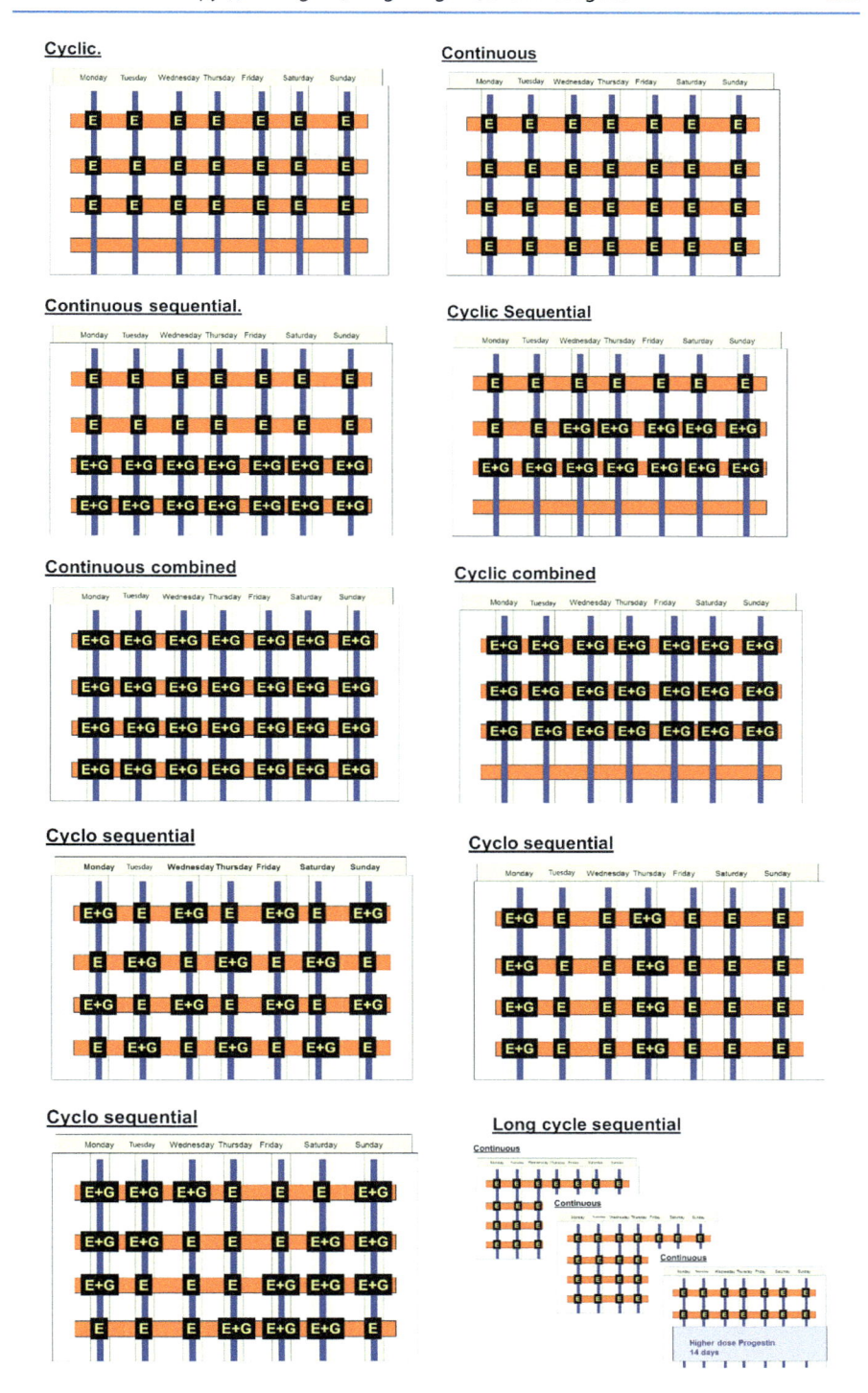

11 Hormone Therapy (I): Estrogens, Progestogens, and Androgens 223

Fig. 11.3 Graphical representation of most usual schemes of treatment for HT. (E: estrogen G: gestagen)

Table 11.4 Characteristics and objectives for different schemes of HT

Scheme of treatment	Characteristics and objectives
Cyclic	To reduce monthly dose of estrogen
	Hormonal variation
	Deprivation bleeding
Continuous	To avoid possible symptomatic periods
	To simplify treatment
	Non hormonal variations
Sequential	Reproduction of physiology
	Hormonal variation
	Deprivation bleeding
Combined	Amenorrhea
	To reduce total progestin dose
	To avoid hormonal variation
	Endometrial atrophy more frequent

decreased libido or depressive tendency, for example), and exactly the opposite might be better for other women, such as when there are premenstrual symptoms.

Therefore, different composition, doses, routes of administration, and schemes of treatment of HT lead to substantial differences that may constitute a main reason for the selection and recommendation of one or the other for a specific woman, in order to increase acceptance and compliance and to minimize side effects and adverse effects.

So, an individual approach, tailored to the wishes and needs of the woman, must be used, and it must be changing according to the response and variations in woman's circumstances and objectives (Fig. 11.4). And therefore, it is necessary for the healthcare providers to know the strategies with proven effectiveness and safety and the differences among them.

Flowchart

Assessment of the status, needs and opportunities of perimenopausal and postmenopausal women
- Current symptoms and foreseeable repercussions
- Assessment of the impact of hormone deprivation on quality of life
- Risk assessment of osteoporosis and cardiovascular disease
- Risk assessment of other common related pathologies

Individualized advice on the use of HT for the specific woman
- Obvious indication of HT
- Contraindication of HT (absolute or relative)
- Preventive option (modification of the foreseeable risk profile)

Treatment selection and proposal
Consider the woman's needs and characteristics and treatment goals.
Woman's agreement
- Composition
- Dose
- Route of administration
- Treatment scheme

Short-term visit
- Response and tolerance assessment
- Possible adjustment or change of treatment
- Setting of goals and horizon of duration plan

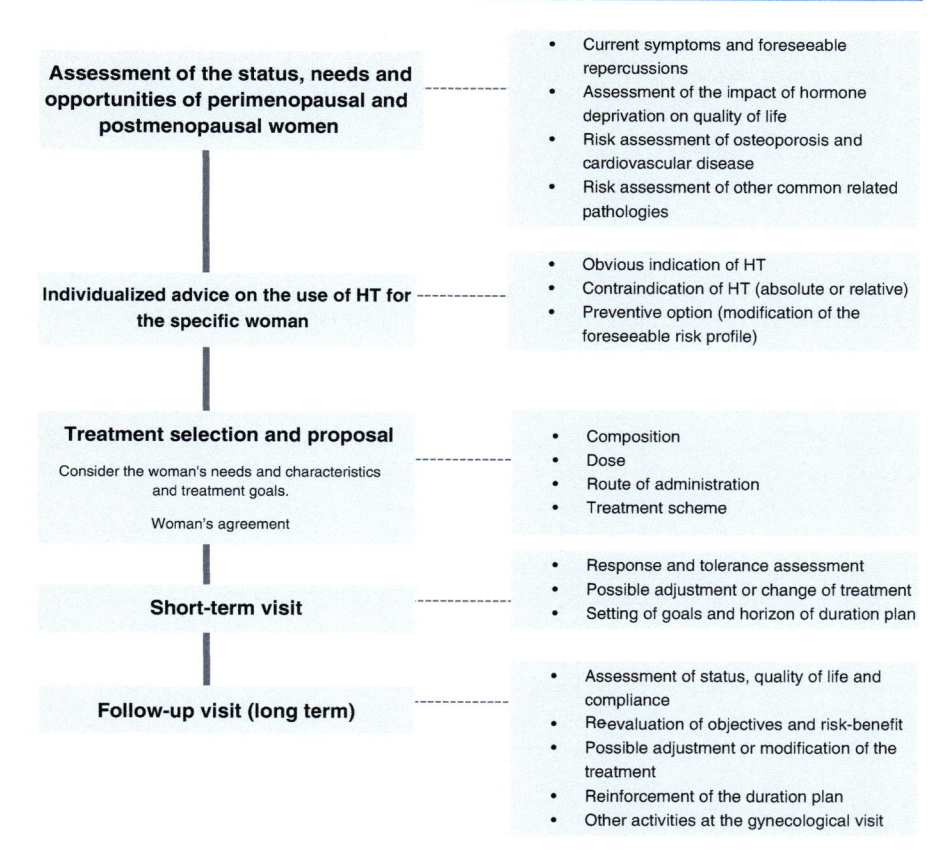

Follow-up visit (long term)
- Assessment of status, quality of life and compliance
- Reevaluation of objectives and risk-benefit
- Possible adjustment or modification of the treatment
- Reinforcement of the duration plan
- Other activities at the gynecological visit

Fig. 11.4 Steps and contents on evaluation and prescription of HT

11.6 HT Follow-Up

Once HT is initiated, a visit in the short term has shown useful for assessment of the effects, adjustment, or change of treatment if required, and to suggest then a plan for the long-term follow-up.

11.6.1 Short-Term Follow-Up Visit

A first visit between the third and the sixth month is not mandatory, but is helpful for verification and reinforcement of compliance. Special attention should be given to detect efficacy and tolerance and absence of adverse effects and, sometimes, to adjust or change the dose or scheme according to results and desires of the user.

Although determination of serum levels of estradiol sometimes may support any decision, a specific threshold never is the target nor is guarantee of good control with HT, so it is not used as a guide. Thus, it is relevant that confirmation of efficacy and adjustment requirements focus on clinical effects, most of them referred by the own woman. Clinical experience has shown that this visit and adequate adjustments improve compliance.

11.6.2 Long-Term Follow-Up

The follow-up of women on HT basically includes the following aspects: prevention and diagnosis of organic pathology, verification of compliance, confirmation of efficacy, and re-evaluation of indication and acceptance of HT and woman's desires and requirements at any time.

After those aspects have been evaluated, a decision based on discussing benefit-risk balance at the moment should be taken. This may result in continuation of HT, modification of dose, route or scheme of treatment, or interruption of treatment.

Each one of these topics deserves some commentaries:

With regard to **prevention and diagnosis of organic pathologies**, women using HT may be followed as untreated women. HT users in general do not require any different strategy, although usually they follow a stricter pattern consisting of higher frequency of regular exams and mammograms, especially women younger of 55 years. In any case, only duration of treatment for longer than 5 years over 55 years of age might be considered as a discrete risk factor for breast cancer and then might be considered for the respective screening.

Of course, any abnormal unexpected uterine bleeding in HT users must be investigated as in non-users. In this sense, both the healthcare provider and the woman should be aware that continuous combined and some cyclo-sequential schemes, despite pursuing amenorrhea, induce occasional bleeding episodes, mainly during the first months of use.

And also, it should be kept in mind that endometrial thickness ultrasound image will be modified depending on the treatment regime and the dose used, and the limits for alert may be higher and more similar to reproductive age in HT users.

With regard to **confirmation of efficacy and adjustment of dose and/or scheme of treatment to women's requirements and desires**, it is in general appropriate to choose the more suitable type, dose, route, and scheme of HT for each particular woman. The target must be the best control of symptomatology, so, when it is not obtained after some months of treatment, the option of modifying treatment should be considered.

Once the objective is obtained, and often after years of use, the target should be to maintain the control with the minimal effective dose. The gradual decrease of dose is a good strategy to prolong the treatment while maintaining a good symptomatic control. And if symptoms recur, consider returning to the previous regimen.

The **review of the indication and acceptance of HT** requires the awareness that a clinically relevant climacteric symptomatology, if no treated, will persist for longer than a few months and often for years. So, the use of HT should be considered as a long-term treatment. However, the benefit-risk ratio should be re-evaluated annually more or less, during the follow-up of each woman. The appearance of a contraindication makes mandatory to withdraw HT, but leaving this aside, it is convenient to inform and discuss benefit-risk at each visit. So, the decision about the persistence of the indication and acceptance to follow HT should be shared between healthcare provider and user. This will require specific information, and the acceptance to continue should take into account each woman's needs and desires. In this context, adjustment of dose and/or scheme of treatment may be done along the time. And in case of doubt, a temporal withdrawal of treatment will clarify if symptoms recur with enough severity to justify the continuation of treatment.

References

1. Brockie J, Lambrinoudaki I, Ceausu I, Depypere H, Erel CT, Pérez-López FR, Schenck-Gustafsson K, van der Schouw YT, Simoncini T, Tremollieres F, Rees M, European Menopause and Andropause Society. EMAS position statement: menopause for medical students. Maturitas. 2014;78(1):67–9.
2. de Villiers TJ, Hall JE, Pinkerton JV, Pérez SC, Rees M, Yang C, Pierroz DD. Revised global consensus statement on menopausal hormone therapy. Maturitas. 2016;91:153–5.
3. "The 2022 Hormone Therapy Position Statement of The North American Menopause Society" Advisory Panel. The 2022 hormone therapy position statement of The North American Menopause Society. Menopause. 2022;29(7):767–794. https://doi.org/10.1097/GME.0000000000002028.
4. Mendoza N, Ramírez I, de la Viuda E, et al. Eligibility criteria for Menopausal Hormone Therapy (MHT): a position statement from a consortium of scientific societies for the use of MHT in women with medical conditions. MHT Eligibility Criteria Group. Maturitas. 2022;166:65–85. https://doi.org/10.1016/j.maturitas.2022.08.008.
5. Alexandersen P, Tanko LB. Algorithm for prescription of HRT or ERT for postmenopausal women. Climacteric. 2006;9(3):238–9.
6. Bastian LA, McBride CM, Fish L, Lyna P, Farrell D, Lipkus IM, et al. Evaluating participants' use of a hormone replacement therapy decision-making intervention. Patient Educ Couns. 2002;48(3):283–91.
7. Castelo-Branco C, Ferrer J, Palacios S, Cornago S. The prescription of hormone replacement therapy in Spain: differences between general practitioners and gynaecologists. Maturitas. 2006;55(4):308–16.
8. Baber RJ, Panay N, Fenton A, IMS Writing Group. 2016 IMS Recommendations on women's midlife health and menopause hormone therapy. Climacteric. 2016;19(2):109–50.
9. Rudy DR. Hormone replacement therapy. How to select the best preparation and regimen. Postgrad Med. 1990;88(8):157–60, 63–4.
10. Purbrick B, Stranks K, Sum C, MacLennan AH. Future long-term trials of postmenopausal hormone replacement therapy—what is possible and what is the optimal protocol and regimen? Climacteric. 2012;15(3):288–93.
11. Gaspard U, Taziaux M, Jost M, Coelingh Bennink HJT, Utian WH, Lobo RA, Foidart JM. A multicenter, randomized, placebo-controlled study to select the minimum effective dose of estetrol in postmenopausal participants (E4Relief): part 2-vaginal cytology, genitourinary syndrome of menopause, and health-related quality of life. Menopause. 2023;30(5):480–9. https://doi.org/10.1097/GME.0000000000002167.
12. Archer DF, Dorin M, Lewis V, Schneider DL, Pickar JH. Effects of lower doses of conjugated equine estrogens and medroxyprogesterone acetate on endometrial bleeding. Fertil Steril. 2001;75(6):1080–7.

13. Lindsay R, Gallagher JC, Kleerekoper M, Pickar JH. Bone response to treatment with lower doses of conjugated estrogens with and without medroxyprogesterone acetate in early postmenopausal women. Osteoporos Int. 2005;16(4):372–9.
14. Fenton A, Panay N. Hormone replacement therapy prescription: a disconnect between personal and patient prescribing. Climacteric. 2012;15(5):409–10.
15. Gambacciani M, Genazzani AR. Hormone replacement therapy: the benefits in tailoring the regimen and dose. Maturitas. 2001;40(3):195–201.
16. Mattsson LA, Skouby SO, Heikkinen J, Vaheri R, Maenpaa J, Timonen U. A low-dose start in hormone replacement therapy provides a beneficial bleeding profile and few side-effects: randomized comparison with a conventional-dose regimen. Climacteric. 2004;7(1):59–69.
17. Panay N, Fenton A. Alternative regimens for endometrial protection? Where are we now? Climacteric. 2011;14(6):607–8.
18. Andersen ML, Alvarenga TF, Mazaro-Costa R, Hachul HC, Tufik S. The association of testosterone, sleep, and sexual function in men and women. Brain Res. 2011;1416:80–104.
19. Bachmann G, Bancroft J, Braunstein G, Burger H, Davis S, Dennerstein L, Goldstein I, Guay A, Leiblum S, Lobo R, Notelovitz M, Rosen R, Sarrel P, Sherwin B, Simon J, Simpson E, Shifren J, Spark R, Traish A, Princeton. Female androgen insufficiency: the Princeton consensus statement on definition, classification, and assessment. Fertil Steril. 2002;77(4):660–5.
20. Howell S, Shalet S. Testosterone deficiency and replacement. Horm Res. 2001;56(Suppl 1):86–92.
21. Penotti M, Sironi L, Cannata L, Vigano P, Casini A, Gabrielli L, et al. Effects of androgen supplementation of hormone replacement therapy on the vascular reactivity of cerebral arteries. Fertil Steril. 2001;76(2):235–40.
22. Shifren JL, Davis SR, Moreau M, Waldbaum A, Bouchard C, DeRogatis L, Derzko C, Bearnson P, Kakos N, O'Neill S, Levine S, Wekselman K, Buch A, Rodenberg C, Kroll R. Testosterone patch for the treatment of hypoactive sexual desire disorder in naturally menopausal women: results from the INTIMATE NM1 Study. Menopause. 2006;13(5):770–9.
23. Gelfand MM, Wiita B. Androgen and estrogen-androgen hormone replacement therapy: a review of the safety literature, 1941 to 1996. Clin Ther. 1997;19(3):383–404.
24. Braunstein GD, Sundwall DA, Katz M, Shifren JL, Buster JE, Simon JA, Bachman G, Aguirre OA, Lucas JD, Rodenberg C, Buch A, Watts NB. Safety and efficacy of a testosterone patch for the treatment of hypoactive sexual desire disorder in surgically menopausal women: a randomized, placebo-controlled trial. Arch Intern Med. 2005;165(14):1582–9.
25. Mendoza N, Abad P, Baró F, Cancelo MJ, Llaneza P, Manubens M, Quereda F, Sánchez-Borrego R. Spanish Menopause Society position statement: use of tibolone in postmenopausal women. Menopause. 2013;20(7):754–60. https://doi.org/10.1097/GME.0b013e31827b18c5.
26. Stute P, Becker HG, Bitzer J, Chatsiproios D, Luzuy F, von Wolff M, Wunder D, Birkhäuser M. Ultra-low dose—new approaches in menopausal hormone therapy. Climacteric. 2015;18(2):182–6. https://doi.org/10.3109/13697137.2014.975198.
27. Johansen OE, Qvigstad E. Rationale for low-dose systemic hormone replacement therapy and review of estradiol 0.5 mg/NETA 0.1 mg. Adv Ther. 2008;25(6):525–51.
28. Burch D, Bieshuevel E, Smith S, Fox H. Can endometrial protection be inferred from the bleeding pattern on combined cyclical hormone replacement therapy. Maturitas. 2000;34(2):155–60.
29. Keller PJ, Hotz E, Imthurn B. A transdermal regimen for continuous combined hormone replacement therapy in the menopause. Maturitas. 1992;15(3):195–8.
30. Simon JA. What's new in hormone replacement therapy: focus on transdermal estradiol and micronized progesterone. Climacteric. 2012;15(Suppl 1):3–10.
31. Sulak PJ, Caubel P, Lane R. Efficacy and safety of a constant-estrogen, pulsed-progestin regimen in hormone replacement therapy. Int J Fertil Womens Med. 1999;44(6):286–96.

32. Rees MC, Kuhl H, Engelstein M, Mattila L, Maenpaa J, Mustonen M. Endometrial safety and tolerability of triphasic sequential hormone replacement estradiol valerate/medroxyprogesterone acetate therapy regimen. Climacteric. 2004;7(1):23–32.
33. Cano A, Tarin JJ, Duenas JL. Two-year prospective, randomized trial comparing an innovative twice-a-week progestin regimen with a continuous combined regimen as postmenopausal hormone therapy. Fertil Steril. 1999;71(1):129–36.
34. Cameron ST, Critchley HO, Glasier AF, Williams AR, Baird DT. Continuous transdermal oestrogen and interrupted progestogen as a novel bleed-free regimen of hormone replacement therapy for postmenopausal women. Br J Obstet Gynaecol. 1997;104(10):1184–90.

Hormone Therapy (II): Tibolone and the TSEC Concept

12

Santiago Palacios and Mariella Lilue

Abstract

Tibolone is a progestin structurally related to norethynodrel. Its mechanism of action is tissue specific. Tibolone, after oral ingestion, is converted to three active metabolites which have different binding affinities to the various sexual steroid receptors. Tibolone has been used in the treatment of climacteric symptoms, improving mood and sexual response, and in the prevention and treatment of osteoporosis. It increases the risk of stroke, and its behavior in the breast is similar to estrogen plus progestin menopause therapy.

Tissue-selective estrogen complex (TSEC) is the combination of a selective estrogen receptor modulator (SERM) with an estrogen. The unique TSEC that we have is the combination of Bazedoxifene (BZA), a SERM of the third generation that is used for osteoporosis management in postmenopausal women at fracture risk, having demonstrated a powerful antiestrogenic effect on the endometrium and conjugated estrogens (CE). This TSEC is designed to not only improve menopausal symptoms and vulvovaginal atrophy but also to prevent bone loss. So it maintains the benefits of estrogen therapy while antagonizes stimulation effects on the endometrium and mammary gland without the effects associated with progestins.

12.1 Tibolone

12.1.1 Introduction

Tibolone ((7α 17)-17-hydroxy-7-methyl-19-norpregnen-5(10)-en-20-In-3-onA, OD14) is a progestin structurally related to norethynodrel. It was developed at the end of 1960s and initially focused on osteoporosis and since then has been shown to

S. Palacios (✉) · M. Lilue
Palacios Clinic of Women's Health, Madrid, Spain
e-mail: spalacios@clinicapalacios.com; mariella.lilue@clinicapalacios.com

have significant effects on other organs and systems, so its use is currently approved primarily for the treatment of vasomotor symptoms in postmenopausal women in more than 70 countries [1].

It is considered that its mechanism of action is tissue specific. This concept has originated as a consequence of three physiological processes:

- Active conversion of molecules leads to differences in the affinity of the metabolites to bind specific receptors.
- As a consequence, physiological tissue or organ responses to a compound are highly dependent on active (local) metabolism, especially when the enzymatic conversion leads to the production of a specific active metabolite.
- A specific response may be expected at the cellular or tissue site.

After oral ingestion, tibolone is converted to three active metabolites: a $\Delta 4$ isomer (especially in endometrial tissue), a 3α-hydroxy metabolite, and a 3β-hydroxy metabolite, which have different binding affinities to the various sexual steroid receptors, which allows them to deploy estrogenic actions, as well as progestational and androgenic actions, both from a basic and clinical point of view [2].

The different metabolites, as well as the original compound, have been tested for their affinity for binding to estrogen, progesterone, or androgen receptors located in the MCF-7 cell nucleus. It has been shown that native tibolone has an affinity for binding to estrogen receptors, as well as progestogen and androgen receptors. Hydroxy metabolites have only affinity to bind to estrogen receptors, whereas the $\Delta 4$-isomer has no affinity for the estrogen receptor [3].

These specific metabolite affinities for binding to sex hormone-specific receptors have led to the prediction of the physiological response of a tissue to a given treatment if known specific tissue metabolism occurs.

For tibolone, this means that, if the tibolone precursor compound is specifically converted to any of the hydroxy metabolites or the $\Delta 4$-isomer, specific tissue hormone activity can be predicted [2, 4].

The main tissue in which the absence or presence of an estrogenic or progestational activity can be demonstrated is, of course, the endometrium. The mechanism, following tissue-specific action (TSA) of tibolone in this tissue, appears to be due to its intrinsic binding properties, in combination with specific endometrial metabolism. In other tissues, such as the bone, breast, or cardiovascular system, different and more complex mechanisms may be involved.

The sum of all these tissue-specific mechanisms of action may explain the interesting clinical profile of this hormone [5], which, like other progestins, can modulate the activity of different enzyme complexes that may influence the in situ production of estradiol, for example, in the breast [6].

We can, however, understand that binding to the receptor is not synonymous with the physiological activity of the product. For example, the affinity of a true antiestrogen to bind to the estrogen receptor is extremely high [7].

Tibolone has been used in the treatment of climacteric symptoms and in the prevention and treatment of osteoporosis for more than 20 years with several trials done (Table 12.1). It effectively controls climacteric symptoms including neuroendocrine, such as hot flashes and night sweats, as well as urogenital symptoms including vaginal dryness and atrophy, but without stimulating the endometrium [8].

As for the breast, it is known that extracellular estrone sulfate (E1S) is the main precursor of estrogen in cancerous mammary cells. E1S reaches the membrane of the tumor cell where it is converted by the action of estrone sulfatase into estrone (E1). Within the cell, E1 is converted to estradiol (E2) by the action of 17β-hydroxysteroid dehydrogenase (17β-HSD). On the other hand, sulfotransferase, on the cell membrane of the tumor cell, converts non-conjugated intracellular estrogens (E1, E2, and estriol) into sulfated estrogens that are secreted into the extracellular medium. Tibolone and its metabolites appear to act via inhibition of enzyme systems, such as sulfatase and 17β-hydroxysteroid dehydrogenase/isomerase (17β-HSD), or via stimulation of cell differentiation and apoptosis. It has been shown that with tibolone these processes occur in both normal and cancerous mammary cells [9–11].

Noting the clinical profile of tibolone, its activity as STEAR (Selective Estrogen Activity Tissue Regulator) is based through the various mechanisms of action mentioned and opening a new therapeutic category.

We know from clinical studies and experience that tibolone is as effective as 1.5 mg of 17β-estradiol, 2 mg of estradiol valerate, or 0.625 mg of conjugated estrogens to control climacteric symptoms, as well as for effects on the bone and in the urogenital tract [12]. However, in a recent systematic review, it was found to be slightly less effective than conventional hormone therapy in the control of vasomotor symptoms [13], but more beneficial in treating symptoms of dizziness and faintness [14].

Table 12.1 Most important tibolone studies: summary

Study	Main purpose	N	Main result
OPAL (2006)	Osteoporosis prevention and lipids in postmenopausal women	866	Tibolone improves bone density and lipids profiles but may alter HDL levels
THEBES (2007)	Tibolone histology of the endometrium and breast endpoints study	3240	Tibolone does not induce endometrial hyperplasia and has a neutral or protective effect on breast tissue
TOTAL (2007)	Tibolone on osteoporosis and total fracture risk	572	Tibolone reduces fracture risk in postmenopausal women
LIFT (2008)	Long-term intervention on fractures with tibolone	4538	Tibolone reduces fracture risk with a low risk of cancer
STEP (2008)	Selective tibolone effects in climacteric symptoms prevention	308	Tibolone alleviates menopausal symptoms, including hot flashes and low libido
LISA (2008)	Livial in sexuality assessment	403	Tibolone improves sexual function in postmenopausal women
LIBERATE (2008)	Livial intervention following breast cancer: efficacy, recurrence, and tolerability endpoints	3058	Tibolone may increase the risk of breast cancer recurrence in women with history of breast cancer

12.1.2 Tibolone and Vasomotor Symptomology

The main indication for the use of hormonal therapy of menopause, whether estrogenic, conventional combined, or tibolone, is the relief of vasomotor symptoms, which has a direct impact on the quality of life of women and, occasionally, those who surround.

Tibolone has demonstrated more or less the same percentage of efficacy over vasomotor symptoms as standard doses of estrogen and gestagen therapy [12–14].

Several authors have shown that the benefits offered by tibolone are not only comparable to those of conventional hormone therapy but are in some respects better. This is reflected in mood, fatigue, or lack of energy and also in improvement in quality of life, probably mediated by its light androgenic effects [12, 13].

12.1.3 Tibolone and Sexuality

There are several aspects of sexuality that have been improved with tibolone, when compared both with placebo and with conventional hormone therapy, that have been well pointed [1, 15, 16].

In relation to placebo: Increase in blood flow and vaginal lubrication; increase in sexual fantasies, desire, and arousal; no differences in coital frequency; sexual activity without penetration or initiation or rejection of sexual activity; and increase in plasma testosterone and sex hormone binding globulin (SHBG).

In relation to conventional hormonal therapy: Increase in sexual desire, orgasms, coital frequency, response, and excitation or satisfaction and increase in plasma testosterone and decrease of SHBG [16, 17].

12.1.4 Tibolone and Bone

Estrogens in preventing or treating osteoporosis act on at least three different levels, according to how the different types of organs that are valued are focused. At skeletal level, they maintain bone mass; at the tissue level, bone remodeling decreases, mainly at the level of bone resorption, due to its cellular and molecular actions, modulating the osteoblast and osteoclast functionality, directly and indirectly affecting the paracrine between these cell strains [18–23].

Because of the importance of the loss of estrogen production in triggering the factors that lead to the development of osteoporosis, it is important to recall the consensus statement published in 1991, which clearly states that osteoporosis can be prevented. The treatment of choice to prevent bone loss in postmenopausal women or with altered ovarian function is hormone therapy at menopause [24].

Tibolone has shown indirect actions on bone, modifying the balance of both calcium and vitamin D3 when compared to non-intervention [25].

Tibolone has an estrogenic effect on bone and prevents postmenopausal bone loss; by selectively blocking the androgen receptor and progesterone receptor in ovariectomized rats, the effect of the drug on bone mineral density is not altered, which is lost when the blocking receptor is estrogen [26]. It has been used in clinical trials for the treatment of climacteric symptoms and in the prevention and treatment of osteoporosis for more than 20 years [27].

In October 2004, a multidisciplinary and international expert panel on menopause management convened at the fourth Menopause Symposium in Amsterdam to determine the specific place for tibolone, a synthetic steroid with a unique clinical profile, among the wide range of therapeutic options for postmenopause available to date [28]. And it was concluded that as regards prevention of bone loss, tibolone is as effective as estrogen therapy (ET)/hormonal therapy (HT), with a level of evidence IA [28, 29]. Subsequently, in the STEP study [30], its superiority to raloxifene was demonstrated in relation to bone mass increase.

Tibolone is able to prevent the development of osteoporosis and also to reduce the risk of fracture, both vertebral (relative risk 0.55, 95% CI 0.41–0.74, $p < 0.001$) and non-vertebral (relative risk 0.74, 95% CI 0.58–0.93, $p < 0.001$) in osteoporotic women as demonstrated in the long intervention fracture trial (LIFT) study at a dose of 1.25 mg daily. The LIFT study [31] was designed as a prospective, randomized, double-blind, placebo-controlled, 3-year (+2 extension), multicenter (worldwide) study. The predictions were intended to include 4000 women with fractures (2000 tibolone and 2000 placebo), and all included patients received between 400–800 IU/day vit. D and 500–1000 mg/day calcium. The main objective of the study was to detect the occurrence of new vertebral fractures. Secondary endpoints included non-vertebral fractures, BMD, bone turnover markers, quality of life, changes in patient height, cognitive function, and economic impact of the intervention.

For a median of 34 months of treatment, the tibolone group, compared to the placebo group, had a decreased risk of vertebral fracture, with 70 cases versus 126 cases per 1000 person-years (relative risk, 0.55; 95% confidence interval [CI]: 0.41–0.74, $p < 0.001$), and a lower risk of non-vertebral fractures, with 122 cases compared to 166 cases per 1000 person-years (relative risk, 0.74, 95% CI, 0.58–0.93, $p = 0.01$). The tibolone group also had a reduction in the risk of invasive breast cancer (RR 0.32, 95% CI, 0.13–0.80, $p = 0.02$) and colon cancer (relative risk, 0.31; 95% CI, 0.10–0.96, $p = 0.04$). However, in the tibolone group, there was an increased risk of stroke (relative risk, 2.19, 95% CI, 1.14–4.23, $p = 0.02$), whereby the study was stopped in February 2006 by recommendation of the data and the safety advice. There were no significant differences in the risk of coronary heart disease or venous thromboembolism between the two groups.

The conclusion of the study was that tibolone reduced the risk of fracture and breast cancer and colon cancer, but increased the risk of stroke in elderly women with osteoporosis [31].

12.1.5 Tibolone and Cardiovascular System

Although tibolone decreases high-density lipoprotein (HDL) cholesterol, unlike the lipid effects of oral estrogens, it also induces a significant decrease in triglycerides, which are an independent risk factor for insulin resistance and for heart disease [32]. Data from a meta-analysis show that tibolone treatment administered in postmenopausal women increased body mass index (BMI) and c-reactive protein [33] but did not change body weight and waist circumference (WC) [33–35].

In the OPAL study [34], annual carotid intima-media thickness (CIMT) values were significantly higher in the tibolone and EEC/AMP groups compared to placebo.

As regards carbohydrate metabolism in women with and without diabetes mellitus, it has been observed that tibolone does not modify blood levels of glucose, insulin, C-peptide, or glycosylated hemoglobin, nor does it modify the glucose tolerance curve [33–35].

The results of the OPAL study [34] and the increased risk of stroke demonstrated in the LIFT study [31] point to tibolone as a hormone with the same cardiovascular risks as estrogen and gestagen therapy.

12.1.6 Tibolone Safety

12.1.6.1 Endometrium

This molecule has been shown to produce no estrogenic effect on the endometrium, either by selective conversion to the $\Delta 4$ tibolone metabolite or by its affinity for progesterone receptors. This leads, from the clinical point of view, to a lower tendency for spotting/bleeding (especially in the first months) than conventional combined hormone therapy, which in the long run is at least as safe as traditional regimens [36, 37], as demonstrated in the THEBES study, comparing face to face with the fixed combination of equine conjugated estrogens + medroxyprogesterone acetate [36].

12.1.6.2 Breast

Although there are discordant results among epidemiological studies, the Million Women Study [38] found that among the 828.923 postmenopausal women included in the main analysis, the risk of breast cancer was significantly higher among hormone therapy users than among non-users (RR = 1.43, 95% CI, 1.36–1.50). This increased risk was largely confined to current users, rather than to users in the past. The RR of breast cancer was significantly higher in current users of E alone (1.30, 95% CI, 1.22–1.38), $E + P$ (2.00, 95% CI, 1.91–2.09), and tibolone (1.45, 95% CI, 1.17–1.76). The magnitude of the increase in risk is very different in these three types of HT and was significantly higher in the current users of $E + P$ ($p < 0.0001$). However, recent data from a South Korean cohort suggests that the risk of breast cancer is not increased by tibolone and the mortality rate from breast cancer is lower [39].

As any preparation with estrogenic action, tibolone is not indicated in the treatment of climacteric syndrome in survivors of breast cancer, as shown by the LIBERATE [40] study. The LIBERATE study [40] was a randomized, controlled, double-blind, multi-center study between tibolone 2.5 mg/day vs. placebo, with a mean follow-up of 3.1 years. The study population was 3058 women with surgical treatment for breast cancer and vasomotor symptoms (mean time of surgery

2.1 years). The results showed a significantly higher rate of recurrence of breast cancer with tibolone than with placebo (RR 1.40). So the study stopped 6 months earlier than planned.

12.1.7 Conclusion

Tibolone, with its different mechanisms of action, has unique characteristics that allow it to approach what has traditionally been considered a good profile of hormonal therapy in menopause, since it allows controlling the climacteric symptoms, improving mood, sexual response, the state of the genitals, and protecting the bone, but without stimulating the endometrium. It also has a beneficial effect on several intermediary indicators of cardiovascular risk, although it increases the risk of stroke and its behavior in the breast is similar to estrogen/progestin hormone therapy.

Tibolone is the first of a new class of compounds, the STEAR, which describe molecules with Selectively Tissue Estrogenic Activity Regulators activity.

12.2 TSEC

12.2.1 Introduction

Tissue selective estrogen complex (TSEC) is a combination of Bazedoxifene (BZA) with conjugated estrogens (CE), and it is a therapeutic option for the management of menopausal symptoms and prevention of postmenopausal osteoporosis [41].

The rationale for TSEC development was that the SERM component would minimize adverse estrogenic effects on the endometrium and breast, while maintaining the beneficial effects of estrogens on menopausal symptoms [42]. BZA was specifically selected as this SERM because it showed favorable preclinical effects on the skeleton, vasomotor activity, and lipid metabolism, as well as mammary and uterine safety [43]. Gene expression profiling of CE in combination with three different SERMs (BZA, raloxifene, and lasoxifene) showed differential patterns of gene expression, indicating that different SERM/CE combinations may have distinct clinical activities [44].

BZA is a third-generation SERM with phenyl rings which act as binding sites for the alpha and beta estrogen receptors but with greater affinity for alpha [45]. This SERM has been extensively studied in preclinical [45, 46] and in clinical studies [45, 47]. In addition to the CE, sex steroid hormones derived from cyclopentanoperhydrophenanthrene also have a great experience with both preclinical [46, 48–51] and clinical studies [52–54].

The efficacy and safety of the combination of BZA/CE for menopausal symptoms and prevention of postmenopausal osteoporosis have also been evaluated in preclinical models. The two points to evaluate for safety were endometrium and breast. Preclinical data have shown that whereas CE alone stimulates proliferation of MCF-7 and T47D human breast cancer cells and reduces cell apoptosis, the addition of BZA at an adequate dose level abrogates these effects [55]. BZA, but not RLX or LAS, antagonized CE-induced increases in uterine wet weight to levels similar to vehicle control [56]. Several studies in rats and monkeys found a safety and efficacy profile while using BZA/CE, different for the one found with estrogen alone, SERMs, and other SERMs with estrogens [44, 48–50].

12.2.2 Clinical Studies

The combination of BZA/CE has been evaluated in different multicenter, randomized, double-blind, placebo control and placebo active, called selective estrogens menopause and response to therapy (SMART) (Table 12.2).

The Study 303, SMART 1 with 3397 patients in 94 sites in the United States, Europe, and Brazil, included healthy postmenopausal women between 40 and 75 years, with uterus, BMI $\leq$32.2 kg/m^2, and normal endometrial biopsy before admission. Its main objective was to evaluate the efficacy of multiple doses of BZA/CE (combination of BZA 10, 40, 20, and 0.45 mg CE or CE 0.625 mg) in endometrial protection, VMS, vulvovaginal atrophy, and osteoporosis prevention. The study duration was 24 months [52, 53, 57, 58].

The Study 305, SMART 2 with 318 patients at 43 sites in the United States, included healthy postmenopausal women aged 40–65 years with a uterus and BMI $\leq$34 kg/m^2. It should have 7 or more hot flashes a day of moderate to severe, or a minimum of 50 a week before starting the study and wishing to start handling them. This study evaluated the effects of BZA 20 mg/CE 0.45 mg and BZA 20 mg/CE 0.625 mg in the improvement of VMS compared with placebo at 12 weeks of treatment. The main result was to see the decrease in intensity and frequency of hot flashes, and secondary were the effects on sleep, quality of life, and satisfaction with treatment [53, 59].

Table 12.2 Selective estrogens menopause and response to therapy (SMART) trials: summary

Studies	Primary objective	Number of subjects	Main result
SMART 1	Evaluate the efficacy and safety of BZA/CE in menopausal symptoms	3397	BZA/CE reduces hot flashes and other menopausal symptoms
SMART 2	Asses the effects on bone density and fracture risk	318	BZA/CE improves bone density
SMART 3	Investigate the impact on the endometrium with BZA/CE	652	BZA/CE helps protect the endometrium from hyperplasia compared to CE alone
SMART 4	Investigate the effects of BZA/CE on the cardiovascular system	1061	BZA/CE does not significantly increase cardiovascular risk
SMART 5	Evaluate the long-term safety of BZA/CE	1843	BZA/CE shows a favorable long-term safety profile

The Study 306, SMART 3 with 652 patients in 66 sites in the United States, included healthy postmenopausal women aged 40–65 years with a uterus and BMI ≤34 kg/m². All had to have vaginal cytological smear with no more than 5% of superficial cells, vaginal pH >5, and VMS least moderate to severe before admission. This study evaluates the effectiveness on vulvovaginal symptoms in women with vulvovaginal atrophy over a period of 12 weeks [60, 61].

SMART 4 (304) study with 1061 patients was a multicenter, double-blind, placebo, and active controlled phase III study in non-hysterectomized postmenopausal women. This study evaluated the effects of BZA 20 mg/CE 0.45 mg and BZA 20 mg/CE 0.625 mg compared with CE/MPA, BZA, and placebo on endometrium and bone mineral density. It lasted for 12 months [62].

The Study 3307, SMART 5 with 1843 patients in 166 sites in the United States, Europe, Latin America, Australia, and New Zealand, included healthy postmenopausal women aged 40–75 years with a uterus and BMI ≤34 kg/m² with normal endometrial biopsy result before admission. It evaluated the efficacy of BZA/CE on endometrial protection, osteoporosis prevention, and effects on breast density. This study evaluated the effects of BZA 20 mg/CE 0.45 mg and BZA 20 mg/CE 0.625 mg compared with CE/MPA, BZA, and placebo. It lasted for 12 months [54, 63].

12.2.3 Effects on Vasomotor Symptoms and Quality of Live

Two clinical studies, SMART 1 and 2, assessed the efficacy of BZA/CE for the treatment of moderate to severe VMS. Both combinations of BZA 20 mg/CE 0.45 mg and BZA 20 mg/CE 0.625 mg were associated with a marked improvement of VMS compared with placebo [53].

SMART 1 showed a decrease in perception of intensity ($p < 0.05$ vs. placebo) and frequency ($p < 0.001$ vs. placebo) of hot flashes at 4 and 12 weeks with BZA 20 mg/CE 0.45 mg and BZA 20 mg/CE 0.625 mg, which indicates the effectiveness for treating VMS even to 2 years of therapy [53].

SMART 2 showed that using BZA 20 mg/CE 0.45 mg and BZA 20 mg/CE 0.625 mg there was a significant decrease ($p < 0.001$) at 2 and 4 weeks in the number of moderate–severe hot flushes (HF) per day compared with placebo. A reduction of 5–6 HF per day with the use of this therapy compared to a decrease of three flushing with placebo and representing a significant improvement in BZA/CE treatment [53].

Data from this two randomized, double-blind, placebo- and active-controlled, phase 3 studies were pooled for nonhysterectomized postmenopausal women with moderate/severe hot flushes (HF) given BZA 20 mg/CE 0.45 mg, BZA 20 mg/CE 0.625 mg, or placebo for 12 weeks. HF frequency and severity were assessed by daily diary [64]. The pooled analysis included 403 participants. At 12 weeks, BZA 20 mg/CE 0.45 mg and BZA 20 mg/CE 0.625 mg significantly (all $p < 0.001$) decreased moderate/severe HF frequency versus placebo (−7.9, −8.2, −4.1), reduced adjusted average daily HF severity score versus placebo (−1.0, −1.3, −0.3), and increased the percentage of women who had a ≥50% (81.2%, 87.1%, 50.6%)

and ≥75% (62.4%, 74.8%, 26.4%) reduction from baseline in daily frequency of moderate/severe HFs. Significantly improved MENQOL vasomotor function versus placebo (adjusted mean change-3.08, −3.69, −1.37). BZA/CE was significantly more effective than placebo irrespective of time since menopause, with some evidence of a lower placebo response in women in later menopause (>5 years) versus early menopause (≤5 years) (65%).

In other analysis of these two studies, the conclusion was that BZA/CE affected the MENQOL vasomotor domain both directly and indirectly, whereas effects on other domains were fully mediated via HF severity reductions [65].

12.2.4 Effects on Vulvovaginal Atrophy

The decrease in estrogen in postmenopausal women can also lead to vulvovaginal symptoms that may associated with sexual dysfunction and alter quality of life. These aspects were evaluated in SMART 1 and 3 [52, 60].

The SMART 3 study evaluated the efficacy of BZA 20 mg/CE 0.45 mg and BZA 20 mg/CE 0.625 mg on vulvovaginal symptoms in women with vaginal maturation index with no more than 5% superficial cells, pH > 5, with moderate to severe vulvovaginal symptoms. Both combinations of BZA 20 mg/CE 0.45 mg and BZA 20 mg/CE 0.625 mg showed an increase in superficial cell compared to placebo ($p < 0.001$) and a decrease in vaginal pH ($p < 0.001$) as well as an improvement in annoying vulvovaginal symptoms for women compared to placebo ($p < 0.05$). Those include dyspareunia, vaginal dryness, and itching [60].

SMART 1 shows similar results in terms of increased superficial cells compared to placebo ($p < 0.001$). These changes on epithelial maturation had had a significant relationship with dyspareunia: decreased compared with placebo during 9–12 weeks of therapy ($p < 0.001$) and improved lubrication compared to placebo ($p < 0.05$) in the Arizona Sexual Experience scale (ASEX), which has a positively impact on quality of life measured by the MENQOL [52].

12.2.5 Effects on Bone Mass

The effect on bone was evaluated by three studies. SMART 1 and where it was found at 12 months of treatment increased lumbar spine BMD using BZA 20 mg/CE 0.45 mg of 1.05% and 0.25% increase in SMART 5, and using BZA 20 mg/CE 0.625 mg, the increase was 1.05% and 0.60% in SMART 1 and 5, respectively, compared to placebo (−1.81% and −1.28%) [54, 57].

In both studies, SMART 1 and 5, significant increases at 12 months in total hip BMD were found compared to the placebo group $p < 0.05$ and $p < 0.001$, respectively [54, 57].

In the 303 study, SMART 1, the increase in BMD at the lumbar spine ($p < 0.001$) and total hip ($p < 0.05$) was observed with the use of BZA 20 mg/CE 0.45 mg and BZA 20 mg/CE 0.625 mg at 12 and 24 months follow-up compared to placebo.

With respect to raloxifene, the BZA/CE at 24 months showed a greater increase in BMD. In women who have been menopausal for less than 5 years, the telopeptide-C levels at 6, 12, 18, and 24 months with BZA 20 mg/CE 0.45 mg and BZA 20 mg/CE 0.625 mg were significantly lower compared to placebo (for all, $p < 0.001$) [57].

These two studies, SMART 1 and SMART 5, were pooled for BMD, and the turnover marker is over 12 months [66]. There were 1172 women, with mean age 54.9 years, mean 6.21 years since menopause, mean lumbar spine, and total hip T scores -1.05 and -0.58; 58.8% had a Fracture Risk Assessment Tool score less than 5% indicating low fracture risk. At 12 months, adjusted differences (vs. placebo) in BMD change in the groups taking conjugated estrogens 0.45 or 0.625 mg plus bazedoxifene 20 mg were 2.3% and 2.4% for lumbar spine, 1.4% and 1.5% for total hip, and 1.1% and 1.5% for femoral neck (all $p < 0.001$ vs. placebo). These increases were unrelated to baseline Fracture Risk Assessment Tool score, age, years since menopause, body mass index, or geographic region. Both doses reduced bone turnover markers ($p < 0.001$) [66].

In the third study, SMART 4 (304) with 1061 patients, both BZA/CE doses (20 mg/CE 0.45 mg and BZA 20 mg/CE 0.625) significantly increased lumbar spine and total hip BMD, versus placebo ($p < 0.001$) [62].

In a small study carried out on 40 postmenopausal women, the combination of BZA/CE has shown improvements in bone strength evaluated by hip structural analysis (HAS) after 12 months [67]. In conclusion, bazedoxifene/conjugated estrogens significantly improved BMD and turnover in a large population of younger postmenopausal women at low fracture risk and are a promising therapy for preventing postmenopausal bone loss.

12.2.6 BZA/CE Safety

Based on the SMART study, doses of BZA 20 mg/CE 0.45 mg and BZA 20 mg/CE 0.625 mg are not only well tolerated but also have a good safety profile which approves its use in healthy postmenopausal patient with uterus [52, 53, 60]. Adverse events and discontinuation of the treatment secondary to these events were similar in all groups.

12.2.6.1 Endometrium
Endometrial protection is the main thing to keep in mind in postmenopausal patients with uterus receiving estrogens. The combination of BZA 20 mg/CE 0.45 mg and BZA 20 mg/CE 0.625 mg showed a low incidence (<1%) for endometrial hyperplasia and cancer similar to placebo during 24 months of treatment. Therefore, the selective activities of SERMs in the combination of BZA/CE are the key to the endometrial protection [52]. At 12 months, in SMART 5, endometrial hyperplasia incidence was low (<1%) and similar with CE/BZA or placebo [54].

Ultrasound reports obtained from transvaginal ultrasounds show with the use of BZA/CE an almost neutral effect on the endometrium at 12 months of treatment (less 1 mm) very similar to what was observed with placebo [52].

Women using CE/medroxyprogesterone acetate (MPA) in SMART 5 had a greater increase in endometrial thickness >5 mm compared with BZA/CE or placebo. Both SMART 1 and 5 evaluated vaginal bleeding and found that using BZA 20 mg/CE 0.45 mg and 0.625 mg was associated with higher cumulative amenorrhea, similar to placebo, in proportion >83%, >87%, >85%, respectively [54, 68]. In SMART 4 study with 1061 patients at 1 year, no cases of endometrial hyperplasia were identified in the BZA 20 mg/CE 0.45 mg group, while 3 cases (1.1%) where confirmed for the BZA 20 mg/CE 0.625 mg group [62].

In a retrospective cohort study including 82 postmenopausal women who received TSEC after switching from another hormone therapy due to adverse events, TSEC proved to be a good option in patients who switched to conventional hormonal therapy due to bleeding disorders [69].

12.2.6.2 Breast

Although the number of patients and the time of treatment were insufficient to draw conclusions across studies, no difference was observed in the incidence of breast cancer 2 years between groups of BZA/CE and placebo (BZA 20 mg/CE 0.45 mg, $n = 1$, BZA 20 mg/CE 0.625 mg, $n = 0$, placebo, $n = 1$) [70]. Data in rodent mammary cells show that CEE stimulates apoptosis (cleaved caspase-3) and BZA exerts very potent antiestrogenic effects by completely blocking the formation of palpable tumors. These data suggest that CEE/BZA is safe for the breast [71].

The effects of BZA/CE on the incidence of pain and breast tenderness were studied in SMART 1, 2, and 5. The pain was evaluated by diaries made by the patient. The use of BZA 20 mg/CE 0.45 mg and 0.625 mg showed no significant difference in pain and breast tenderness compared to placebo, raloxifene, or BZA 20 mg alone [52].

In SMART 5, the incidence of pain and tenderness using BZA/CE was significantly lower compared with women treated with CE 0.45 mg/MPA 1.5 mg ($p < 0.001$). BZA 20 mg/CE 0.45 mg and BZA 20 mg/CE 0.625 mg did not show inferiority compared to placebo in terms of changes in breast density, different from what was found in patients using CE/MPA [52, 59]. The results show that using BZA 20 mg/CE 0.45 mg and BZA 20 mg/CE 0.625 mg have neutral effect (similar to placebo) in breast density [54].

12.2.6.3 Cardiovascular Disease

In a recent study [72], it was pooled in cardiovascular adjudicated safety data from healthy, non-hysterectomized, postmenopausal women who received ≥1 dose of CE 0.45 mg/BZA 20 mg ($n = 1585$), CE 0.625 mg/BZA 20 mg ($n = 1583$), any CE/BZA dose ($n = 4868$), or placebo ($n = 1241$) for up to 2 years in 5 trials. Venous thromboembolic events (VTEs), coronary heart disease (CHD), and cerebrovascular events were reviewed using a meta-analytic approach.

The rate of VTEs per 1000 woman-years (95% confidence interval, CI) was 0.3 (0.0–2.0) in women taking BZA 20 mg/CE 0.45 mg, 0 (0.0–1.5) in those taking BZA 20 mg/CE 0.625, 0.7 (0.0–1.5) among women taking any BZA/CE dose, and 0.6 (0.0–2.9) with placebo. The incidence of stroke per 1000 woman-years (95% CI) was 0.4 (0.0–2.4), 0.2 (0.0–1.9), 0.44 (0.0–1.1), and 0.0 (0.0–1.7), respectively. The CHD rate per 1000 woman-years was 2.6 (0.0–5.6), 1.4 (0.0–3.9), 2.4 (1.00–3.7), and 2.0 (0.0–5.2). Compared with placebo, relative risk (95% CI) with any BZA/CE dose was 0.5 (0.1–1.8) for VTE, 0.5 (0.1–2.6) for stroke, and 0.63 (0.23–1.74) for CHD [69].Up to 2 years, BZA/CECE had an acceptable cardiovascular safety profile, with rates of stroke and CHD comparable to placebo in healthy postmenopausal women. VTE risk was low [72].

12.2.6.4 Lipids and Coagulation Factors

In the SMART 5 trial, evaluated lipid ($n = 1843$) and coagulation ($n = 590$) variables were assessed in women receiving daily BZA 20 mg/CE 0.45 mg, BZA 20 mg/CE 0.625 mg, BZA 20 mg, CE 0.45 mg/medroxyprogesterone acetate (MPA) 1.5 mg, or placebo for 12 months [73].

At 12 months, BZA 20 mg/CE 0.45 mg, BZA 20 mg/CE 0.625 mg, BZA 20 mg, and CE 0.45 mg/MPA 1.5 mg decreased total cholesterol and low-density lipoprotein cholesterol compared with placebo ($p < 0.01$ for all). Both BZA/CE doses and CE/MPA increased high-density lipoprotein cholesterol compared with placebo ($p < 0.05$ for all). BZA 20 mg/CE had a neutral effect on triglycerides. Both BZA/CE doses were associated with small but significant effects on hemostasis variables, including reductions in antithrombin, plasminogen activator inhibitor-1, and fibrinogen activity and an increase in plasminogen activity relative to placebo at 12 months [73].

Although recent data indicate that in mouse models, chronic treatment with CE + BZA protects against thrombosis induced in vivo, also without significant functional alterations in the levels of coagulation factors [74]. However, it would be important to have data from real-life observations in postmenopausal women who have consumed TSEC for more than 5 years.

12.2.7 Conclusion

The TSEC is a new therapy and an alternative for the management of menopausal symptoms and bone loss with the protective effect up to 2 years in the breast and endometrium.

Treatment with BZA/CE has been shown in preclinical and clinical studies of its safety profile and tolerability making a significant change in improving VMS, VVA, and osteoporosis prevention in postmenopausal women as well as security in lipid and as cardiovascular profile. Thrombotic events do not show a higher incidence compared to placebo, being able to compare them with estrogens or SERMs.

Author's Contribution Both authors declare that they have jointly carried out an exhaustive examination of the topic and have contributed equally to the writing of the text.

References

1. Mendoza N, Abad P, Baró F, Cancelo MJ, et al. Spanish Menopause Society position statement: use of tibolone in postmenopausal women. Menopause. 2013;20:754–60.
2. Palacios S. Tibolone: what does tissue specific activity mean? Maturitas. 2001;37(3):159–65. Review.
3. Kloosterboer HJ. Tibolone and its metabolites: pharmacology, tissue specificity and effects in animal models of tumors. Gynecol Endocrinol. 1997;11(Suppl 1):63–8.
4. Rymer JM. The effects of tibolone. Gynecol Endocrinol. 1998;12:213–20.
5. Genazzani AR, Benedek-Jaszmann LJ, Hart DM, Andolsek L, Kicovic PM, Tax L. Org OD 14 and the endometrium. Maturitas. 1991;13:243–51.
6. Lello S, Capozzi A, Scambia G, Franceschini G. Tibolone and breast tissue: a review. Reprod Sci. 2023;30(12):3403–9.
7. Brzozowski AM, Pike CWA, Dauter Z, et al. Molecular basis of agonism and antagonism in the oestrogen receptor. Nature. 1997;389:753–8.
8. Formoso G, Perrone E, Maltoni S, Balduzzi S, Wilkinson J, Basevi V, Marata AM, Magrini N, D'Amico R, Bassi C, Maestri E. Short-term and long-term effects of tibolone in postmenopausal women. Cochrane Database Syst Rev. 2016;10(10):CD008536. https://doi.org/10.1002/14651858.CD008536.pub3. PMID: 27733017; PMCID: PMC6458045.
9. Gompel A, Somai S, Chaouat M, et al. Hormonal regulation of apoptosis in breast cells and tissues. Steroids. 2000;65:593–8.
10. Chetrite G, Kloosterboer HJ, Pasqualini JR. Effect of 'tibolone' (Org OD14) and its metabolites on estrone sulphatase activity in MCF-7 and T-47D mammary cáncer cells. Anticancer Res. 1997;17:135–40.
11. de Gooyer ME, Overklift Vaupel Kleyn GT, Smits KC, et al. Tibolone: a compound with tissue specific inhibitory effects on sulfatase. Mol Cell Endocrinol. 2001;183:55–62.
12. Moore RA. Livial—a review of clinical studies. Br J Obstet Gynaecol. 1999;106(Suppl 19):1–21.
13. Formoso G, Perrone E, Maltoni S, et al. Short and long terms effects of tibolone in postmenopausal women. Cochrane Database Syst Rev. 2012;2:CD008536.
14. Hsiao SM, Liao SC. Effect of tibolone versus hormone replacement therapy on climacteric symptoms and psychological distress. J Chin Med Assoc. 2024;87(2):189–95. https://doi.org/10.1097/JCMA.0000000000001012.
15. Palacios S, Menendez C, Jurado AR, Castaño R, Vargas JC. Changes in sex behaviour after menopause: effects of tibolone. Maturitas. 1995;22(2):155–61.
16. Nijland EA, Weijmar Schultz WC, Nathorst-Boös J, Helmond FA, Van Lunsen RH, Palacios S, Norman RJ, Mulder RJ, Davis SR, LISA Study Investigators. Tibolone and transdermal E2/NETA for the treatment of female sexual dysfunction in naturally menopausal women: results of a randomized active-controlled trial. J Sex Med. 2008;5(3):646–56.
17. Hsiao SM, Chang SR. Effect of tibolone versus hormone replacement therapy on lower urinary tract symptoms and sexual function. J Formos Med Assoc. 2024;123(6):710–5. S0929-6646(23)00487-4.
18. Srivastava S, Weitzmann MN, Kimble RB, et al. Estrogen blocks M-CSF gene expression and osteoclast formation by regulating phosphorylation of Egr-1 and its interaction with Sp-1. J Clin Invest. 1998;102:1850–9.
19. Srivastava S, Weitzmann MN, Cenci S, Ross FP, Adler S, Pacifici R. Estrogen decreases TNF gene expression by blocking JNK activity and the resulting production of c-Jun and JunD. J Clin Invest. 1999;104:503–13.
20. Sunyer T, Lewis J, Collin-Osdoby P, Osdoby P. Estrogen's bone-protective effects may involve differential IL-1 receptor regulation in human osteoclast-like cells. J Clin Invest. 1999;103:1409–18.
21. Simonet WS, Lacey DL, Dunstan CR, et al. Osteoprotegerin: a novel secreted protein involved in the regulation of bone density. Cell. 1997;89:309–19.

22. Srivastava S, Toraldo G, Weitzmann MN, Cenci S, Ross FP, Pacifici R. Estrogen decreases osteoclast formation by down-regulating receptor activator of NF-kB ligand (RANKL)-induced JNK activation. J Biol Chem. 2001;276:8836–40.
23. Manolagas SC, Kousteni S, Jilka RL. Sex steroids and bone. Recent Prog Horm Res. 2002;57:385–409.
24. Battacharya SM, Gosh M. Changes in calcium and vitamin D3 levels after tibolone treatment and their correlations with health-related quality of life. Int J Gynaecol Obstet. 2015;128:174–6.
25. Consensus development conference, prophylaxis and treatment of osteoporosis. Am J Med. 1991;90:107.
26. Ederveen AGH, Kloosterboer HJ. The protective effect of tibolone, a tissue-specific steroid, on ovariectomy-induced bone loss is blocked by an anti-estrogen. Presented at the first Amsterdam menopause symposium, Amsterdam, The Netherlands, 1998.
27. Rymer J, Robinson J, Fogelman I. 10 years of treatment with tibolone 2.5 mg daily: effects on bone loss in postmenopausal women. Climacteric. 2002;5:390–8.
28. Kenemans P, Speroff L. Clinical recommendations and practical guides. Maturitas. 2005;51:21–8.
29. Roux C, Pelissier C, Fechtenbaum J, Loiseau-Peres S, Benhamou CL. Randomized, double-blind, 2-year comparison of tibolone with 17b-estradiol and norethindrone acetate in preventing postmenopausal bone loss. Osteoporosis Int. 2002;13:241–8.
30. Delmas PD, Davis SR, Hensen J, Adami S, van Os S, Nijland EA. Effects of tibolone and raloxifene on bone mineral density in osteopenic postmenopausal women. Osteoporos Int. 2008;19(8):1153–60.
31. Cummings SR, Ettinger B, Delmas PD, et al. The effects of tibolone in older postmenopausal women. N Engl J Med. 2008;359:697–708.
32. Clarkson TB. Does tibolone exacerbate atherosclerosis? Eur Heart J. 2006;27:635–7.
33. Li C, Wei M, Mo L, Velu P, Prabahar K, Găman MA, Chen M. The effect of tibolone treatment on apolipoproteins and lipoprotein (a) concentrations in postmenopausal women: a meta-analysis of randomized controlled trials. Eur J Obstet Gynecol Reprod Biol. 2024;292:8–16.
34. Bots ML, Evans GW, Riley W, McBride KH, Paskett ED, Helmond FA, Grobbee DE, OPAL Investigators. The effect of tibolone and continuous combined conjugated equine estrogens plus medroxyprogesterone acetate on progression of carotid intima/media thickness: the Osteoporosis Prevention and Arterial effects of tibolone (OPAL) study. Eur Heart J. 2006;27:746–55.
35. Yuan Q, Santos HO, Alshahrani MS, Baradwan S, Ju H. Does tibolone treatment have favorable effects on obesity, blood pressure, and inflammation? A meta-analysis of randomized controlled trials. Steroids. 2022;178:108966. https://doi.org/10.1016/j.steroids.2022.
36. Archer D, Hendrix S, Ferenczy A, et al. Tibolone histology of the endometrium and breast endpoints study: design of the trial and endometrial histology at baseline in postmenopausal women. Fertil Steril. 2007;88:866–78.
37. Hammar ML, van de Weijer P, Franke HR, Pornel B, von Mauw EM, Nijland EA, TOTAL Study Investigators Group. Tibolone and low-dose continuous combined hormone treatment: vaginal bleeding pattern, efficacy and tolerability. BJOG. 2007;114:1522–9.
38. Beral V, Million Women Study Collaborators. Breast cancer and hormone replacement therapy in Million Women Study. Lancet. 2003;362:419–27.
39. Yuk JS, Kim T, Cho H, Gwak G. Breast cancer risk association with postmenopausal hormone therapy: Health Insurance Database in South Korea-based cohort study. Eur J Endocrinol. 2024;190(1):1–11.
40. Kenemans P, Bundred NJ, Foidart JM, et al. LIBERATE study groups. Safety and efficacy of tibolone in breast cancer patients with vasomotor symptoms: a double blind, randomized, non inferiority trial. Lancet Oncol. 2009;10:135–46.
41. Palacios S, Mejía RA. Bazedoxifene/conjugated estrogens combination for the treatment of the vasomotor symptoms associated with menopause and for prevention of osteoporosis in postmenopausal women. Drugs Today (Barc). 2015;51(2):107–16.

42. Komm BS, Mirkin S. Evolution of the tissue selective estrogen complex (TSEC). J Cell Physiol. 2013;228:1423–7.
43. Komm BS, Kharode YP, Bodine PV, Harris HA, Miller CP, Lyttle CR. Bazedoxifene acetate: a selective estrogen receptor modulator with improved selectivity. Endocrinology. 2005;146:3999–4008.
44. Pickar JH, Boucher M, Morgenstern D. Tissue selective estrogen complex (TSEC): a review. Menopause. 2018;25(9):1033–45.
45. Palacios S. Bazedoxifene acetate for the management of postmenopausal osteoporosis. Drugs Today (Barc). 2011;47(3):187–95.
46. Ethun KF, Wood CE, Register TC, Cline JM, Appt SE, Clarkson TB. Effects of bazedoxifene acetate with and without conjugated equine estrogens on the breast of postmenopausal monkeys. Menopause. 2012;19:1242–52.
47. Palacios S, Silverman SL, de Villiers TJ, Levine AB, Goemaere S, Brown JP, De Cicco Nardone F, Williams R, Hines TL, Mirkin S, Chines AA, Bazedoxifene Study Group. A 7-year randomized, placebo-controlled trial assessing the long-term efficacy and safety of bazedoxifene in postmenopausal women with osteoporosis: effects on bone density and fracture. Menopause. 2015;22(8):806–13.
48. Kharode Y, Bodine PV, Miller CP, Lyttle CR, Komm BS. The pairing of a selective estrogen receptor modulator, bazedoxifene, with conjugated estrogens as a new paradigm for the treatment of menopausal symptoms and osteoporosis prevention. Endocrinology. 2008;149:6084–91.
49. Komm BS, Vlasseros F, Samadfam R, Chouinard L, Smith SY. Skeletal effects of bazedoxifene paired with conjugated estrogens in ovariectomized rats. Bone. 2011;49:376–86.
50. Song Y, Santen RJ, Wang JP, Yue W. Effects of the conjugated equine estrogen/bazedoxifene tissue-selective estrogen complex (TSEC) on mammary gland and breast cancer in mice. Endocrinology. 2012;153:5706–15.
51. Peano BJ, Crabtree JS, Komm BS, Winneker RC, Harris HA. Effects of various selective estrogen receptor modulators with or without conjugated estrogens on mouse mammary gland. Endocrinology. 2009;150:1897–903.
52. Lobo RA, Pinkerton JV, Gass ML, et al. Evaluation of bazedoxifene/conjugated estrogens for the treatment of menopausal symptoms and effects on metabolic parameters and overall safety profile. Fertil Steril. 2009;92:1025–38.
53. Pinkerton JV, Utian WH, Constantine GD, Olivier S, Pickar JH. Relief of vasomotor symptoms with the tissue-selective estrogen complex containing bazedoxifene/conjugated estrogens: a randomized, controlled trial. Menopause. 2009;16:1116–24.
54. Pinkerton JV, Harvey JA, Lindsay R, Pan K, Chines AA, Mirkin S, Archer DF, SMART-5 Investigators. Effects of bazedoxifene/conjugated estrogens on the endometrium and bone: a randomized trial. J Clin Endocrinol Metab. 2014;99(2):E189–98. https://doi.org/10.1210/jc.2013-1707.
55. Song Y, Santen RJ, Wang JP, Yue W. Inhibitory effects of a bazedoxifene/conjugated equine estrogen combination on human breast cancer cells in vitro. Endocrinology. 2013;154:656–65.
56. Kulak J Jr, Ferriani RA, Komm BS, Taylor HS. Tissue selective estrogen complexes (TSECs) differentially modulate markers of proliferation and differentiation in endometrial cells. Reprod Sci. 2013;20(2):129–37.
57. Lindsay R, Gallagher JC, Kagan R, Pickar JH, Constantine G. Efficacy of tissue-selective estrogen complex of bazedoxifene/conjugated estrogens for osteoporosis prevention in at-risk postmenopausal women. Fertil Steril. 2009;92:1045–52.
58. Pickar JH, Yeh I-T, Bachmann G, Speroff L. Endometrial effects of a tissue selective estrogen complex containing bazedoxifene/conjugated estrogens as a menopausal therapy. Fertil Steril. 2009;92:1018–24.
59. Utian W, Yu H, Bobula J, Mirkin S, Olivier S, Pickar JH. Bazedoxifene/conjugated estrogens and quality of life in postmenopausal women. Maturitas. 2009;63:329–35.
60. Kagan R, Williams RS, Pan K, Mirkin S, Pickar JH. A randomized, placebo-and active-controlled trial of bazedoxifene/conjugated estrogens for treatment of moderate to severe vulvar/vaginal atrophy in postmenopausal women. Menopause. 2010;17:281–9.

61. Bachmann G, Bobula J, Mirkin S. Effects of bazedoxifene/conjugated estrogens on quality of life in postmenopausal women with symptoms of vulvar/vaginal atrophy. Climacteric. 2010;13:132–40.
62. Mirkin S, Komm BS, Pan K, Chines AA. Effects of bazedoxifene/conjugated estrogen on endometrial safety and bone in postmenopausal women. Climacteric. 2013;16(3):338–46.
63. Yu H, Racketa J, Chines AA, Mirkin S. Hot flush symptom-free days with bazedoxifene/conjugated estrogens in postmenopausal women. Climacteric. 2013;16:252–7.
64. Archer DF, Freeman EW, Komm BS, Ryan KA, Yu CR, Mirkin S, Pinkerton JV. Pooled analysis of the effects of conjugated estrogens/bazedoxifene on vasomotor symptoms in the selective estrogens, menopause, and response to therapy trials. J Womens Health (Larchmt). 2016;25(11):1102–11.
65. Abraham L, Bushmakin AG, Dragon E, Komm BS, Pinkerton JV. Direct and indirect effects of conjugated estrogens/bazedoxifene treatment on quality of life in postmenopausal women. Maturitas. 2016;94:173–9.
66. Gallagher JC, Palacios S, Ryan KA, Yu CR, Pan K, Kendler DL, Mirkin S, Komm BS. Effect of conjugated estrogens/bazedoxifene on postmenopausal bone loss: pooled analysis of two randomized trials. Menopause. 2016;23(10):1083–91.
67. Kim BM, Kim SE, Lee DY, Choi D. Effect of tissue-selective estrogen complex on hip structural geometry in postmenopausal women: a 12-month study. Front Endocrinol (Lausanne). 2021;12:649952. https://doi.org/10.3389/fendo.2021.649952.
68. Archer DF, Lewis V, Carr BR, Olivier S, Pickar JH. Bazedoxifene/conjugated estrogens (BZA/CE): incidence of uterine bleeding in postmenopausal women. Fertil Steril. 2009;92:1039–44.
69. Kim SE, Lee DY, Choi D. Tissue-selective estrogen complex for women who experience breast discomfort or vaginal bleeding when on hormone therapy. Menopause. 2019;26(4):383–6.
70. Harvey JA, Pinkerton JV, Baracat EC, Shi H, Chines AA, Mirkin S. Breast density changes in a randomized controlled trial evaluating bazedoxifene/conjugated estrogens. Menopause. 2013;20:138–45.
71. Yue W, Wang J, Atkins KA, Bottalico L, Mesaros C, Blair IA, Santen RJ. Effect of a tissue selective estrogen complex on breast cancer: role of unique properties of conjugated equine estrogen. Int J Cancer. 2018;143(5):1259–68.
72. Komm BS, Thompson JR, Mirkin S. Cardiovascular safety of conjugated estrogens plus bazedoxifene: meta-analysis of the SMART trials. Climacteric. 2015;18(4):503–11.
73. Skouby SO, Pan K, Thompson JR, Komm BS, Mirkin S. Effects of conjugated estrogens/bazedoxifene on lipid and coagulation variables: a randomized placebo- and active-controlled trial. Menopause. 2015;22(6):640–9.
74. Noirrit E, Buscato M, Dupuis M, Payrastre B, Fontaine C, Arnal JF, Valera MC. Effects of conjugated estrogen and bazedoxifene on hemostasis and thrombosis in mice. Endocr Connect. 2019;8(6):788–95.

The Effect of Menopause Hormone Therapy on Climacteric Symptoms

Camil Castelo-Branco, Laura Ribera, and Claudio Hernández-Angeles

Abstract

Healthy women have menopause at a mean age of 51 years, becoming 95% of them menopausal between 45 and 55 years. Oestrogen is the most effective available treatment for the relief of menopausal symptoms, most importantly hot flashes. Menopausal hormone therapy (MHT; oestrogen alone or combined with a progestin) is currently indicated for the management of menopausal symptoms. Its long-term use for the prevention of disease is no longer recommended. The treatment of menopausal symptoms with MHT will be reviewed in this chapter. An overview of the risks and benefits of oestrogens, available hormone preparations, and menopausal therapies for women who choose not to or cannot take oestrogens are discussed separately.

13.1 General Principles

Many women experience a range of symptoms during the menopause and perimenopause, and these symptoms are often shortly lived and lessen or disappear over time. The most common include vasomotor symptoms (e.g. hot flashes and sweats), effects on mood (e.g. low mood), and urogenital symptoms (e.g. vaginal dryness). Postmenopausal women are at an increased risk of a number of long-term conditions, such as osteoporosis, cardiovascular disease, and changes in the vagina and bladder, which occur because of natural aging as well as oestrogen depletion [1].

During the latter part of the last century, hormone replacement therapy (HRT), also known as hormone therapy (HT) and menopausal hormone therapy (MHT), was advocated for both symptom relief and chronic disease prevention. MHT is the broad term used to describe unopposed oestrogen therapy (ET) for women who have undergone hysterectomy or combined oestrogen-progestin therapy (EPT) for women with an intact uterus who need a progestin to prevent oestrogen-associated endometrial hyperplasia [2]. For menopausal women aged less than 60 years, being menopausal for less than 10 years, and who suffer from bothersome vasomotor symptoms (with or without additional climacteric symptoms) without contraindications or an excess of risk of cardiovascular pathology or breast cancer, MHT can be initiated according to the patient's preferences.

Variations in consultation patterns for menopausal symptoms depend on many factors, including cultural, ethnic, educational, and psychosocial factors, as well as the impact of the symptoms on the women. However, it is thought that more than one-third of all women want more support for managing menopausal symptoms from their general practitioner or practice nurse [1].

13.2 Goals of the Therapy

The goal of MHT is to relieve menopausal symptoms, most importantly hot flashes (vasomotor symptoms). Other symptoms associated with perimenopause and menopause that respond to MHT include mood lability/depression, vaginal atrophy, sleep disturbances (when related to hot flashes), and, in some cases, joint pain.

Women who are treated for menopausal symptoms such as hot flashes require the use of systemic oestrogen. Women being only treated for vulvovaginal atrophy (now referred to as "genitourinary syndrome of menopause" [GSM]) should be treated with low-dose vaginal oestrogen rather than systemic oestrogen.

In the past, MHT was also used by some clinicians to prevent coronary heart disease [CHD] and osteoporosis. However, MHT is not currently recommended for the prevention of disease given the results of the Women's Health Initiative (WHI), a set of two large randomized trials that demonstrated an unfavourable risk-benefit profile of MHT.

13.3 Importance of Patient's Age

While the WHI clearly demonstrated adverse effects of MHT in older postmenopausal women (over 60 years of age), this is not the most frequent collective who suffers from new onset menopausal symptoms. Almost all women who seek medical therapy for menopausal symptoms do so in their late 40s or middle 50s. Women in this age group should be reassured that the absolute risk of complications for healthy, young postmenopausal women taking MHT for 5 years is very low [2].

13.4 Benefits of Menopausal Hormone Therapy

13.4.1 Vasomotor Symptoms

Hot flashes are the classic symptom of the menopausal transition, experienced by more than 70% of women at some point during the menopausal transition. Hot flashes are associated with impairments in quality of life (QoL) and depressed mood and reported sleep disturbance and possibly even poorer memory function. Despite their prevalence and impact on women's lives, the understanding of the physiology of hot flashes remains incompletely understood. Leading models conceptualize hot flashes as originating in the central nervous system. Some data support acute changes in the brain regions associated with awareness of bodily sensation, such as the insula and prefrontal cortex, during hot flashes and the involvement of brainstem areas in the triggering of hot flashes [3, 4].

Hot flashes occur in the context of oestrogen (E) withdrawal, and the effects of E on brain structure and function in humans remain controversial. Hot flashes often begin as the sudden sensation of heat centred on the upper chest and face. In some instances, this will become generalized, lasting for several minutes, and can be associated with profuse perspiration, palpitations, or anxiety, which may be very distressing and limit activities of the daily living, particularly when they occur repeatedly during the day and at night. At night, hot flushes and night sweats will often cause insomnia that leads to fatigue.

Treatment for VMS may include HRT, since symptoms occur at a time when oestrogen levels are dropping and "replacement" leads to relief. HRT comprises synthetic hormones that may be identical to those produced from the ovaries during the reproductive years (oestradiol and progesterone) although other similar compounds (such as conjugated equine oestrogens, oestradiol valerate and several synthetic progestogens) are widely used. Although there are alternative therapies for vasomotor symptoms, none are as effective as oestrogen, which is the most effective treatment for vasomotor symptoms, thus improving women's quality of life (QoL). In a dose-dependent manner, MHT reduces hot flash frequency by approximately 75% and severity by 87%, compared with the 50% reduction with placebo [4].

In this field, a new drug is emerging. Fezolinetant (posology: 45 mg/day) is a neurokinin 3 receptor antagonist that has shown to significantly reduce the frequency and severity of VMS (from severe to moderate) in comparison with placebo in two phase 3 randomized controlled trials. Changes in VMS have not significantly differed between fezolinetant and different HRT regimens, although it could be an option for patients who are unwilling to take HRT (or have contraindications for such treatment) [5].

13.4.2 Anxiety and Depressive Symptoms

Depression and mood change is common at times of hormonal change, such as during the menstrual cycle, after pregnancy, and in the perimenopausal period. There is a robust relationship between gonadal hormones such as oestrogens and mood disorders in women. There are several known female-specific depressive disorders that are linked to changes in hormonal status. Premenstrual disorders, postpartum depression, and perimenopausal depression are all characterized by a sharp decrease in estradiol associated with the symptom onset. This association reinforces the role of oestrogens in the maintenance of the mood. Studying these disorders both in humans and in animal models will provide opportunities for the development of more successful treatment options and will clarify the relationship between oestrogens and depression.

Anxiety symptoms increase during the menopause transition and are associated with an increased likelihood of a major depressive disorder. MHT, alone or in combination with an antidepressant such as a selective serotonin reuptake inhibitor (SSRI), is effective for women who experience mood lability or depression during the menopausal transition. ET may improve mild to moderate depressive symptoms during or shortly after the menopause transition, whereas antidepressant therapy remains the appropriate treatment for major depression [6].

Mood disorders are common during the menopausal transition, often coexisting with vasomotor symptoms. Two small, short duration clinical trials assessed MHT in women with depression or depressive symptoms during the menopausal transition. After 3 weeks, depression scores improved significantly in depressed women treated with transdermal estradiol (0.05 mg/day) compared to placebo [7]. After 12 weeks, depressive disorders were significantly more likely to remit with transdermal estradiol (0.1 mg/day) compared to placebo [8].

The present approach is to choose initial therapy based upon the woman's predominant symptom. If her main concern is depression and hot flashes are not severe, an SSRI should be started. On the other hand, if vasomotor symptoms are the major symptom and depression or mood symptoms are mild, MHT should be the recommended beginning. For women in whom depression and vasomotor symptoms are both severe, starting with both MHT and a SSRI may be an option, which does not exclude the reference of the patient to a mental health specialist [9].

13.4.3 Skin, Cartilage, and Connective Tissues

Oestrogen receptors have been detected in many skin elements including keratinocytes, melanocytes, fibroblasts, hair follicles, and sebaceous glands so it is likely that the withdrawal of oestrogen at menopause will have measurable effects on skin health. The skin surface texture, its water-holding capacity, the collagen content of the dermis, and its viscoelasticity have proven to be improved with the use of oestrogen [10]. A recent meta-analysis on the topic including 1589 postmenopausal patients has shown MHT increases in elasticity and collagen content in the skiing, thereby reducing the severity of wrinkles and increasing skin thickness [11].

A spectrum of musculoskeletal symptoms follows estrogen deficiency in large numbers of women, from arthralgia to osteoarthritis. The effects of estrogen in bone are well characterized, but data on the impact of oestrogen on cartilage, skin, and connective tissues have been slower to emerge. Oestrogen is synthesized by aromatases in most connective tissues. Critically, oestrogen receptors are present in all joint tissues including articular cartilage, subchondral bone and synovium.

Although no clear association has been found between lifetime oestrogen exposure and the risk of osteoarthritis, generalized muscle and joint aches are among the most common symptoms experienced by women at menopause. Furthermore, arthritis in women is more likely to be progressive and symptomatic [10]. Oestrogen receptors ERa and ERb have both been identified in chondrocytes, and recent studies have also demonstrated oestrogen receptors in synoviocytes [12].

It is unclear whether arthralgia is related to oestrogen deficiency or constitutes a rheumatologic disorder by itself, but in the WHI, women with joint pain or stiffness at baseline got a 45% reduction of symptoms with MHT in comparison to placebo [10, 13]. Joint pain increased slightly after discontinuation of treatment [14]. In the absence of specific studies, three related mechanisms have been proposed as possible oestrogen effects:

- **Inflammation**. There is a large amount of data that suggest oestrogens are anti-inflammatory and mildly immunosuppressive.
- **Bone**. The effects of MHT on the bone are well-known. Targeting bone turnover may be one mechanism by which MHT could interfere with osteoarthritis.
- **Pain. O**estrogen receptors and aromatase are present in the hypothalamus, limbic system, neurone, and joint. ET has been shown to decrease synovial nerve fibre substance P in a rat model of osteoarthritis. Oestrogen is antinociceptive, activating inhibitory pain pathways in the spinal cord, whilst progestins are pro-nociceptive.

13.4.4 Genitourinary Syndrome of Menopause

The female genital and lower urinary tracts share a common embryological origin, arising from the urogenital sinus and being both sensitive to the effects of female sex steroid hormones throughout life. The epithelial linings of the vagina and urethra are very sensitive to oestrogen, and oestrogen deficiency leads to the thinning of the vaginal epithelium. Oestrogen is known to have an important role in the function of the lower urinary tract, and oestrogen and progesterone receptors have been found in the vagina, urethra, bladder, and pelvic floor musculature [15].

Oestrogen deficiency results in the genitourinary syndrome of menopause (also called vaginal atrophy or atrophic vaginitis), causing symptoms of vaginal dryness, itching, dyspareunia, and, sometimes, urinary symptoms. Both systemic and vaginal oestrogen are effective for genitourinary atrophy symptoms, but vaginal oestrogen therapy is preferred for women who suffer from GSM without other menopausal symptoms such as hot flashes [16].

Low-dose vaginal oestrogen therapy is effective for the treatment of vaginal symptoms with some evidence of additive benefit against recurrent urinary tract infections and dysuria. Several vaginal preparations are available, including vaginal creams, tablets, and a silastic ring that releases E2 locally over a 3-month period. Of these, the 10 mg E2 tablet and the 7.5 mg vaginal ring result in the least amount of systemic oestrogen absorption. When low-dose vaginal oestrogen therapies are used according to labelling, it is unlikely that endometrial stimulation will occur, and progestogen therapy is therefore not routinely recommended for women using only vaginal oestrogen therapy.

Regarding the specific situation of GSM in breast cancer survivors, there is a need to limit the underdiagnosis and undertreatment of GSM in this collective [17]. The primary goal of physicians treating breast cancer survivors regarding this issue has to be the provision of information of what to expect regarding genital and sexual symptoms and to counsel on early first-line treatments that may help prevent more severe GSM. Due to safety concerns on oestrogen-based treatments for GSM in breast cancer survivors, new options are appearing, such as androgen-based treatments, which according to proprieties would not be transformed systemically to oestrogens in patients receiving aromatase inhibitors. In this way, a pilot study was conducted to assess the security and efficacy of vaginal prasterone (dehydroepiandrostenedione [DHEA]) in ten breast cancer survivors treated with aromatase inhibitors who complained of severe GSM [18]. Participants were instructed to use one ovule containing 7.5 mg of DHEA every night during the first month and one ovule every two nights for the entire 5 remaining months. Mean serum estradiol remained low after 6 months of follow-up; the visual analogue scale of dyspareunia improved from 8.5 to mean values after treatment of 0.4. The Vaginal Health Index (VHI) scale and Female Sexual Function Index improved from 9.75 to 15.8 ($p = 0.0277$) and from an initial score of 11.2 to 20.6 ($p = 0.0277$), respectively. Vaginal pH changed from basal 8.1 to final 6.5 ($p = 0.0330$). Also oral options are available. On the one hand, tibolone is a synthetic steroid with selective tissue estrogenic activity approved for the treatment of menopausal symptoms. Despite its oestrogen effects, tibolone has shown to have no effect on breast tumour cell proliferation in oestrogen receptor negative tumours, by contrast with patients with oestrogen receptor positive tumours [19]. On the other hand, systemic SERM therapy is also available for treating dyspareunia due to menopause, also in breast cancer survivors (having ended adjuvancy). Oral ospemifene, 60 mg daily, improves dyspareunia, vaginal dryness, and female sexual function. Ospemifene seems well suited for women who prefer oral rather than vaginal therapy. Cost, accessibility, and individual preferences should dictate the choice of the treatment formulation for the management of the GSM, which should be established in an informed decision process [20].

13.4.5 Urinary Incontinence

The role of systemic oestrogens in the management of postmenopausal women with lower urinary tract symptoms has been investigated in three large epidemiological studies examining the use of combined oestrogen/progestogen and oestrogen-only systemic HRT [12–14]. In all of these trials, systemic ET was found to increase the risk of developing both stress and urgency urinary incontinence, and in those women who complained of urinary incontinence at baseline, the symptoms were found to deteriorate. This was also reflected in deterioration in quality of life.

A recent systematic review was conducted to study the effects of HRT for urinary symptoms in perimenopausal and postmenopausal women and reinforced the relationship between systemic HRT use and urinary incontinence beginning or worsening, even though vaginal oestrogen use was shown to improve dysuria, frequency, urge and stress incontinence, and recurrent UTI in menopausal women [21].

13.4.6 Cardiovascular Disease

Cardiovascular disease (CVD) is the major cause of death in women in all European countries; below 75 years, 42% of women die from CVD compared with 38% of men. The lower rates of CVD in premenopausal women—but not of stroke—may be interpreted as a protective effect of endogenous oestrogens. However, exploration of trends over time and between countries shows that the relationship varies [22].

Major primary prevention measures are smoking cessation, weight loss, blood pressure reduction, regular aerobic exercise, and diabetes and lipid control [10]. There is strong and consistent evidence that oestrogen therapy may be cardioprotective if started around the time of menopause (often referred to as the 'window of opportunity' or 'timing' hypothesis) and may be harmful if started more than 10 years after menopause.

The American Heart Association (AHA) [23] published an update of its guidelines for the prevention of CVD in women, which emphasize that recommendations are the same for both men and women, with few exceptions. The use of the Framingham score is recommended and nowadays includes a category of "ideal cardiovascular health" comprising absence of raised risk factors, BMI <25 kg/m^2, regular moderate-to-vigorous physical activity, and a healthy diet.

The Endocrine Society guideline suggests calculating cardiovascular and breast cancer risks before initiating MHT [24]. They suggest the use of nonhormonal therapies for symptomatic women who are at high risk (>10% at 10-year risk) for CVD or moderate (1.67–5% at 5-year risk) to high risk (>5%) for breast cancer. For women at moderate risk of CVD (5–10% at 10-year risk), they suggest transdermal rather than oral oestrogen, with micronized progesterone for those with a uterus. They note that a population-based CVD risk calculator should be used to estimate CVD risk.

Although this represents the ideal approach, a formal CVD calculation may not be necessary in a thin, healthy, nonhypertensive patient who is well-known to the clinician. For women at increased risk of venous thromboembolism (VTE), they also suggest transdermal oestrogen with a progestin that has a neutral effect on coagulation parameters (e.g. micronized progesterone) [24].

A recent meta-analysis on the use of MHT and cardiovascular impact in postmenopausal women, which included 33 RCTs involving 44,639 postmenopausal women, concluded that MHT lowers the risk of all-cause death and cardiovascular events, while it increases the risk of stroke and venous thrombosis in postmenopausal women. No difference was found in the outcome of cardiovascular system endpoints between mono-oestrogen therapy and combination therapy of oestrogen and progesterone [25].

Therefore, MHT should not be used for CVD prevention, even in young postmenopausal women. Although the risk profile appears to be more favourable in young women taking ET, its use with this indication is still not warranted [12]. The hormone regimen studied in the WHI was conjugated oestrogens and medroxyprogesterone acetate (MPA). While it is possible that other oestrogen or progestin formulations or doses might not have the same negative cardiovascular effects as conjugated oestrogen and MPA, data to support their use for prevention are not available. Nevertheless, HRT utilized in appropriately selected younger postmenopausal women close to the onset of menopause is safe from a cardiovascular perspective, in line with consensus recommendations [26].

13.4.7 Osteoporosis

Osteoporosis is a systemic skeletal disease characterized by diminished bone strength with the risk of sustaining a fracture when falling from the own body height (fragility fracture) [27]. Bone strength is determined by a combination of bone density and microarchitectural integrity. Postmenopausal osteoporosis results from a failure to attain peak bone density, accelerated bone loss after menopause, age-related bone loss, or a combination of factors. Accelerated postmenopausal bone loss is induced by oestrogen deprivation [10].

Assessment of Bone Mineral Density is not a cost-effective population screening tool but is best applied on a selective basis, based on age and other risk factors such as a personal or family history of fractures, history of amenorrhea, primary ovarian insufficiency, low body mass, diet, smoking, alcohol abuse, the use of bone toxic medication, and rheumatoid arthritis [10].

MHT is the only available therapy with proven efficacy of fracture reduction in patients with osteopenia. Although MHT prevents fractures at any age after the menopause, age at the initiation of MHT is important [23]. In the age group 50–60 years or within 10 years after menopause, the benefits of MHT are most likely to outweigh any risk and can be considered as first-line therapy [28]. Initiation of MHT in the age group 60–70 years requires individually calculated benefit/risk, consideration of other available drugs, and the use of the lowest effective dose [28]. MHT should not be initiated after age 70 years.

Non-oestrogen-based treatments for osteoporosis include bisphophonates, denosumab, selective oestrogen receptor modulators (SERMs), parathyroid hormone (PTH), and strontium ranelate. Bisphosphonates (such as alendronate, risedronate, ibandronate, and zoledronic acid) inhibit bone resorption by inducing apoptosis of osteoclasts, thus preventing age-related bone loss and deterioration of bone microarchitecture. They are the most widely prescribed drugs, mainly due to their low cost and the generally favourable safety profile. Denosumab is a human monoclonal antibody to the receptor activator of nuclear factor-kappaB ligand (RANKL), a bone resorbing cytokine. It is administered as a subcutaneous injection every 6 months. All anti-resorptive agents are associated with an increased risk of osteonecrosis of the jaw and atypical femoral fracture. But both conditions are rare [29].

The two SERMS approved for the treatment of postmenopausal osteoporosis are raloxifene and bazedoxifene. Both reduce the risk of vertebral but not hip fracture and increase the risk of venous thromboembolism and hot flushes. They are both associated with a decreased risk of breast cancer in postmenopausal women with osteoporosis. Future treatments for osteoporosis include cathepsin K inhibitors which appear to have mixed antiresorptive and anabolic actions as they inhibit one of the major osteoclast digestive enzymes without suppressing bone formation, thereby leading to anabolic effects in the bone [30].

13.4.8 Cognitive Function and Dementia

Numerous studies have reported an effect of estradiol on memory ability. It appears that estradiol improves hippocampal dependent memory performance through activation of Erβ. Despite current knowledge of the memory impairments associated with depression, little effort has been placed on the exploration of cognitive deficits and hippocampal changes related to postpartum depression and perimenopausal depression. Human research on memory impairments has produced conflicting results [31].

Currently, the routine use of MHT for peri- and postmenopausal women who are experiencing cognitive symptoms (memory loss and difficulty concentrating) is not recommended. Although there is substantial biologic evidence supporting the importance of oestrogens for the cognitive function, clinical trial evidence has generally ruled out any global (but not domain specific) cognitive benefit.

Additionally, MHT is not recommended for the prevention of dementia. Although some epidemiologic data has suggested that oestrogens may be beneficial, clinical trials of MHT administered to women aged 65 years or older have shown to cause harm [32].

A recent case-control study [33] including 29,104 women aged 50–60 years with hysterectomy and without dementia nor contraindications for HRT showed that oestrogen-only vs. never use was associated with increased dementia rate (hazard ratio [HR], 1.55; 95% CI, 1.25–1.93); HR was 1.49 (95% CI, 1.15–1.93) for 5 years use or less and 1.62 (95% CI, 1.25–2.09) for greater than 5 years' use. Increasing daily estradiol dose yielded increasing HRs, and oral estradiol HR was 1.62 (95% CI, 1.28–2.05) and transdermal 1.39 (95% CI, 0.97–1.99). The association persisted in women using oestrogen only until a maximum of aged 55 years (HR, 1.58; 95% CI, 1.06–2.35). Studies are warranted to ascertain whether findings represent a causal link between oestrogen-only use and dementia risk or predisposition among women needing therapy.

13.4.9 Sexual Disorders

Psychological, relational, and environmental factors are regarded as being of paramount importance for the sexual function and behaviour. Indeed, a comprehensive approach to women's sexuality requires more than the mere understanding of a physiological process. The most relevant variables are the duration and quality of the partnership (if present), age, general and mental health, achievement of reproductive goals, education, body image, self-esteem, and personal experiences.

The known decrease in ovarian androgen production rates and serum androgen concentrations has caused concern that menopause might be associated with a libido decline. An age-associated decline in sexual desire has been observed in both men and women. However, it is unclear whether the decline in libido in women is age or menopause related, since studies in women have not shown a significant correlation between libido and the serum estradiol or testosterone levels.

Clinical trials of exogenous testosterone replacement suggest modest benefits of testosterone therapy in postmenopausal women. However, there are potential risks associated with androgen replacement, and the use of testosterone is limited by the lack of approved and commercially available products for women. Until the beneficial effects of androgen replacement are better established, it cannot be routinely recommended to postmenopausal women.

13.4.10 Extended Use of MHT

Both the North American Menopause Society [2] and the International Menopause Society [10] agree that the use of MHT should be individualized and not discontinued solely based upon the patient's age. They suggest that extended use of MHT (beyond age 60 or even 65 years) may be reasonable when the clinician and patient agree that the benefits of symptom relief outweigh the risks. As noted, over 40% of women aged 60–65 years have persistent hot flashes that can impair sleep and quality of life.

For women who choose an extended use of MHT (more than 5 years or beyond 60 years of age), oestrogen should be used at the lowest possible dose and for the shortest period of time.

13.5 Summary and Recommendations

- The goal of menopausal hormone therapy (MHT) is to relieve menopausal symptoms, most importantly hot flashes (vasomotor symptoms). Other symptoms associated with perimenopause and menopause that respond to oestrogen therapy (ET) include mood lability/depression, genitourinary syndrome of menopause (GSM; vaginal atrophy), and sleep disturbances (when related to hot flashes).
- Healthy symptomatic women in their 50s should be reassured that the absolute risk of complications for healthy, postmenopausal women taking MHT for 5 years is very low.

- For healthy, peri-/postmenopausal women within 10 years of menopause (or <age 60 years) with moderate-to-severe vasomotor symptoms, we suggest MHT as the treatment of choice (Grade 2B). Exceptions include women with a history of breast cancer, coronary heart disease (CHD), a previous venous thromboembolic event or stroke, active liver disease, or those at high risk for these complications.
- We suggest transdermal 17-beta estradiol for many women starting MHT (Grade 2C). The transdermal route is particularly important in women with hypertriglyceridemia or risk factors for thromboembolism. However, the baseline risk of both venous thromboembolism (VTE) and stroke is very low in otherwise healthy, young postmenopausal women. Therefore, if a patient prefers an oral preparation over a transdermal one (cost or personal preference), we consider oral oestrogen to be safe. All types and routes of oestrogen are equally effective for hot flashes.
- For women who experience recurrent, bothersome hot flashes after stopping oestrogen, we initially suggest nonhormonal options. However, if this approach is unsuccessful and symptoms persist, we resume MHT at the lowest dose possible in carefully selected women.
- For women with an intact uterus who choose ET, progestin therapy must be added to prevent endometrial hyperplasia and carcinoma.
- We suggest micronized progesterone as a first-line progestin because it is effective for endometrial hyperplasia, is metabolically neutral, and does not appear to increase the risk of either breast cancer or CVD, although data are limited (Grade 2C).
- Recommendations for women who choose not to take systemic oestrogen, have contraindications to oestrogen, or have stopped their MHT and are having recurrent symptoms are found elsewhere.
- We currently suggest not using MHT for the prevention of chronic disease (osteoporosis, CVD, or dementia) (Grade 2B). However, women who cannot tolerate other options for osteoporosis may be reasonable candidates.

References

1. National Collaborating Centre for Women's and Children's Health. Menopause clinical guideline. 2015;V1.5.
2. North American Menopause Society. The 2012 hormone therapy position statement of: The North American Menopause Society. Menopause. 2012;19:257.
3. Freedman RR. Menopausal hot flashes: mechanisms, endocrinology, treatment. J Steroid Biochem. 2014;142:115–20.
4. Thurston RC, Maki PM, Derby CA, Sejdic E, Aizenstein HJ. Menopausal hot flashes and the default mode network. Fertil Steril. 2015;103(6):1573–8.
5. Morga A, Ajmera M, Gao E, Patterson-Lomba O, Zhao A, Mancuso S, Siddiqui E, Kagan R. Systematic review and network meta-analysis comparing the efficacy of fezolinetant with hormone and nonhormone therapies for treatment of vasomotor symptoms due to menopause. Menopause. 2024;31(1):68–76.
6. Santen RJ, Allred DC, Ardoin SP, et al. Postmenopausal hormone therapy: an Endocrine Society scientific statement. J Clin Endocrinol Metab. 2010;95:s1–s66.

7. Schmidt PJ, Nieman L, Danaceau MA, et al. Estrogen replacement in perimenopause-related depression: a preliminary report. Am J Obstet Gynecol. 2000;183:414–20.
8. Soares CD, Almeida OP, Joffe H, Cohen LS. Efficacy of estradiol for the treatment of depressive disorders in perimenopausal women: a double-blind, randomized, placebo-controlled trial. Arch Gen Psychiatry. 2001;58:529–34.
9. Soares CN. Mood disorders in midlife women: understanding the critical window and its clinical implications. Menopause. 2014;21:198–206.
10. Baber RJ, Panay N, Fenton A, IMS Writing Group. 2016 IMS Recommendations on women's midlife health and menopause hormone therapy. Climacteric. 2016;19(2):109–50.
11. Pivazyan L, Avetisyan J, Loshkareva M, Abdurakhmanova A. Skin rejuvenation in women using menopausal hormone therapy: a systematic review and meta-analysis. J Menopausal Med. 2023;29(3):97–111.
12. Karsdal MA, Bay-Jensen AC, Henriksen K, Christiansen C. The pathogenesis of osteoarthritis involves bone, cartilage and synovial inflammation: may estrogen be a magic bullet? Menopause Int. 2012;18:139–46.
13. Chlebowski RT, Cirillo DJ, Eaton CB, et al. Estrogen alone and joint symptoms in the Women's Health Initiative randomized trial. Menopause. 2013;20:600.
14. Marjoribanks J, Farquhar C, Roberts H, Lethaby A. Long term hormone therapy for perimenopausal and postmenopausal women. Cochrane Database Syst Rev. 2012;(7):CD004143.
15. Hendrix SL, Cochrane BR, Nygaard IE, et al. Effects of estrogen with and without progestin on urinary incontinence. JAMA. 2005;293:935–48.
16. Castelo-Branco C, Biglia N, Nappi RE, Schwenkhagen A, Palacios S. Characteristics of postmenopausal women with genitourinary syndrome of menopause: implications for vulvovaginal atrophy diagnosis and treatment selection. Maturitas. 2015;81(4):462–9.
17. Castelo-Branco C, Mension E, Torras I, Cebrecos I, Anglès-Acedo S. Treating genitourinary syndrome of menopause in breast cancer survivors: main challenges and promising strategies. Climacteric. 2023;26(4):296–301.
18. Mension E, Alonso I, Cebrecos I, Castrejon N, Tortajada M, Matas I, Gómez S, Ribera L, Anglès-Acedo S, Castelo-Branco C. Safety of prasterone in breast cancer survivors treated with aromatase inhibitors: the VIBRA pilot study. Climacteric. 2022;25(5):476–82.
19. Garrido Oyarzún MF, Castelo-Branco C. Use of hormone therapy for menopausal symptoms and quality of life in breast cancer survivors. Safe and ethical? Gynecol Endocrinol. 2017;33(1):10–5.
20. Oyarzún MFG, Castelo-Branco C. Local hormone therapy for genitourinary syndrome of menopause in breast cancer patients: is it safe? Gynecol Endocrinol. 2017;33(6):418–20.
21. Christmas MM, Iyer S, Daisy C, Maristany S, Letko J, Hickey M. Menopause hormone therapy and urinary symptoms: a systematic review. Menopause. 2023;30(6):672–85.
22. Lawlor DA, Ebrahim S, Davey SG. Sex matters: secular, geographical trends in sex differences in coronary heart disease mortality. BMJ. 2001;323:541–5.
23. Mosca L, Benjamin EJ, Berra K, Bezanson JL, Dolor RJ, Lloyd-Jones DM, et al. Effectiveness-based guidelines for the prevention of cardiovascular disease in women-2011 update: a guideline from the American Heart Association. Circulation. 2011;123:1243–62.
24. Stuenkel CA, Davis SR, Gompel A, et al. Treatment of symptoms of the menopause: an endocrine society clinical practice guideline. J Clin Endocrinol Metab. 2015;100:3975.
25. Gu Y, Han F, Xue M, Wang M, Huang Y. The benefits and risks of menopause hormone therapy for the cardiovascular system in postmenopausal women: a systematic review and meta-analysis. BMC Womens Health. 2024;24(1):60.
26. Nudy M, Buerger J, Dreibelbis S, Jiang X, Hodis HN, Schnatz PF. Menopausal hormone therapy and coronary heart disease: the roller-coaster history. Climacteric. 2024;27(1):81–8.
27. Castelo-Branco C. Calcium-collagen chelate supplementation reduces bone loss in osteopenic postmenopausal women. Climacteric. 2015;18:105–6.
28. Manson JE, Chlebowski RT, Stefanick ML, et al. Menopausal hormone therapy and health outcomes during the intervention and extended poststopping phases of the Women's Health Initiative randomized trials. JAMA. 2013;310:1353–68.

29. de Villiers TJ, Gass MLS, Haines CJ, et al. Global consensus statement on menopausal hormone therapy. Climacteric. 2013;16:203–4.
30. de Villiers TJ, Stevenson JC. The WHI: the effect of hormone replacement therapy on fracture prevention. Climacteric. 2012;15:263–6.
31. Mueller SC, Grissom EM, Dohanich GP. Assessing gonadal hormone contributions to affective psychopathologies across humans and animal models. Psychoneuroendocrinology. 2014;46:114–28.
32. Borrow AP, Cameron NM. Estrogenic mediation of serotonergic and neurotrophic systems: implications for female mood disorders. Prog Neuropsychopharmacol Biol Psychiatry. 2014;54:13–25.
33. Pourhadi N, Mørch LS, Holm EA, Torp-Pedersen C, Meaidi A. Dementia in women using estrogen-only therapy. JAMA. 2024;331(2):160–2.

14

The Impact of Hormone Therapy on Other Noncommunicable Diseases: Central Nervous System, Cardiovascular Tree, Osteoarthritis, and Cancer

Esperanza Navarro-Pardo, Tomi S. Mikkola, Tommaso Simoncini, Marta Millán, María Dolores Juliá, and Antonio Cano

Abstract

The main indication for the use of hormone therapy is to control symptoms during the years around menopause. However, and because estrogens have receptors spread over many systems in the body, the use of hormones may have consequences on health. Hormone therapy consists of estrogens essentially, since

E. Navarro-Pardo
Department of Developmental and Educational Psychology, University of Valencia, Valencia, Spain
e-mail: esperanza.navarro@uv.es

T. S. Mikkola
Department of Obstetrics and Gynecology, Helsinki University Central Hospital, Helsinki, Finland
e-mail: tomi.mikkola@hus.fi

T. Simoncini
Division of Obstetrics and Gynecology, Department of Clinical and Experimental Medicine, University of Pisa, Pisa, Italy
e-mail: tommaso.simoncini@med.unipi.it

M. Millán
Hospital Universitario Marqués Valdecilla, University of Cantabria, Santander, Spain
e-mail: martamartinm@scsalud.es

M. D. Juliá
Department of Pediatrics, Obstetrics and Gynecology, University of Valencia, Valencia, Spain

Section of Gynecology and Reproduction, University and Polytechnic Hospital La Fe, Valencia, Spain
e-mail: M.Dolores.Julia@uv.es

A. Cano (✉)
Full Professor of Obstetrics and Gynecology, Salus Vitae Women's Health Clinical Center, Valencia, Spain
e-mail: Antonio.cano@uv.es

menopausal symptoms mainly derive from estrogen deprivation at different target tissues. Progesterone has a neutralizing effect over endometrial proliferation, this being the reason for adding progestogens to hormone therapy formulations. Because of that, the impact of hormone therapy on health should also consider the specific effects of both estrogens and progestogens in addition to those of only estrogens. While this has turned to be of minor importance in some areas, it is not so in others, for example, the breast. This chapter analyzes the effect of estrogens, with or without progestogens, on tissues of interest for health. The analysis includes the central nervous system, the cardiovascular tree, the joints, the breast, and the genital organs, uterus, and ovary.

14.1 Introduction

Hormone therapy (HT) has menopausal symptom control as the main indication. However, and because estrogens have receptors spread over many systems in the body, the use of hormones may have consequences on health. Hormone therapy consists of estrogens essentially, since menopausal symptoms mainly derive from estrogen deprivation at different target tissues. However, the normal ovarian cycle includes the regular secretion of progesterone during the days of the luteal phase. Progesterone has a neutralizing effect over endometrial proliferation, this being the reason for adding progestogens to HT formulations in order to protect endometrium. So, guidelines recommend that women with uterus use estrogen plus progestogens, which may be combined in different forms. And because of that, the impact of HT on health should also consider the specific effects of both estrogens and progestogens in addition to those of only estrogens.

14.2 The Impact of Hormone Therapy on Cognition and Mood

14.2.1 Introduction

The impact of the reduction of circulating estrogens on cognitive deterioration after menopause is being an area widely investigated. There is a considerable amount of experimental data favoring an interaction of estrogens with cognitive functions [1]. The issue, however, remains controversial at clinical level. For example, some investigators have found that users of HT performed better on specific tasks such as psychomotor speed, visual memory, non-verbal memory and attention, and digit span-forward and recall [2–5]. In contrast, other studies could not find a significant association with global function or with specific domains (verbal memory, verbal fluency, working memory, attention, or executive functions) [6, 7].

Memory has been the most studied domain within the cognitive universe, perhaps because it is more clearly affected and because it has a potential to predict the development of Alzheimer's disease (AD) [8, 9].

14.2.2 Psychobiological Feasibility

The background supporting the estrogen action arises from molecular evidences and from observations obtained in different experimental models. There is, for example, abundance of estrogen receptors (ER) at different areas related with cognition in the central nervous system (CNS). This is the case of the hippocampus and the frontal lobes, which subserve verbal memory, working memory, and retrieval [10]. Also, outside the hypothalamus, ER have been described in cortical and limbic areas that are involved in the processes of learning and memory [1].

In parallel, cell culture experiments have shown that estrogens alter synaptic circuitry in the hypothalamus, hippocampus, and, more recently, neocortex [reviewed in [11]].

14.2.3 Studies in Animal Models

The availability of different types of animal models has facilitated the intensive study of the impact of estrogens on different cognitive functions.

Work in mice has shown that treatment with estrogens is followed by dramatic increases in hippocampal spine synapse density within minutes and that this is accompanied by improved general discrimination learning, probably through increasing formation of silent or immature synapses within hippocampus via ERα activation [12]. Other studies in rodents have focused on learning and working memory performance and have shown that ovarian hormones affect both cognitive processes and neural substrates that underlie those tasks [13–15]. Deficiencies in spatial learning capabilities and increases in the myelin sheath volume of the white matter were demonstrated by treatment with estrogens in ovariectomized (OVX) rats [16].

So, exogenous estradiol seems to behave as a crucial regulator of hippocampal morphology and plasticity and also of memory in rodents. Of interest, some groups have obtained similar findings in nonhuman primates [17–19].

However, data from animal studies are not unanimous. The positive effects described above were also accompanied by detrimental actions in some cases. Pompili et al. [15] described that estrogens selectively improved working memory but had a negative effect in spatial reference memory. As for any work with experimental models, it is possible that methodological differences may explain the discrepant findings.

The impact of progestogens has received some attention as well. The association of progesterone to estradiol was neutral when assessed on visual and spatial recognition memory in older monkeys [20]. However, a study in OVX rats obtained different outcomes depending on the type of progestogen; so, whereas levonorgestrel enhanced learning, two other synthetic progestogens, medroxyprogesterone acetate (MPA) and norethisterone acetate, impaired learning and memory [21].

14.2.4 Clinical Studies

14.2.4.1 Effects of HT on Cognition
The current clinical knowledge has been obtained from observational studies and, more recently, randomized controlled trials. Some attention has been paid to the specific form of HT, including hormone preparations, either estrogen alone or combined with progestogens, and route, either oral or transdermal.

The cross-sectional results obtained in the cohort followed in The Study of Women Across the Nation (SWAN) are a landmark because a substantial number of participants were analyzed and also because information on circulating hormones was obtained. A total of 1657 community-based midlife women were stratified according to menopause stage, and their cognitive function was evaluated. When adjusting for covariates, no association was found between the measured cognitive performance tests and menopause stage or hormonal level, estradiol, and follicle-stimulating hormone (FSH) [22].

One main intervention study has been the Women's Health Initiative Memory Study (WHIMS). Conceived as an ancillary study of the Women's Health Initiative (WHI) randomized controlled trial, WHIMS aimed at evaluating the effect of estrogen plus progestogen on the incidence of dementia or mild cognitive impairment compared with placebo [23]. At the early termination of the study after an average follow-up of 4.05 years, 40 women were diagnosed of probable dementia in the treatment group versus 21 in the placebo. The hazard ratio was 2.05. The incidence of mild cognitive impairment did not differ between groups. Of interest, a subset of 1403 women were measured regional brain volumes, including hippocampal and frontal regions by magnetic resonance at an average of 3.0 years post-trial (WHIMS-MRI study). The use of hormones, either conjugated equine estrogens (CEE) alone or associated with MPA, was associated with greater brain atrophy, the effects being more evident in women who already suffered cognitive deficits before initiating hormones [24].

As for other outcomes of the WHI study, there has been debate on whether the unfavorable impact might be due to the relatively advanced age, 65 years or older, of participants in the WHIMS. A decrease in the responsiveness of neurons to estrogen with increasing age or the inability of the hormone to reverse neural loss and/or dysfunction, which may have occurred during the interim between menopause and the initiation of treatment, cannot be discarded. This caveat was one reason to design the Kronos Early Estrogen Prevention Study (KEEPS), another randomized controlled trial that had an ancillary study, the KEEPS-Cog. Women were now younger, 52.6 years average age, and 1.4 years since menopause. A total of 693 women were randomized to daily oral CEE or transdermal estradiol, in both cases associated with micronized progesterone (12 days per month), or placebo. The primary outcome was the effect on the Modified Mini-Mental State examination. Again, HT was not associated with clear benefit, although against the results in the WHIMS, no harm was found this time [25].

The Women's Health Initiative Memory Study of Younger Women (WHIMSY) study had a similar purpose. Cognition was assessed in women who had enrolled in the WHI study when they were 50–55 years of age. When 7.2 years had elapsed since the end of the trial, women were assessed by telephone, their mean age being

67.2 at that moment. As for the KEEPS-Cog, no substantial difference was found between women receiving hormones and the placebo-treated controls [6].

Some investigators have claimed that, despite the consistent evidence obtained in randomized studies, the duration of therapy might have been missed as a variable, since none of them followed participants for longer than few years. In response of this uncertainty, a cohort of women in France was assessed for cognitive function, and the reported duration of HT was used as a variable. HT was associated with better performance in certain cognitive domains, and the associations were dependent on the duration of treatment [26]. This conclusion is further supported in another recent study in Finland [27].

To summarize, and in consistence with the conclusion from experienced groups [7], the most solid evidence seems to favor the notion that HT does not have a clear impact on cognition, including episodic memory or executive functions. The neutral effect extends for a reasonable number of years. There is not enough evidence to support the existence of a window of opportunity in the immediate post-menopause. However, studies are still insufficient and late-life cognitive consequences are still poorly addressed.

14.2.4.2 Effects of HT on Mood

Mood disorders are prevalent during the menopausal transition, with figures that attain a 16.5% for depressed mood in midlife women [28]. The SWAN study found that women were two to four times more likely to suffer a depressive episode during the menopausal transition [29]. Other investigators have reported similar findings [30]. The known interaction of estrogens with serotonin and other monoamines provides biochemical rationality to the clinical findings [31]. Mood problems have been found to increase in those with a history of mood continuum disorders, but can also occur de novo as a consequence of the hormonal changes. In most cases, the period of vulnerability to mood problems [32] subsides when the hormonal levels stabilize and women enter full menopause. It is understood that it is hormonal fluctuations that more directly determine the mood changes [33].

The clear hormonal influence has prompted the postulation of HT as an efficacious remedy. One recent central study has been the previously mentioned KEEPS-Cog, a multicenter randomized trial that, in addition to cognitive effects, assessed the impact on mood, including depression and anxiety. Oral CEE, but not transdermal estradiol, effectively reduced scores of depression and anxiety over the 48 months of treatment [25]. The reasons for the difference remain elusive, although it is against the well-known stable levels provided by the estradiol patches. This effect of estrogens in KEEPS-Cog further confirms previous studies of different sizes and relevance, as shown in several reviews [32–34].

14.3 Cardiovascular Disease

Cardiovascular disease (CVD) remains the most common killer of women worldwide. After menopause, with the decline of ovarian function, the incidence of CVD in women increases rapidly until it equals that of men. Postmenopausal HT has been

Table 14.1 Mechanisms by which estrogen may exert beneficial cardiovascular effects

Direct effects	Indirect effects
Nitric oxide production and release↑	Total cholesterol↓, LDL↓, HDL↑
Prostacyclin production and release↑	Antioxidant effects: oxidation of LDL↓
Endothelin-1 production and release ↓	Blood pressure↓
Cytokine release ↓	Insulin sensitivity↑
Inflammation ↓	Homocysteine ↓
Smooth-muscle cell growth↓	Ischemia/reperfusion injury↓, cardiac hypertrophy↓
Atherosclerotic plaque progression↓	

used for more than 80 years mainly to alleviate vasomotor symptoms (VMS) and other menopausal symptoms. However, during the past couple decades, the health benefits and risks of HT have been under vigorous debate, particularly focusing on the impact of HT on the cardiovascular health.

Estrogen has various well-established direct effects on the vascular wall resulting to vasodilation and prevention of occlusive events (Table 14.1) [35, 36]. Furthermore, estrogen mediates a number of secondary changes in the vasculature that slow down the initiation and progression of atherosclerosis (Table 14.1). However, these beneficial vascular effects of estrogen are lost at later stages of more complicated atherosclerosis and may lead to propensity of plaque rupture and thrombosis [37]. This is in line with the recent clinical data indicating that HT is beneficial to the cardiovascular health if initiated soon after the onset of menopause but not anymore if started in elderly women with advanced atherosclerosis [38, 39].

The majority of observational studies assessing the effect of HT on CVD comes from women who have chosen to initiate HT close to menopause to alleviate various menopausal symptoms [40]. Overall, these data suggest a 30–50% reduction in CVD in HT users compared with nonusers. This dogma was challenged by the WHI randomized trial, where HT failed to provide primary prevention of CVD events in women who started HT at a mean age of 63 years [41]. This led to rapid decline in HT use and change in guidelines worldwide and, most importantly, ended the use of HT for primary prevention of CVD.

14.3.1 New Evidence to Support the Benefit of HT in Cardiovascular Health

There is a strong evidence that the discrepancy between the results of the large body of epidemiological studies and the primary results of the WHI-study can mainly be explained by the "timing-hypothesis," i.e., HT initiation is beneficial for the cardiovascular health in healthy recently menopausal women but not in elderly women with various CVD risk factors [37–39, 42, 43]. This has been confirmed by several sub-analyses of the WHI study [44]. Also the most recent clinical trials and epidemiological studies suggest that HT reduces the incidence of CVD in recently menopausal women [45]. In a Danish trial (DOPS study), women who received HT

7 months after the onset of menopause suffered half as many myocardial infarctions, heart failure, and death as women who did not receive treatment [46]. In the Early versus Late Intervention Trial (ELITE-study) estradiol-based HT resulted in a significantly slower progression of carotid artery intima media thickness compared to placebo, but only among women who initiated HT less than 6 years after menopause [39]. These data suggest that HT impairs the development of atherosclerosis and CVD when initiated early after menopause.

A study in Finland detected that myocardial infarction attack-related death risk was 38% smaller in estradiol-based HT users compared to nonusers, and this may indicate HT-induced cardiac benefits before and/or during the myocardial infarction [47]. Furthermore, HT has been shown to reduce cardiac death risk the earlier the HT is initiated [38]. These data suggest that 60 years of age at the initiation of HT is not necessarily a threshold age, but the earlier the HT had been started, the smaller was the cardiac mortality risk. This is supported by the fact that atherosclerotic changes start to develop already in premenopausal age, and thus, the findings are in line with the "timing-hypothesis."

Many women choose to discontinue HT due to recommendations that HT should be used for the shortest possible time, and furthermore, annual or bi-annual HT pause has become a routine practice to evaluate if a woman could manage without HT. In a recent large-scale population-based study, women who discontinued estradiol-based hormone therapy compared with women who continued it had a 2.3-fold increased risk of CVD mortality during the first year after hormone therapy [48]. Furthermore, these risk elevations were markedly higher in women who had been younger than 60 years at the initiation of HT use. Although the mechanisms behind these findings are not established, it is possible that acute withdrawal of vasodilatory estrogen, as in discontinuation of HT, may result in constriction of coronary arteries and even fatal thrombogenic events. Thus, these findings strongly question the safety of the annual discontinuation practice, particularly in recently menopausal women.

14.3.2 Effect of Type and Route of HT in Cardiovascular Health

In the USA, most studies have been conducted with CEE, whereas estradiol has been used almost exclusively in Europe. Some data indicate that CEE could be more prothrombotic than estradiol [49]. Thus, more studies comparing head to head CEE and estradiol are needed, and for now comparisons between clinical CVD outcomes obtained with CEE or estradiol should be done with caution.

The progestogen component of HT, and particularly MPA, has often been associated with the failure of HT in primary prevention of CVD [50]. In a large study MPA, norethisterone acetate and a number of other progestogens used with estradiol were accompanied with overall comparable reductions in CVD mortality risk [38]. However, dydrogesterone, a less androgenic progestogen than, e.g., MPA, showed a tendency of being more beneficial than other progestogens when HT was initiated before 60 years of age [38]. Thus, although there might be some differences in the cardiovascular effects of the different progestogens used in HT, they do not appear to fully antagonize the beneficial cardiovascular effects of estrogen.

Oral and transdermal administration results in different estrogenic milieus; oral route causes higher circulating levels of estrone than transdermal use of estradiol. By avoiding the hepatic first-pass metabolism, the transdermal route results in fewer adverse effects on coagulation markers compared to oral estrogens, and thus, the transdermal route is devoid of increased risk of deep vein thromboembolism [51, 52]. However, comparisons between oral and transdermal estradiol with other CVD events as primary endpoints are needed. Interestingly, the use of local estradiol to alleviate vaginal atrophy leads to slight increases in circulating estradiol levels [53], and this estradiol rise appears to benefit heart; the risk of CVD mortality was significantly decreased in a study with 330,000 women using local estradiol [54]. Thus, even the very low levels of nonoral estradiol appear to provide cardiac benefits and perhaps particularly in elderly women.

14.3.3 Conclusions

After the primary WHI publications, new research data have been accumulated that uniformly support the beneficial effects of estradiol-based HT in cardiovascular health primary prevention of CVD. Control of VMS should remain the primary indication for prescribing HT; however, to obtain concomitant cardiac benefit, HT use should be initiated soon after the onset of menopause.

14.4 Osteoarthritis

14.4.1 Introduction

The increase in the incidence of osteoarthritis (OA) after menopause [55], together with the identification of ER in diverse joint tissues [56, 57], supports the hypothesis that estrogens have a role in the development of the disease. This fact has posed the possibility of including estrogen therapy (ET) as an option in the treatment of OA. Despite the large number of studies postulating the chondroprotective effect of estrogens (Table 14.2), the mechanisms by which estrogens act appear complex [58]

Table 14.2 Possible mechanisms of the chondroprotective effect of estrogens

Increases glycosaminoglycan synthesis
Prevents chondrocytes apoptosis
Decreases NF-KB, iNOS, COX 2, and ROS
Reduces prostaglandins
Decreases metalloproteinases 3 and 13
Prevents type II collagen degradation
Decreases subchondral bone turnover

and are not fully understood. Yet, experimental observations point to both direct and indirect effects on the articular cartilage; indirect effects seem to occur via inhibition of subchondral bone turnover [59], while direct effects include cell-autonomous actions on the articular chondrocyte. Herein we will only focus on the latter ones.

The experimental observations have been paralleled by clinical studies examining the effect of the treatment with estrogens on OA [60, 61]. More recently, selective estrogen receptor modulators (SERMs) have received some interest too.

14.4.2 Experimental Evidence

14.4.2.1 Beneficial Effect of Estrogens on the Cartilage

There are several actions of estrogens that have been considered beneficial for cartilage health. Previous studies established that estrogen deprivation decreases glycosaminoglycans (GAG) synthesis. Further, cartilage compression increased significantly GAG release and induced chondrocytes apoptosis. Against those observations, physiological concentrations of estradiol prevented the injury-related cell death and reduced the GAG release significantly in a receptor-mediated manner, suggesting that HT could be an option for OA [62]. Molecular studies have shown the implication of ERα in preserving the functional performance of chondrocytes [63].

Also, chondrocytes display a metabolism adapted to anaerobic conditions. Indeed, oxygen tension in synovial fluid can change and lead to ischemia-reperfusion phenomena. These changes can abnormally accelerate tissue metabolism and produce anomalous levels of reactive oxygen species (ROS) that have been described to increase the risk for OA development [64]. Estradiol has been postulated to affect oxidative stress. Claassen et al. [65] showed how the addition of estrogen to articular chondrocytes in vitro provided an antioxidant effect, which protects chondrocytes from ROS-induced damage.

Estrogens can also decrease the production of some pro-inflammatory cytokines [66]. The expression of MMP-13 and IL-1β in the chondrocyte was downregulated by the interaction of 17β-estradiol with its receptor through the induction of miR-140 [67]. Moreover, the effects of IL-1α and TNF-α on the production of prostaglandin E2 are mainly due to an increase in cyclooxygenase-2 (COX-2) activity. Morisset et al. [68] found that 17β-estradiol reduced prostaglandins through a decrease in the mRNA steady-state levels of COX-2 in bovine articular chondrocytes. This effect has been claimed to provide protection against ROS-induced chondrocyte damage. Figure 14.1 shows morphological features of cultured chondrocytes when attacked by the artificially generated oxygen radicals and the protective effect of estrogen.

Other in vitro experiments performed in chondrocytes suggested that not only estrogens but also raloxifene, one well-known SERM, might have a potential chondroprotective role. Decrease in proteoglycan levels and increase in both metalloproteinase-3 (MMP-3) and nitric oxide (NO) have been observed when cultured human

Fig. 14.1 Morphological features of chondrocytes in culture without (**a**) and with (**b**) estradiol and attacked by the artificial generation of oxygen radicals. Unprotected chondrocytes were characterized by the production of vesicles (arrows) representing damaged plasma membranes and cell organelles. In some areas (stars), chondrocytes were disintegrated. Chondrocytes exposed to estradiol (**b**) had a healthy morphology, without vesicles, indicating that estradiol protects them against ROS-induced membrane damage. Bars, 20 μm. (With permission of Springer Verlag from Claassen H et al. Cell Tissue Res (2005) 319: 439–445. Permission obtained through Copyright Clearance Center, Inc.)

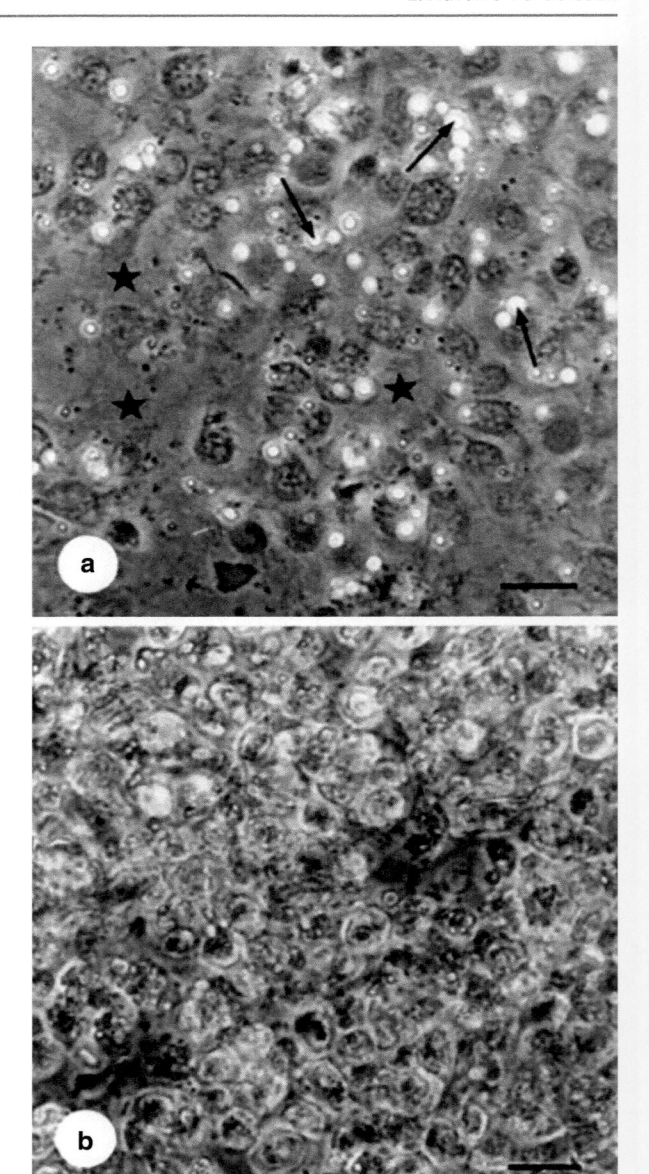

chondrocytes are treated with interleukin-1β (IL-1β). Raloxifene, in a way not too different to estrogens, blunts the decrease in proteoglycan levels and the increase of both MMP-3 and NO, a deleterious effect induced by IL-1β on cultured human chondrocytes. In addition, raloxifene decreased the gene expression of the inducible nitric oxide synthase (iNOS), which was noticeably expressed in IL-1β stimulated chondrocytes [69].

14.4.2.2 Deleterious Effects of Estrogen Therapy on the Cartilage

In contrast with the beneficial effects reported by some studies, a deleterious effect on cartilage by estrogen therapy has been documented as well. The data were obtained in an experimental model of young OVX rabbits receiving either systemic [70] or intra-articular estrogen [71]. Surprisingly, both models developed the typical OA changes. At the cellular level, some authors found that high doses of estrogens induced proteoglycan degradation and MMP production, suggesting that estrogen might exert a dual effect on the joints, either positive or negative, depending on the final concentration achieved within the cartilage microenvironment [72].

14.4.2.3 A Possible Timing Process

Estrogen deficiency increases the erosion of the articular surface and accelerates the renewal of matrix molecules. Oestergaard et al. [73] showed how estrogen supplementation in OVX rats blunts the enzymatic degradation of type II collagen induced by sex hormone loss and decreases the cartilage damage induced by acute loss of estrogens. However, delayed initiation of estrogen therapy after OVX resulted in diminished efficacy in terms of preventing cartilage damage, as compared with early hormone intervention. It seemed that the beneficial effects of HT required a therapeutic window opportunity.

Taking all these data together, it can be concluded that, although more research is needed to understand how estrogens influence chondrocytes homeostasis, both optimal dose concentration and timing of administration after sexual hormone deficiency are two important factors to promote the beneficial effects of estrogens.

14.4.3 Clinical Evidence

The effect of estrogens on OA has been investigated in studies including both radiological imaging and clinical end points. As for the experimental studies, the impact seems mixed, with both protective and deleterious results on the disease.

14.4.3.1 Hormone Therapy and OA in Large Joints

Two classical cross-sectional studies gave favorable results for postmenopausal women using estrogens. The Chingford study in the UK general population showed that women using estrogens for longer than 12 months were significantly less affected by knee and distal interphalangeal OA [74]. Also, the Framingham Osteoarthritis Study in the USA found an inverse relationship between the use of estrogens and radiographic knee OA, although the effect was weak and nonsignificant [75]. Another cross-sectional study examined the possible association between drugs with a bone anti-resorptive effect (estrogens, raloxifene, and alendronate) with structural features of OA, as assessed by magnetic resonance. Both alendronate and estrogen are associated with significantly less OA-related subchondral lesions [76].

The relationship between estrogen therapy and OA in large joints has been also examined in some case-control studies performed some years ago. Denninson et al.

[77] found a protective effect of long-term estrogens on hip OA. However, another study of similar design could not find any effect of life estrogen exposure, as assessed by age at menarche or menopause, contraceptive use, or postmenopausal HT and the diagnosis of OA [78].

Similarly, both the long-term follow-up of the Chingford and the Framingham Osteoarthritis Study found a protective effect of treatment with estrogens on radiographic knee OA, but the effect was weak and, importantly, nonsignificant [79, 80]. Furthermore, a nested case-control study examining the association of estrogen therapy and incident symptomatic OA (hand, hip, and knee) found that the new use of estrogen was associated with a higher incidence of OA [81].

14.4.3.2 Hormone Therapy and Risk for Joint Replacement in Large Joints

Some investigators have looked at the issue from a different angle and examined the possible association between HT and joint replacement because of OA. One important piece of evidence came from the WHI study, in which women receiving only CEE had a lower rate of hip arthroplasty, although the finding could not be reproduced in the group of women receiving estrogens plus progestogen [82]. In the same line, the Nurse's Health Study, a cohort observational study, found that HT was a neutral factor for risk of total hip replacement [83]. A more recent study concluded that, possibly because the bone anti-resorptive effect of HT, the revision rates of hip and knee arthroplasty were reduced in hormone users [84].

However, some discrepant studies have been published as well. A case-control study in Sweden found that the use of estrogens after age 50 increased the risk for OA prosthetic surgery [85]. Another observational study including 1.3 million women found that the use of HT associated with increased risk for hip and knee replacement [86].

14.4.3.3 Hormone Therapy and Hand OA

The effect of HT on hand OA has received insufficient attention. The initial cross-sectional Chingford study, previously mentioned because of the beneficial effect detected for knee OA in hormone users, could not find a similar protective effect on the hand [74]. Similar neutral effects were found in another cross-sectional study [87].

Again, there is also some data suggesting that hormones might be deleterious for hand OA. For example, ever or current use of HT was associated with increased prevalence and severity of Heberden's nodes and distal interphalangeal OA in 348 Tasmanian women [88].

14.4.3.4 Studies on Biological Markers

Some investigators have looked at the impact of hormone use on biological indicators of cartilage health. The cartilage volume, as measured by magnetic resonance, and the changes in the serum or urinary levels of some biomarkers have been selected.

A study involving 81 women treated with hormones for longer than 5 years found that hormone users had more cartilage at the knee joint than untreated controls [89]. The same group could not reproduce the findings when examining the cartilage at the patella [90] or at the tibia when women were followed longitudinally for approximately 2.5 years [91].

Concerning circulating biomarkers, the cartilage oligomeric matrix protein (COMP) is considered an indicator of joint destruction that can be measured in serum. A case-control study found that estrogen therapy significantly decreased the levels of COMP after 6 months. This observation led investigators to suggest a role for estrogens in the prevention of joint damage [92]. In a different approach, the changes in the urinary levels of C-telopeptides of type II collagen (uCTX-II), a marker of cartilage degradation, were found to be decreased by oral or transdermal estrogen when using samples from two randomized, double-blind, placebo-controlled trials in Denmark [93].

14.4.4 Other Agents Interacting with Estrogen Receptors: SERMs

An alternative approach is provided by the selective estrogen receptor modulators (SERMs), a class of compounds different to estrogens but with the ability to interact with the ER. There is high-quality evidence showing the protective effect of SERMs in osteoporosis, and the hypothesis has been raised that a similar effect might be extended to the joint and the cartilage. Some data support this contention. For example, levormeloxifene, a SERM from the triphenylethylene family, reduced by approximately 50% the urinary excretion of CTX-II [94]. There is an additional information from animal models that suggest a protective role for SERMs [95], but clinical studies are still insufficient.

14.4.5 Conclusion

There is some evidence in favor of a protective effect of estrogens on the joints, but there are also neutral studies at both experimental and clinical level. Because there is also some evidence, though sparse, showing deleterious effects, the best judgement should be that the issue is controversial at present. Further, the favorable studies are not unanimous in what refers to the dose of estrogens, the length of treatment, or the optimal therapeutic window. More evidence is, therefore, required. This insufficiency also includes the needed clarification of the potential impact of SERMs.

14.5 Hormone Therapy and Cancer Risk

14.5.1 Introduction

The impact of menopause on the risk of cancer is tightly related with the role of ovarian steroids in the risk for malignancies of genital tract and breast. Indeed, cancerophobia has been one of the most frequently argued reasons for rejecting or abandoning

HT [96]. While no particular oncogenic risk has been detected with the decline in estrogens during menopause, HT has been associated with increased risk of breast and endometrial cancer and, after more recent clinical data, also with ovarian cancer.

14.5.2 Biological Plausibility

The physiological changes of breast and endometrium in response to the oscillations of the circulating levels of estrogens are clearly perceived by women as a proof of the hormonal sensitivity of both tissues. Symptoms like cyclical breast tenderness and the own development of the gland during puberty strengthen the notion. The endometrial cycle, with menstruation as the final phase, is an obvious correlate at the level of the uterus. Estrogens have been considered the main responsible of the observed clinical changes, and only after more careful work, has become apparent the role of progesterone. This all, in any case, has resulted from work performed several years ago.

The differential roles of estrogens and progesterone on the endometrium were unveiled by work on endometrial specimens [97] that was performed in the UK by Roger King and collaborators. According to the information provided by biopsies obtained during the menstrual cycle, it became clear that estradiol promotes endometrial proliferation while progesterone stops the process and induces differentiation in glands and stroma. The preparation of the endometrium for an eventual embryo implantation was the biological result of this finely tuned coordination between estradiol and progesterone during the human menstrual cycle, as described in classical papers [98]. The mechanisms underlying these changes, and the corresponding fluctuations in the population of estrogen and progesterone receptors, have been exquisitely well described by investigators using basic biochemistry or immunohistochemistry.

The breast follows a different pattern. The role of progesterone, which was assumed to be antiproliferative like in the endometrium, turned to be opposite. The finding that breast biopsies during the luteal phase of the cycle [99] showed increased proliferation and mitoses puzzled clinicians and investigators. It is now evident, as confirmed in rodents, that progestogens increase proliferative activity in the breast. Moreover, more recent work has shown that progestogens might act through interaction with the pathway of the receptor activator of nuclear factor κ (RANK), a receptor that binds RANK ligand (RANKL), a cytokine. This proliferative action of progestogens may convey the increased risk for breast cancer associated with hormones [100, 101]. The role of progesterone in breast cancer risk, nonetheless, is complex and still poorly understood [102].

14.5.3 Hormones and Risk for Specific Types of Cancer

14.5.3.1 Endometrial Cancer
The early observation that the use of estrogens for HT in women with a uterus was associated with an increased risk for endometrial cancer [103] led to the use of combined estrogen plus progestogen regimes. Abundant literature has reproduced

the association in subsequent years [104], and more refined studies have detected an association with the lifetime exposure to estrogens, even in premenopausal women [105]. This is the interpretation given to the increased risk for women with early menarche or late menopause, or high body mass index [106]. The promotion of proliferation and reduction of apoptosis by estrogens are taken as factors influencing the association.

The well-established antiproliferative action of progesterone was the argument to include the generalized use of combined treatments in women with a uterus. Two combinations have been in use since then, the cyclic and the continuous combined. The difference between them relies in the mode of progestogen administration, which accumulated for only some days of the cycle, usually 12–14 days, in the case of the cyclic formulations, or daily, together with the estrogen, in the continuous combined option. While the cyclic protocols use to leave a few hormone-free days to allow for withdrawal bleeding, the continuous combined regimes are prolonged uninterrupted to achieve amenorrhea. The daily progestogen dose is lower in continuous regimes, although the more prolonged use makes that the total dose per month does not differ significantly between them. The continuous combined formulations are not free of unscheduled bleeding episodes, particularly during the first year of use.

It is worth mentioning that the regular use of progestogens with estrogens in HT actually reduces the risk of endometrial cancer [107]. Because of this reduction in the risk for endometrial cancer, together with the unwanted bleeding episodes, the hypothesis was raised of whether using less progestogen might diminish side effects while maintaining a good endometrial control. One alternative protocol has consisted of the use of vaginal progesterone, which is less potent than synthetic molecules as a progestogen. Vaginal dosing allows for selective accumulation of progesterone in the uterus and reduced systemic concentration [108]. In a further step, the use of interrupted formulations, in which the progestogen is given twice-a-week, has shown very competitive effectiveness [108]. Moreover, this formulation may be used with success with the use of micronized vaginal progesterone [109]. However, the issue needs to be investigated further, as some data suggest that protection may be reduced in the case of sequential combinations, where progestogens are used for 12–14 days per month, or when micronized progesterone is used [110].

14.5.3.2 Breast Cancer

Whereas the risk of endometrial cancer has been apparently abrogated by the inclusion of a progestogen in the hormonal formulations, breast cancer has consistently arisen as an adverse effect of HT. In an almost unanimous form, the early evidence emerged in observational studies. Together with the biological plausibility and the social impact of breast cancer, the issue has arisen as a deterrent against the use of hormones by postmenopausal women [96, 111]. The association was detected for both estrogen and estrogen plus progestogen regimes, although the responsible role of estrogens was considered as granted. More solid conclusion was obtained when stronger evidence, as provided by randomized controlled trials, was available. A landmark in this sequence was provided by the WHI study, which confirmed an approximately 30% increase in risk in hormone users after approximately 5 years of treatment. Of interest in the WHI, the division of the trial in two arms, estrogens only and estrogen plus progestogen depending on whether women were, or were not, hysterectomized, disclosed that while increased risk was found in women with combined treatments, women receiving only estrogen did not show increased risk [112]. The findings were consistent with the earlier and somewhat unexpected observations of a mitogenic role of progesterone on the breast, as described in breast biopsies taken during the luteal phase of the cycle [99].

A more refined perspective has arisen since then. The oncogenic role of estrogens remains supported by experimental studies and also by the consistent epidemiological association with features shared with endometrial cancer. Good examples are early menarche, late menopause, or high body mass index. Also, there is a relationship of breast cancer risk with the circulating levels of endogenous estrogens and estrogen metabolites [53]. And there are indirect data, yet inconclusive, suggesting association of the levels of circulating estrogens with breast density, a notable risk factor for breast cancer incidence and, perhaps, also progression [113]. And finally, the risk decrease provided by drugs reducing the estrogen exposure, like aromatase inhibitors and SERMs, is an additional argument. And to further reinforce these evidences, epidemiological data published subsequently to the WHI study keep confirming an increased risk associated with the use of estrogens in HT.

Having said so, the principal responsibility of progestogens seems warranted. It is not only the data of the WHI but also the confirmation provided by subsequent studies [114] and by more recent meta-analyses [115, 116]: They all are unanimous in showing increased risk with combination therapies, the risk being consistently higher than that of estrogens. To further support the role of progestogens, there is biological evidence showing that the RANK/RANKL pathway may convey the action of progestogens [100] (Fig. 14.2). Consequently, the present view is that it is progestogen that mostly increases the risk of breast cancer, albeit a lower estrogen-mediated risk seems warranted as well.

There is also some debate on whether there is a class effect in the risk mediated by estrogens and progestogens. The topic is of high interest, because it raises the point of whether some variants of estrogens may be used with minor or undetectable risk. The debate has included estradiol [117, 118], but also estriol, and the more recent estetrol.

Estriol is considered a weak estrogen because of the poor potential for inducing proliferation in target tissues. The main source of natural estriol is the placenta. No definitive conclusion can be offered at present, mainly because most of the data have been originated in experimental models and results are controversial [119, 120]. Clinical studies with systemically used estriol are sparse [121], since most available preparations have been designed for local vaginal use. The case of estetrol is slightly different. Estetrol is originated also during pregnancy. Considered initially as a weak estrogen due to its weak affinity for the receptor, recent research has evidenced that it is a potent estrogen with agonistic actions in most target tissues, with the exception of the breast [122]. This attractive profile makes estetrol a

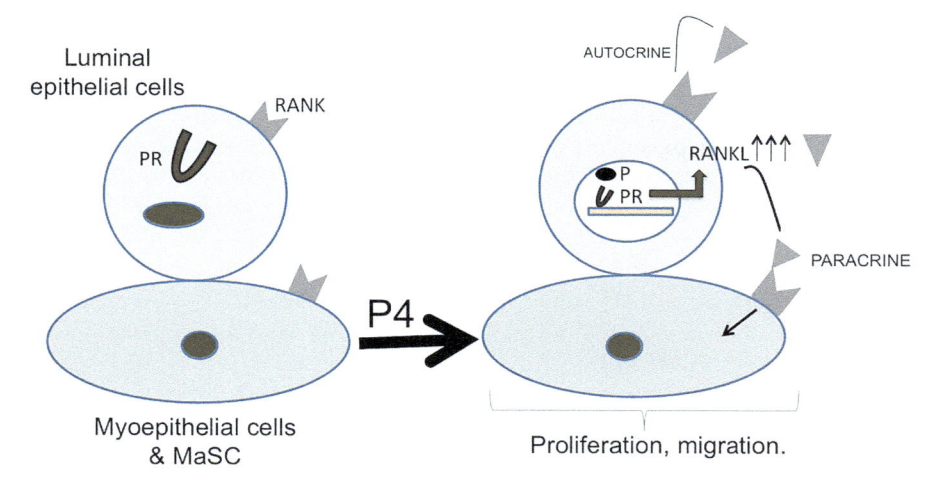

Fig. 14.2 Role of RANK/RANKL in progestogen-mediated proliferation of breast epithelium. Mammary stem cells (MaSC) and luminal cells express RANK at their membranes. Progesterone receptors (PR), however, are expressed only in luminal cells. The activation of PR by progesterone (P4) increases the expression of RANKL in luminal cells. Then, the cytokine acts through two possible ways, either autocrine, which further increases the production of RANKL, or paracrine, which increases proliferation, migration, and differentiation of MaSC. (With permission of Taylor & Francis from González Ricarte M, et al. Gynecol Endocrinol. (2016); 32: 6–8. Permission obtained through Copyright Clearance Center, Inc.)

potentially valid agent for HT [123–126] and contraception [127], but the clinical experience is still sparse.

There is also some debate in what regards progestogens. Micronized progesterone, for example, and also some synthetic progestogens like dydrogesterone have been ascribed a more neutral role than other progestogens as inducers of breast cancer. The weakness of this claim is that the information is still sparse and comes from observational studies [128, 129].

Finally, there are also some data about tibolone, one synthetic compound vastly used in some European countries as an efficacious form of HT. A recent Cochrane systematic review could not detect an increased risk in women with no history of breast cancer, but the quality of the evidence was described as very low [130]. A study in Norway followed a cohort of 178,383 women who were prescribed HT for an average of 4.8 years. A total of 7910 invasive breast cancers were detected, tibolone being associated with a relative risk of 1.91, which was slightly lower than that of combined estradiol and norethisterone acetate, a synthetic progestogen [114]. An increased risk was also found in two meta-analyses [115, 116].

There is a debate on whether HT only promotes the growth of cancers that were already in the breast, in a quiescent state, and that, perhaps because of so, the mortality of cases associated with the use of hormones would be lower. Investigators from the WHI trial found that survival after breast cancer was similar in users and nonusers of hormones. This finding made them to conclude that, because the prognosis was not different, increased diagnosis should translate into higher mortality [131]. In addition, a subsequent long-term follow-up analysis showed a decreased risk of breast cancer mortality in women randomized to estrogen alone, while no change in breast cancer-associated mortality was detected in women using the estrogen/progestogen combination [132]. Also, the analysis of the nationwide reimbursement register in Finland, which followed HT users till death because of breast cancer (n = 1578 women), found that the cancer-associated mortality was approximately 50% of that in breast cancer nonusers of hormones [133]. Of further interest in this regard, and most probably because of other reasons too, global mortality seems reduced in users of HT from early postmenopause [134].

14.5.3.3 Ovarian Cancer

Ovarian cancer is first among the gynecological malignancies in terms of mortality. The possible association with HT has been highlighted relatively late, as compared with breast or endometrial cancer.

The link between HT and increased risk for ovarian cancer was first detected in observational studies, but the potential recall or selective participation bias blurred the consistence of the results [135–137]. The WHI study, a randomized controlled study, detected an increase in risk, but did not reach statistical significance [138]. Two subsequent meta-analyses agreed in an increased risk [139, 140], and similarly the Million Women Study, which found an increase in both incident and fatal cancer in women using HT in the UK. Investigators advanced that since 1991, roughly 1300 cases of ovarian cancer and 1000 additional deaths from the disease could be attributed to the use of HT in the UK [141]. Additional arguments provided the observed reduction in incidence in the USA after the drastic decline in the use of hormones in the years following the publication of the WHI study [142]. Information, however, is not unanimous, since a study based on the data from the Finnish Cancer Registry could only find an association with estrogen plus progestogen combinations [143].

More recent meta-analyses agree in that the evidence, albeit obtained in observational studies, unanimously suggests the association. Specifically, the increased risk in current users, even if for less than 5 years, attained a 43% (RR 1.43, 95% CI 1.31–1.56; $p < 0.0001$). The risk was similar for estrogen-only or estrogen-progestogen formulations and, when considering the tumor type, was clearly increased in the most common forms, serous (RR 1.53, 95% CI 1.40–1.66) and endometrioid (1.42, 1.20–1.67). Translating the risk to absolute figures, authors indicate that women who use HT for 5 years have about one extra ovarian cancer per 1000 users and about one extra ovarian cancer death per 1700 users [144]. Risk of similar size was found in another meta-analysis, which reproduced the increased risk for serous, but not for endometrioid tumors [145]. Similar results were obtained in a more recent meta-analysis [146] and in cohort studies in Sweden [147] or in France [148]. The French E3N cohort followed 75,606 postmenopausal women for an average of 15.3 years. The hazard ratio for every use of estrogens combined with progesterone or dydrogesterone is 1.28 (95% CI = 1.04–1.57). Studies on potential racial disparities in risk do not seem to be substantiated, although the data are still sparse [149].

References

1. Pompili A, Arnone B, Gasbarri A. Estrogens and memory in physiological and neuropathological conditions. Psychoneuroendocrinology. 2012;37:1379–96.
2. Gorenstein C, Rennó J, Vieira Filho A, Gianfaldoni A, Gonçalves M, Halbe H, et al. Estrogen replacement therapy and cognitive functions in healthy postmenopausal women: a randomized trial. Arch Womens Ment Health. 2011;14:367–73.
3. MacLennan A, Henderson V, Paine B, Mathias J, Ramsay E, Ryan P, et al. Hormone therapy, timing of initiation, and cognition in women aged older than 60 years: the REMEMBER pilot study. Menopause. 2006;13:28–36.
4. Ryan J, Carrière I, Scali J, Ritchie K, Ancelin M. Life-time estrogen exposure and cognitive functioning in later life. Psychoneuroendocrinology. 2009;34:287–98.
5. Smith Y, Giordani B, Lajiness-O'Neill R, Zubieta J. Long-term estrogen replacement is associated with improved nonverbal memory and attentional measures in postmenopausal women. Fertil Steril. 2001;76:1101–7.
6. Espeland M, Shumaker S, Leng I, Manson J, Brown C, LeBlanc E, et al. Long-term effects on cognitive function of postmenopausal hormone therapy prescribed to women aged 50 to 55 years. JAMA Intern Med. 2013;173:1429–36.
7. Henderson V, Popat R. Effects of endogenous and exogenous estrogen exposures in midlife and late-life women on episodic memory and executive functions. Neuroscience. 2011;191:129–38.
8. Parikh M, Hynan L, Weiner M, Lacritz L, Ringe W, Cullum C. Single neuropsychological test scores associated with rate of cognitive decline in early Alzheimer disease. Clin Neuropsychol. 2014;28:926–40.
9. Mueller K, Koscik R, LaRue A, Clark L, Hermann B, Johnson S, et al. Verbal fluency and early memory decline: results from the Wisconsin Registry for Alzheimer's Prevention. Arch Clin Neuropsychol. 2015;30:448–57.
10. Sherwin B. Estrogen and cognitive aging in women. Neuroscience. 2006;138:1021–6.
11. Hara Y, Waters E, McEwen B, Morrison J. Estrogen effects on cognitive and synaptic health over the lifecourse. Physiol Rev. 2015;95:785–807.
12. Phan A, Suschkov S, Molinaro L, Reynolds K, Lymer J, Bailey C, et al. Rapid increases in immature synapses parallel estrogen-induced hippocampal learning enhancements. Proc Natl Acad Sci U S A. 2015;112:16018–23.
13. Velazquez-Zamora D, Garcia-Segura L, Gonzalez-Burgos I. Effects of selective estrogen receptor modulators on allocentric working memory performance and on dendritic spines in medial prefrontal cortex pyramidal neurons of ovariectomized rats. Horm Behav. 2012;61:512–7.
14. Frick K, Kim J, Tuscher J, Fortress A. Sex steroid hormones matter for learning and memory: estrogenic regulation of hippocampal function in male and female rodents. Learn Mem. 2015;22:472–93.
15. Pompili A, Tomaz C, Arnone B, Tavares M, Gasbarri A. Working and reference memory across the estrous cycle of rat: a long-term study in gonadally intact females. Behav Brain Res. 2010;213:10–8.
16. Luo Y, Xiao Q, Chao F, He Q, Lv F, Zhang L, et al. 17β-estradiol replacement therapy protects myelin sheaths in the white matter of middle-aged female ovariectomized rats: a stereological study. Neurobiol Aging. 2016;47:139–48.
17. Hara Y, Yuk F, Puri R, Janssen W, Rapp P, Morrison J. Estrogen restores multisynaptic boutons in the dorsolateral prefrontal cortex while promoting working memory in aged rhesus monkeys. J Neurosci. 2016;36:901–10.
18. Gasbarri A, Pompili A, D'Onofrio A, Tostes-Abreu C, Tavares M. Working memory for emotional facial expressions: role of estrogen in humans and non-human primates. Rev Neurosci. 2008;19:129–48.

19. Hara Y, Yuk F, Puri R, Janssen W, Rapp P, Morrison J. Presynaptic mitochondrial morphology in monkey prefrontal cortex correlates with working memory and is improved with estrogen treatment. Proc Natl Acad Sci U S A. 2014;111:486–91.
20. Voytko M, Higgs C, Murray R. Differential effects on visual and spatial recognition memory of a novel hormone therapy regimen of estrogen alone or combined with progesterone in older surgically menopausal monkeys. Neuroscience. 2008;154:1205–17.
21. Braden B, Andrews M, Acosta J, Mennenga S, Lavery C, Bimonte-Nelson H. A comparison of progestins within three classes: differential effects on learning and memory in the aging surgically menopausal rat. Behav Brain Res. 2017;322:258–68.
22. Luetters C, Huang M, Seeman T, Buckwalterm G, Meyer P, Avis N, et al. Menopause transition stage and endogenous estradiol and follicle-stimulating hormone levels are not related to cognitive performance: cross-sectional results from the study of women's health across the nation (SWAN). J Womans Health. 2007;16:331–44.
23. Shumaker S, Legault C, Rapp S, Thal L, Wallace R, Ockene J, et al. Estrogen plus progestin and the incidence of dementia and mild cognitive impairment in postmenopausal women: the Women's Health Initiative Memory Study: a randomized controlled trial. JAMA. 2003;289:2651–62.
24. Resnick S, Espeland M, Jaramillo S, Hirsch C, Stefanick M, Murray A, et al. Postmenopausal hormone therapy and regional brain volumes: the WHIMS-MRI study. Neurology. 2009;72:135–42.
25. Gleason C, Dowling N, Wharton W, Manson J, Miller V, Atwood C, et al. Effects of hormone therapy on cognition and mood in recently postmenopausal women: findings from the randomized, controlled KEEPS-cognitive and affective study. PLoS Med. 2015;12:e1001833.
26. Ryan J, Carrière I, Scali J, Dartigues J, Tzourio C, Poncet M, et al. Characteristics of hormone therapy, cognitive function, and dementia: the prospective 3C Study. Neurology. 2009;73:1729–37.
27. Imtiaz B, Taipale H, Tanskanen A, Tiihonen M, Kivipelto M, Heikkinen A, et al. Risk of Alzheimer's disease among users of postmenopausal hormone therapy: a nationwide case-control study. Maturitas. 2017;98:7–13.
28. Prairie B, Wisniewski S, Luther J, Hess R, Thurston R, Wisner K, et al. Symptoms of depressed mood, disturbed sleep, and sexual problems in midlife women: cross-sectional data from the study of women's health across the nation. J Womens Health. 2015;24:119–26.
29. Bromberger J, Kravitz H, Chang Y, Cyranowski J, Brown C, Matthews K. Major depression during and after the menopausal transition: study of women's health across the nation (SWAN). Psychol Med. 2011;41:1879–88.
30. Soares C. Can depression be a menopause-associated risk? BMC Med. 2010;8:79.
31. Warnock J, Cohen L, Blumenthal H, Hammond J. Hormone-related migraine headaches and mood disorders: treatment with estrogen stabilization. Pharmacotherapy. 2017;37:120–8.
32. Alexander J, Dennerstein L, Woods NKK, Halbreich U, Burt V, et al. Neurobehavioral impact of menopause on mood. Expert Rev Neurother. 2007;7:S81–91.
33. Wharton W, Gleason C, Olson S, Carlsson C, Asthana S. Neurobiological underpinnings of the estrogen - mood relationship. Curr Psychiatr Rev. 2012;8:247–56.
34. Toffol E, Heikinheimo O, Partonen T. Hormone therapy and mood in perimenopausal and postmenopausal women: a narrative review. Menopause. 2015;22:564–78.
35. Mendelsohn M, Karas R. Molecular and cellular basis of cardiovascular gender differences. Science. 2005;308:1583–7.
36. Menazza S, Murphy E. The expanding complexity of estrogen receptor signaling in the cardiovascular system. Circ Res. 2016;118:994–1007.
37. Mikkola T, Clarkson T. Estrogen replacement therapy, atherosclerosis, and vascular function. Cardiovasc Res. 2002;53:605–19.
38. Savolainen-Peltonen H, Tuomikoski P, Korhonen P, et al. Cardiac death risk in relation to the age at initiation or the progestin component of hormone therapies. J Clin Endocrinol Metab. 2016;101:2794–801.

39. Hodis H, Mack W, Henderson V, et al. Vascular effects of early versus late postmenopausal treatment with estradiol. N Engl J Med. 2016;374:1221–31.
40. Grady D, Rubin S, Petitti D, Gox C, Black D, Ettinger B, et al. Hormone therapy to prevent disease and prolong life in postmenopausal women. Ann Intern Med. 1992;117:1016–37.
41. Rossouw J, Anderson G, Prentice R, et al. Risks and benefits of estrogen plus progestin in healthy postmenopausal women: principal results from the women's health initiative randomized controlled trial. JAMA. 2002;288:321–33.
42. Manson JE, Crandall CJ, Rossouw JE, Chlebowski RT, Anderson GL, Stefanick ML, et al. The women's health initiative randomized trials and clinical practice: a review. JAMA. 2024;331:1748–60. https://doi.org/10.1001/jama.2024.6542.
43. Nudy M, Buerger J, Dreibelbis S, Jiang X, Hodis HN, Schnatz PF. Menopausal hormone therapy and coronary heart disease: the roller-coaster history. Climacteric. 2024;27:81–8. https://doi.org/10.1080/13697137.2023.2282690.
44. Rossouw J, Prentice R, Manson J, et al. Postmenopausal hormone therapy and risk of cardiovascular disease by age and years since menopause. JAMA. 2007;297:1465–77.
45. Boardman H, Hartley L, Eisinga A, Main C, Roqué i Figuls M, Bonfill Cosp X, et al. Hormone therapy for preventing cardiovascular disease in post-menopausal women. Cochrane Database Syst Rev. 2015;3:CD002229.
46. Schierbeck L, Rejnmark L, Tofteng C, et al. Effect of hormone replacement therapy on cardiovascular events in recently postmenopausal women: randomised trial. BMJ. 2012;345:e6409.
47. Tuomikoski P, Salomaa V, Havulinna A, Airaksinen J, Ketonen M, Koukkunen H, et al. Decreased mortality risk due to first acute coronary syndrome in women with postmenopausal hormone therapy use. Maturitas. 2016;94:106–9.
48. Mikkola T, Tuomikoski P, Lyytinen H, et al. Increased cardiovascular mortality risk in women discontinuing postmenopausal hormone therapy. J Clin Endocrinol Metab. 2015;100:4588–94.
49. Smith N, Blondon M, Wiggins K, et al. Lower risk of cardiovascular events in postmenopausal women taking oral estradiol compared with oral conjugated equine estrogens. JAMA Intern Med. 2014;174:25–31.
50. Stanczyk F, Hapgood J, Winer S, Mishell D. Progestogens used in postmenopausal hormone therapy: differences in their pharmacological properties, intracellular actions, and clinical effects. Endocr Rev. 2013;34:171–208.
51. Canonico M. Hormone therapy and hemostasis among postmenopausal women: a review. Menopause. 2014;21:753–62.
52. Booyens RM, Engelbrecht AM, Strauss L, Pretorius E. To clot, or not to clot: the dilemma of hormone treatment options for menopause. Thromb Res. 2022;218:99–111. https://doi.org/10.1016/j.thromres.2022.08.016.
53. Santen R, Yue W, Wang J. Estrogen metabolites and breast cancer. Steroids. 2015;99:61–6.
54. Mikkola T, Tuomikoski P, Lyytinen H, et al. Vaginal estradiol use and the risk for cardiovascular mortality. Hum Reprod. 2016;31:804–9.
55. Srikanth V, Fryer J, Zhai G, Winzenberg T, Hosmer D, Jones G. A meta-analysis of sex differences prevalence, incidence and severity of osteoarthritis. Osteoarthr Cartil. 2005;13:769–81.
56. Ushiyama T, Ueyama H, Inoue K, Ohkubo I, Hukuda S. Expression of genes for estrogen receptors alpha and beta in human articular chondrocytes. Osteoarthr Cartil. 1999;7:560–6.
57. Sciore P, Frank C, Hart D. Identification of sex hormone receptors in human and rabbit ligaments of the knee by reverse transcription-polymerase chain reaction: evidence that receptors are present in tissue from both male and female subjects. J Orthop Res. 1998;16:604–10.
58. Ge Y, Zhou S, Li Y, Wang Z, Chen S, Xia T, et al. Estrogen prevents articular cartilage destruction in a mouse model of AMPK deficiency via ERK-mTOR pathway. Ann Transl Med. 2019;7(14):336. https://doi.org/10.21037/atm.2019.06.77. PMID: 31475206; PMCID: PMC6694256.
59. Sniekers Y, Weinans H, van Osch G, van Leeuwen J. Oestrogen is important for maintenance of cartilage and subchondral bone in a murine model of knee osteoarthritis. Arthritis Res Ther. 2010;12:R182–94.

60. De Klerk B, Schiphof D, Groeneveld F, Koes B, van Osch G, van Meurs J, et al. Limited evidence for a protective effect of unopposed oestrogen therapy for osteoarthritis of the hip: a systematic review. Rheumatology. 2009;48:104–12.
61. Mei Y, Williams JS, Webb EK, Shea AK, MacDonald MJ, Al-Khazraji BK. Roles of hormone replacement therapy and menopause on osteoarthritis and cardiovascular disease outcomes: a narrative review. Front Rehabil Sci. 2022;3:825147. https://doi.org/10.3389/fresc.2022.825147.
62. Imgenberg J, Rolauffs B, Grodzinsky A, Schünke M, Kurz B. Estrogen reduces mechanical injury-related cell death and proteoglycan degradation in mature articular cartilage independent of the presence of the superficial zone tissue. Osteoarthr Cartil. 2013;21:1738–45.
63. Wang N, Zhang X, Rothrauff BB, Fritch MR, Chang A, He Y, et al. Novel role of estrogen receptor-α on regulating chondrocyte phenotype and response to mechanical loading. Osteoarthr Cartil. 2022;30:302–14. https://doi.org/10.1016/j.joca.2021.11.002.
64. Yudoh K, Nguyen V, Nakamura H, Hongo-Masuko K, Kato T, Nishioka K. Potential involvement of oxidative stress in cartilage senescence and development of osteoarthritis: oxidative stress induces chondrocyte telomere instability and downregulation of chondrocyte function. Arthritis Res Ther. 2005;7:R380–91.
65. Claassen H, Schünke M, Kurz B. Estradiol protects cultured articular chondrocytes from oxygen-radical-induced damage. Cell Tissue Res. 2005;319:439–45.
66. Straub R. The complex role of estrogens in inflammation. Endocr Rev. 2007;28:521–74.
67. Liang Y, Duan L, Xiong J, Zhu W, Liu Q, Wang D, et al. E2 regulates MMP-13 via targeting miR-140 in IL-1β-induced extracellular matrix degradation in human chondrocytes. Arthritis Res Ther. 2016;18:105–15.
68. Morisset S, Patry C, Lora M, de Brum-Fernandes A. Regulation of cyclooxygenase-2 expression in bovine chondrocytes in culture by interleukin 1alpha, tumor necrosis factor alpha, glucocorticoids, and 17beta-estradiol. J Rheumatol. 1998;25:1146–53.
69. Tinti L, Niccolini S, Lamboglia A, Pascarelli N, Cervone R, Fioravanti A. Raloxifene protects cultured human chondrocytes from IL-1β induced damage: a biochemical and morphological study. Eur J Pharmacol. 2011;670:67–73.
70. Rosner I, Goldberg V, Getzy L, Moskowitz R. Effects of estrogen on cartilage and experimentally induced osteoarthritis. Arthritis Rheum. 1979;22:52–8.
71. Tsai C, Liu T. Estradiol-induced knee osteoarthrosis in ovariectomized rabbits. Clin Orthop Relat Res. 1993;291:295–302.
72. Richette P, Dumontier M, François M, Tsagris L, Korwin-Zmijowska C, Rannou F, et al. Dual effects of 17beta-oestradiol on interleukin 1beta-induced proteoglycan degradation in chondrocytes. Ann Rheum Dis. 2004;63:191–9.
73. Oestergaard S, Sondergaard B, Hoegh-Andersen P, Henriksen K, Qvist P, Christiansen C, et al. Effects of ovariectomy and estrogen therapy on type II collagen degradation and structural integrity of articular cartilage in rats: implications of the time of initiation. Arthritis Rheum. 2006;54:2441–51.
74. Spector T, Nandra D, Hart D, Doyle D. Is hormone replacement therapy protective for hand and knee osteoarthritis in women? The Chingford Study. Ann Rheum Dis. 1997;56:432–4.
75. Hannan M, Felson D, Anderson J, Naimark A, Kannel W. Estrogen use and radiographic osteoarthritis of the knee in women. The Framingham Osteoarthritis Study. Arthritis Rheum. 1990;33:525–32.
76. Carbone L, Nevitt M, Wildy K, Barrow K, Harris F, Felson D, et al. Health, aging and body composition study: the relationship of antiresorptive drug use to structural findings and symptoms of knee osteoarthritis. Arthritis Rheum. 2004;50:3516–25.
77. Dennison E, Arden N, Kellingray S, Croft P, Coggon D, Cooper C. Hormone replacement therapy, other reproductive variables and symptomatic hip osteoarthritis in elderly white women: a case-control study. Br J Rheumatol. 1998;37:1198–202.
78. Samanta A, Jones A, Regan M, Wilson S, Doherty M. Is osteoarthritis in women affected by hormonal changes or smoking? Br J Rheumatol. 1993;32:366–70.

79. Hart D, Doyle D, Spector T. Incidence and risk factors for radiographic knee osteoarthritis in middle-aged women: the Chingford Study. Arthritis Rheum. 1999;42:17–24.
80. Zhang Y, McAlindon T, Hannan M, Chaisson C, Klein R, Wilson P, et al. Estrogen replacement therapy and worsening of radiographic knee osteoarthritis: the Framingham Study. Arthritis Rheum. 1998;41:1867–73.
81. Oliveria S, Felson D, Cirillo P, Reed J, Walker A. Body weight, body mass index, and incident symptomatic osteoarthritis of the hand, hip, and knee. Epidemiology. 1999;10:161–6.
82. Cirillo D, Wallace R, Wu L, Yood R. Effect of hormone therapy on risk of hip and knee joint replacement in the women's health initiative. Arthritis Rheum. 2006;54:3194–204.
83. Karlson E, Mandl L, Aweh G, Sangha O, Liang M, Grodstein F. Total hip replacement due to osteoarthritis: the importance of age, obesity and other modifiable risk factors. Am J Med. 2003;114:93–8.
84. Prieto-Alhambra D, Javaid M, Judge A, Maskell J, Cooper C, Arden N, On Behalf of the COASt Study Group. Hormone replacement therapy and mid-term implant survival following knee or hip arthroplasty for osteoarthritis: a population-based cohort study. Ann Rheum Dis. 2015;74:557–63.
85. Sandmark H, Hogstedt C, Lewold S, Vingard E. Osteoarthrosis of the knee in men and women in association with overweight, smoking, and hormone therapy. Ann Rheum Dis. 1999;58:151–5.
86. Liu B, Balkwill A, Cooper C, Roddam A, Brown A, Beral V, et al. Reproductive history, hormonal factors and the incidence of hip and knee replacement for osteoarthritis in middle-aged women. Ann Rheum Dis. 2009;68:1165–70.
87. Maheu E, Dreiser RL, Guillou G, Dewailly J. Hand osteoarthritis patients characteristics according to the existence of a hormone replacement therapy. Osteoarthr Cartil. 2000;8(Suppl A):S33–7.
88. Cooley H, Stankovich J, Jones G. The association between hormonal and reproductive factors and hand osteoarthritis. Maturitas. 2003;45:257–65.
89. Wluka A, Davis S, Bailey M, Stuckey S, Cicuttini F. Users of oestrogen replacement therapy have more knee cartilage than nonusers. Ann Rheum Dis. 2001;60:332–6.
90. Cicuttini F, Wluka A, Wang Y, Stuckey S, Davis S. Effect of estrogen replacement therapy on patella cartilage in healthy women. Clin Exp Rheumatol. 2003;21:79–82.
91. Wluka A, Wolfe R, Davis S, Stuckey S, Cicuttini F. Tibial cartilage volume change in healthy postmenopausal women: a longitudinal study. Ann Rheum Dis. 2004;63:444–9.
92. Seo S, Yang H, Lim K, Jeon Y, Choi Y, Cho S, et al. Changes in serum levels of cartilage oligomeric matrix protein after estrogen and alendronate therapy in postmenopausal women. Gynecol Obstet Investig. 2012;74:143–50.
93. Ravn P, Warming L, Christgau S, Christiansen C. The effect on cartilage of different forms of application of postmenopausal estrogen therapy: comparison of oral and transdermal therapy. Bone. 2004;35:1216–21.
94. Christgau S, Tanko L, Cloos P, Mouritzen U, Christiansen C, Delaisse J, et al. Suppression of elevated cartilage turnover in postmenopausal women and in ovariectomized rats by estrogen and a selective estrogen-receptor modulator (SERM). Menopause. 2004;11:508–18.
95. Lugo L, Villalvilla A, Largo R, Herrero-Beaumont G, Roman-Blas J. Selective estrogen receptor modulators (SERMs): new alternatives for osteoarthritis? Maturitas. 2014;77:380–4.
96. Cano A. Compliance to hormone replacement therapy in menopausal women controlled in a third level academic centre. Maturitas. 1994;20:91–9.
97. Whitehead M, Townsend P, Pryse-Davies J, Ryder T, King R. Effects of estrogens and progestins on the biochemistry and morphology of the postmenopausal endometrium. N Engl J Med. 1981;305:1599–605.
98. Lessey B, Killam A, Metzger D, Haney A, Greene G, McCarty KJ. Immunohistochemical analysis of human uterine estrogen and progesterone receptors throughout the menstrual cycle. J Clin Endocrinol Metab. 1988;67:334–40.
99. Ferguson D, Anderson T. Morphological evaluation of cell turnover in relation to the menstrual cycle in the "resting" human breast. Br J Cancer. 1981;44:177–81.

100. González Ricarte M, de Castro PA, Tarín J, Cano A. Progestogens and risk of breast cancer: a link between bone and breast? Gynecol Endocrinol. 2016;32:6–8.
101. Monzó-Miralles A, Martín-González V, Smith-Ballester S, Iglesias-Miguel V, Cano A. The RANKL/RANK system in female reproductive organ tumors: a preclinical and clinical overview. Adv Clin Exp Med. 2021;30:879–83. https://doi.org/10.17219/acem/140422.
102. Trabert B, Sherman ME, Kannan N, Stanczyk FZ. Progesterone and breast cancer. Endocr Rev. 2020;41:320–44. https://doi.org/10.1210/endrev/bnz001.
103. Grady D, Gebretsadik T, Kerlikowske K, Ernster V, Petitti D. Hormone replacement therapy and endometrial cancer risk: a meta-analysis. Obstet Gynecol. 1995;85:304–13.
104. Brinton L, Trabert B, Anderson G, Falk R, Felix A, Fuhrman B, et al. Serum estrogens and estrogen metabolites and endometrial cancer risk among postmenopausal women. Cancer Epidemiol Biomarkers Prev. 2016;25:1081–90.
105. Setiawan V, Yang H, Pike M, McCann S, Yu H, Xiang Y, et al. Type I and II endometrial cancers: have they different risk factors? J Clin Oncol. 2013;31:2607–18.
106. Brown S, Hankinson S. Endogenous estrogens and the risk of breast, endometrial, and ovarian cancers. Steroids. 2015;99:8–10.
107. Chlebowski R, Anderson G, Sarto G, Haque R, Runowicz C, Aragaki A, et al. Continuous combined estrogen plus progestin and endometrial cancer: the women's health initiative randomized trial. J Natl Cancer Inst. 2015;108:djv350.
108. Cano A, Tarín J, Dueñas J. Two-year prospective, randomized trial comparing an innovative twice-a-week progestin regimen with a continuous combined régimen as postmenopausal hormone therapy. Fertil Steril. 1999;71:391–405.
109. Fernández-Murga L, Hermenegildo C, Tarín J, García-Pérez M, Cano A. Endometrial response to concurrent treatment with vaginal progesterone and transdermal estradiol. Climacteric. 2012;15:455–9.
110. Tempfer CB, Hilal Z, Kern P, Juhasz-Boess I, Rezniczek GA. Menopausal hormone therapy and risk of endometrial cancer: a systematic review. Cancers (Basel). 2020;12:2195. https://doi.org/10.3390/cancers12082195.
111. Corrado F, D'Anna R, Caputo F, Cannata M, Zoccali M, Cancellieri F. Compliance with hormone replacement therapy in postmenopausal Sicilian women. Eur J Obstet Gynecol Reprod Biol. 2005;118:225–8.
112. Chlebowski R, Anderson G, Aragaki A, Prentice R. Breast cancer and menopausal hormone therapy by race/ethnicity and body mass index. J Natl Cancer Inst. 2015;108:djv327.
113. Folkerd E, Dowsett M. Sex hormones and breast cancer risk and prognosis. Breast. 2013;S2:S38–43.
114. Román M, Sakshaug S, Graff-Iversen S, Vangen S, Weiderpass E, Ursin G, et al. Postmenopausal hormone therapy and the risk of breast cancer in Norway. Int J Cancer. 2016;138:584–93.
115. Collaborative Group on Hormonal Factors in Breast Cancer. Type and timing of menopausal hormone therapy and breast cancer risk: individual participant meta-analysis of the worldwide epidemiological evidence. Lancet. 2019;394:1159–68. https://doi.org/10.1016/S0140-6736(19)31709-X.
116. Vinogradova Y, Coupland C, Hippisley-Cox J. Use of hormone replacement therapy and risk of breast cancer: nested case-control studies using the QResearch and CPRD databases. BMJ. 2020;371:m3873. https://doi.org/10.1136/bmj.m3873.
117. Yang Z, Hu Y, Zhang J, Xu L, Zeng R, Kang D. Estradiol therapy and breast cancer risk in perimenopausal and postmenopausal women: a systematic review and meta-analysis. Gynecol Endocrinol. 2017;33:87–92. https://doi.org/10.1080/09513590.2016.1248932.
118. Holder EX, Houghton SC, Sanchez SS, Eliassen AH, Qian J, Bertone-Johnson ER, et al. Estrogenic activity and risk of invasive breast cancer among postmenopausal women in the nurses' health study. Cancer Epidemiol Biomarkers Prev. 2022;31:831–8. https://doi.org/10.1158/1055-9965.EPI-21-1157.
119. Diller M, Schüler S, Buchholz S, Lattrich C, Treeck O, Ortmann O. Effects of estriol on growth, gene expression and estrogen response element activation in human breast cancer cell lines. Maturitas. 2014;77:336–43.

120. Girgert R, Emons G, Gründker C. Inhibition of GPR30 by estriol prevents growth stimulation of triple-negative breast cancer cells by 17β-estradiol. BMC Cancer. 2014;14:935.
121. Brusselaers N, Tamimi RM, Konings P, Rosner B, Adami HO, Lagergren J. Different menopausal hormone regimens and risk of breast cancer. Ann Oncol. 2018;29:1771–6. https://doi.org/10.1093/annonc/mdy212.
122. Visser M, Coelingh Bennink H. Clinical applications for estetrol. J Steroid Biochem Mol Biol. 2009;114:85–9.
123. Coelingh Bennink H, Verhoeven C, Zimmerman Y, Visser M, Foidart J, Gemzell-Danielsson K. Pharmacodynamic effects of the fetal estrogen estetrol in postmenopausal women: results from a multiple-rising-dose study. Menopause. 2017;24:677–85.
124. Gallez A, Blacher S, Maquoi E, Konradowski E, Joiret M, Primac I, et al. Estetrol combined to progestogen for menopause or contraception indication is neutral on breast cancer. Cancers (Basel). 2021;13:2486. https://doi.org/10.3390/cancers13102486.
125. Gérard C, Arnal JF, Jost M, Douxfils J, Lenfant F, Fontaine C, et al. Profile of estetrol, a promising native estrogen for oral contraception and the relief of climacteric symptoms of menopause. Expert Rev Clin Pharmacol. 2022;15:121–37. https://doi.org/10.1080/17512433.2022.2054413.
126. Gaspard U, Taziaux M, Jost M, Coelingh Bennink HJT, Utian WH, Lobo RA, et al. A multicenter, randomized, placebo-controlled study to select the minimum effective dose of estetrol in postmenopausal participants (E4Relief): part 2-vaginal cytology, genitourinary syndrome of menopause, and health-related quality of life. Menopause. 2023;30:480–9. https://doi.org/10.1097/GME.0000000000002167.
127. Kluft C, Zimmerman Y, Mawet M, Klipping C, Duijkers I, Neuteboom J, et al. Reduced hemostatic effects with drospirenone-based oral contraceptives containing estetrol vs. ethinyl estradiol. Contraception. 2017;95:140–7.
128. Fournier A, Fabre A, Mesrine S, Boutron-Ruault M, Berrino F, Clavel-Chapelon F. Use of different postmenopausal hormone therapies and risk of histology- and hormone receptor-defined invasive breast cancer. J Clin Oncol. 2008;26:1260–8.
129. Fournier A, Berrino F, Clavel-Chapelon F. Unequal risks for breast cancer associated with different hormone replacement therapies: results from the E3N cohort study. Breast Cancer Res Treat. 2008;107:103–11.
130. Formoso G, Perrone E, Maltoni S, Balduzzi S, Wilkinson J, Basevi V, et al. Short-term and long-term effects of tibolone in postmenopausal women. Cochrane Database Syst Rev. 2016;10:CD008536.
131. Chlebowski R, Manson J, Anderson G, Cauley J, Aragaki A, Stefanick M, et al. Estrogen plus progestin and breast cancer incidence and mortality in the women's health initiative observational study. J Natl Cancer Inst. 2013;105:526–35.
132. Chlebowski RT, Anderson GL, Aragaki AK, Manson JE, Stefanick ML, Pan K, et al. Association of menopausal hormone therapy with breast cancer incidence and mortality during long-term follow-up of the women's health initiative randomized clinical trials. JAMA. 2020;324:369–80. https://doi.org/10.1001/jama.2020.9482.
133. Mikkola T, Savolainen-Peltonen H, Tuomikoski P, Hoti F, Vattulainen P, Gissler M, et al. Reduced risk of breast cancer mortality in women using postmenopausal hormone therapy: a Finnish nationwide comparative study. Menopause. 2016;23:1199–203.
134. Benkhadra K, Mohammed K, Al Nofal A, Carranza Leon B, Alahdab F, Faubion S, et al. Menopausal hormone therapy and mortality: a systematic review and meta-analysis. J Clin Endocrinol Metab. 2015;100:4021–8.
135. Weiss N, Lyon J, Krishnamurthy S, Dietert S, Liff J, Daling J. Noncontraceptive estrogen use and the occurrence of ovarian cancer. J Natl Cancer Inst. 1982;68:95–8.
136. Purdie D, Bain C, Siskind V, Russell P, Hacker N, Ward B, et al. Hormone replacement therapy and risk of epithelial ovarian cancer. Br J Cancer. 1999;81:559–63.
137. Riman T, Dickman P, Nilsson S, Correia N, Nordlinder H, Magnusson C, et al. Hormone replacement therapy and the risk of invasive epithelial ovarian cancer in Swedish women. J Natl Cancer Inst. 2002;94:497–504.

138. Anderson G, Judd H, Kaunitz A, Barad D, Beresford S, Pettinger M, et al. Women's Health Initiative Investigators. Effects of estrogen plus progestin on gynecologic cancers and associated diagnostic procedures: the women's health initiative randomized trial. JAMA. 2003;290:1739–48.
139. Greiser C, Greiser E, Dören M. Menopausal hormone therapy and risk of ovarian cancer: systematic review and meta-analysis. Hum Reprod Update. 2007;13:453–63.
140. Zhou B, Sun Q, Cong R, Gu H, Tang N, Yang L, et al. Hormone replacement therapy and ovarian cancer risk: a meta-analysis. Gynecol Oncol. 2008;108:641–51.
141. Beral V, MWS Collaborators, Bull D, Green J, Reeves G. Ovarian cancer and hormone replacement therapy in the Million Women Study. Lancet. 2007;369:1703–10.
142. Yang H, Anderson W, Rosenberg P, Trabert B, Gierach G, Wentzensen N, et al. Ovarian cancer incidence trends in relation to changing patterns of menopausal hormone therapy use in the United States. J Clin Oncol. 2013;31:2146–51.
143. Koskela-Niska V, Pukkala E, Lyytinen H, Ylikorkala O, Dyba T. Effect of various forms of postmenopausal hormone therapy on the risk of ovarian cancer—a population-based case control study from Finland. Int J Cancer. 2013;133:1680–8.
144. Collaborative Group on Epidemiological Studies of Ovarian Cancer. Menopausal hormone use and ovarian cancer risk: individual participant meta-analysis of 52 epidemiological studies. Lancet. 2015;385:1835–42.
145. Shi L, Wu Y, Li C. Hormone therapy and risk of ovarian cancer in postmenopausal women: a systematic review and meta-analysis. Menopause. 2016;23:417–24.
146. Liu Y, Ma L, Yang X, Bie J, Li D, Sun C, et al. Menopausal hormone replacement therapy and the risk of ovarian cancer: a meta-analysis. Front Endocrinol (Lausanne). 2019;10:801. https://doi.org/10.3389/fendo.2019.00801.
147. Simin J, Tamimi RM, Callens S, Engstrand L, Brusselaers N. Menopausal hormone therapy treatment options and ovarian cancer risk: a Swedish prospective population-based matched-cohort study. Int J Cancer. 2020;147:33–44. https://doi.org/10.1002/ijc.32706.
148. Fournier A, Cairat M, Severi G, Gunter MJ, Rinaldi S, Dossus L. Use of menopausal hormone therapy and ovarian cancer risk in a French cohort study. J Natl Cancer Inst. 2023;115:671–9. https://doi.org/10.1093/jnci/djad035.
149. Petrick JL, Joslin CE, Johnson CE, Camacho TF, Peres LC, Bandera EV, et al. Menopausal hormone therapy use and risk of ovarian cancer by race: the ovarian cancer in women of African ancestry consortium. Br J Cancer. 2023;129:1956–67. https://doi.org/10.1038/s41416-023-02407-7.

Nonhormonal Management of the Menopause

15

Jenifer Sassarini and Mary Ann Lumsden

Abstract

Menopause is the permanent cessation of menstrual periods that occurs naturally or is induced by surgery, chemotherapy, or radiation. With improved healthcare and increased life expectancy, women may spend 30 years on average after the menopause. There are several symptoms associated with menopausal transition, and 75% of women will experience some of these.

Vasomotor symptoms (VMS) are the most commonly reported, and often the most difficult to manage effectively with non-hormonal therapies. The most commonly used alternatives will be covered in this chapter. Among them, the effectiveness of the lifestyle measures to improve vasomotor symptoms, the alternatives to hormone therapy most often prescribed, the recently incorporated antagonists of the neurokinin receptors, the non-pharmacological therapies, and the non-hormonal management of vulvovaginal symptoms.

Menopause is defined by the World Health Organisation (WHO) and STRAW Working Groups as the permanent cessation of menstrual periods that occurs naturally or is induced by surgery, chemotherapy, or radiation [1].

With improved healthcare and increased life expectancy, women spend a considerable proportion of their lives (30 years on average) after the menopause, and it is estimated that within the next 25 years, more than one billion women worldwide will be older than 50 years, and approximately two million will reach menopause annually.

J. Sassarini (✉)
Glasgow Royal Infirmary, University of Glasgow, Glasgow, UK
e-mail: Jenifer.sassarini@glasgow.ac.uk

M. A. Lumsden
University of Glasgow, Glasgow, UK
e-mail: Maryann.lumsden@glasgow.ac.uk

There are several symptoms associated with menopausal transition, and it is estimated that approximately 75% of women will experience some symptoms related to oestrogen deficiency during this time, although some women will experience none of these.

Symptoms include hot flushes and night sweats (vasomotor symptoms), vaginal symptoms, depression, anxiety, irritability and mood swings (psychological effects), joint pains, migraines or headaches, sleeping problems, and urinary incontinence.

Vasomotor symptoms (VMS) are the most commonly reported and often the most difficult to manage effectively with nonhormonal therapies; we have attempted to cover the most commonly used alternatives in this chapter. We will also briefly touch on vulvovaginal symptoms, but it is simply not possible, within the remit of this chapter, to cover all possible treatments for mood disturbance.

15.1 Vasomotor Symptoms

The most commonly reported symptoms are vasomotor symptoms, characterised by a feeling of intense warmth, often accompanied by profuse sweating, anxiety, skin reddening palpitations, and sometimes followed by chills. It was previously thought that they resolve spontaneously in most women after 2 years, but may persist for up to 15 years; however, recent research suggests that median duration is in fact 7.4 years [2]. The sleep disturbance, fatigue, and decreased cognitive function associated with hot flushes and night sweats have been shown to lead to a significant reduction in HRQoL and an increased use of medical resources.

Flushes generally occur at times of relative oestrogen withdrawal, and replacing it will result in improvement in most women; however, circulating levels of oestrogen do not differ significantly between symptomatic and asymptomatic postmenopausal women. And, whilst oestrogen concentrations remain low after the menopause, most vasomotor symptoms will diminish with time, and therefore a fall in oestrogen concentration does not seem to provide the complete answer.

Furthermore, it is thought that withdrawal of oestrogen, rather than low circulating oestrogen levels, is the central change that leads to hot flushes, and there are several observations to support this theory. The abrupt oestrogen withdrawal due to bilateral oophorectomy in premenopausal women is associated with an increased prevalence of flushes when compared with women who experience a gradual physiological menopause. Also, young women with gonadal dysgenesis, who have low levels of endogenous oestrogen, do not experience hot flushes unless they receive several months of oestrogen therapy and then abruptly discontinue its use.

A hot flush closely resembles a heat dissipation response (sweating and peripheral vasodilation), and as such, dysfunction in the central control of thermoregulation remains our best understanding of the mechanism of flushing [3]. Freedman's hypothesis of a narrowed thermoneutral zone is well known; however, the trigger is incompletely characterised.

Changes in core temperature may also be associated with alterations in neuroendocrine pathways involving steroid hormones, noradrenaline (NA), the endorphins, and serotonin. Noradrenaline and serotonin, particularly, appear to play a key role.

It is well accepted that reduced secretion of oestrogen at the time of menopause is associated with increased GnRH secretion from the hypothalamus, resulting in high luteinising hormone (LH) and follicle-stimulating hormone (FSH) concentrations. Flushes also seem to coincide with pulses of LH in peripheral plasma [4], but neither LH nor GnRH is required for hot flush symptoms [5]. The close timing of flush episodes with LH pulses suggests that the onset of flushes is related to the hypothalamic circuitry controlling pulsatile GnRH secretion [6].

The proximate and obligate stimulus to GnRH secretion is the neurokinin system, also called the kisspeptin/neurokinin B/dynorphin (KNDy) signalling system, found in the hypothalamus, and with projections to the median preoptic are of the hypothalamus and or the thermoregulatory centre [7].

Neurokinin B (NKB) gene expression is markedly increased in the infundibular (arcuate) nucleus of postmenopausal women [8] and is modulated by oestrogen withdrawal and replacement in multiple species [9]. And although the exact mechanism remains unclear, the decline in oestrogen at menopause results in an increase in NKB signalling at the KNDy neurons, with resultant increases in hot flushes.

NKB administration has also been shown to cause induction of hot flushes in healthy premenopausal women [10].

The NICE guideline (NG23) [11] has recommended that women should be offered HRT for vasomotor symptoms after a discussion of the short-term (up to 5 years) and longer-term benefits and risks. However, there are of course a group of women for whom hormonal therapy is not suitable. Fifty percent of the more than half million women living with breast cancer in the UK will not adhere to the recommended 10 years of tamoxifen, often as a result of the severity of the hot flushes that are associated with taking this drug. They are also generally advised against taking HRT. It is essential that we are able to safely and accurately advise women on treatment alternatives for symptoms of the menopause, particularly for these women to help them continue a potentially life-saving treatment.

15.1.1 Cooling Techniques and Avoiding Triggers

Hot flushes can be triggered by small increases in core body temperature, and therefore, it seems logical to suggest practices that lower body temperature or prevent it from rising. These might include loose clothing, made from natural fibres, fans, and cool packs. There is no clinical evidence for either these interventions or the avoidance of triggers, which might be reported by some spicy or hot food and drinks and alcohol.

15.1.2 Lifestyle Modifications

There is evidence that body mass index (BMI), smoking, alcohol consumption, and sedentary lifestyle are associated with reports of vasomotor symptoms; however, there are few papers reporting the direct effect modifications have on flushes.

It may be safe to assume, though, that there will be an improvement in symptoms if a risk factor for exacerbation of those symptoms is removed. Smoking cessation and weight loss have numerous other health benefits, not exclusively alterations in endothelial function, which may be involved in the hot flush mechanism.

15.1.3 Exercise

As well as having significant physiological benefits (e.g., cardiovascular and bone health), exercise may be one of the promising alternatives to HRT and if demonstrated to be effective in the treatment of vasomotor symptoms is an inexpensive intervention that typically has few known side effects.

The Cochrane Collaboration carried out a systematic review [12] to examine the effectiveness of any type of exercise intervention in the management of vasomotor symptoms in symptomatic perimenopausal and postmenopausal women. Only one very small trial was considered suitable for inclusion, which found, not unexpectedly, that HRT was more effective than exercise. There is no available evidence examining whether exercise is an effective treatment relative to other interventions or no intervention.

15.1.4 Weight Loss

Studies have found that women who are obese are more likely to report more frequent and severe hot flashes than women of normal weight. Randomised, controlled trials have found that weight loss from behavioural interventions is associated with a decrease in VMS. Additionally, reducing hot flashes was a major motivator for losing weight [13].

15.1.5 Pharmacological Preparations

15.1.5.1 Clonidine

Monoamines have been shown to play an important role in the control of thermoregulation, and animal studies have shown that noradrenaline (NA) acts to narrow the thermoregulatory zone. Noradrenergic stimulation of the medial preoptic area of the hypothalamus in monkeys and baboons causes peripheral vasodilation, heat loss, and a drop in core temperature, similar to changes which occur in women during hot flushes.

It has also been shown that plasma levels of a noradrenaline metabolite are significantly increased both before and during hot flush episodes in postmenopausal women.

Clonidine is an alpha$_2$-adrenergic agonist licensed for the treatment of hypertension, migraines, and postmenopausal vasomotor symptoms. It is also used for postoperative shivering because it is thought that, like general anaesthetic agents and sedatives, it decreases shivering thresholds by a generalised impairment of central thermoregulatory control. It has also been demonstrated to increase the sweating threshold.

When used for the treatment of flushing, it has been shown to be more effective than placebo, but less effective than SSRIs, SNRIs, and gabapentin [14, 15]. However, it is not well tolerated, because of adverse effects, including dry mouth, insomnia, and drowsiness.

15.1.5.2 Selective Serotonin (and Noradrenaline) Reuptake Inhibitors

Serotonin is involved in many bodily functions including mood, anxiety, sleep, sexual behaviour, and thermoregulation. Oestrogen withdrawal is associated with decreased blood serotonin levels, and short-term oestrogen therapy has been shown to increase these levels.

Selective serotonin reuptake inhibitors (SSRIs) are a group of drugs typically used as antidepressants, which are thought to function by blocking the reuptake of serotonin to the presynaptic cell. This increases the amount of serotonin in the synaptic cleft available to bind to the postsynaptic cell. SSRIs were commonly prescribed for the treatment of depression in women undergoing treatment for breast cancer. Anecdotally, these same women were noted to have an improvement in their vasomotor symptoms, which occurred as a side effect of treatment. Studies were then carried out to determine the efficacy of these as an effective treatment for flushing.

Meta-analyses [14, 16, 17] and a Cochrane review [14, 15] have demonstrated mild to moderate improvements in flush frequency and severity in symptomatic postmenopausal (surgical and natural) women. Statistically significant reductions in flushing were seen with paroxetine [18], escitalopram, citalopram, venlafaxine, and desvenlafaxine. Sertraline and fluoxetine appear to be less consistent, although there was still a trend towards improvement.

SNRIs may produce significant nausea, but this typically improves in 2–3 days and can be reduced by titrating the dose slowly.

Use of these drugs in women with breast cancer using tamoxifen is common; therefore, consideration must be given to potential interactions. Tamoxifen must be metabolised by the cytochrome P450 enzyme system, predominantly cytochrome P450 isoenzyme 2D6 (CYP2D6), to become active, and CYP2D6 is inhibited to varying degrees by SSRIs. Paroxetine is an exceptionally potent inhibitor, whereas sertraline inhibits to a lesser degree and citalopram and escitalopram are only weak inhibitors. Evidence is conflicting on the success rates of tamoxifen in preventing recurrence of breast cancer when using a concurrent SSRI. For those women who need to begin treatment with an SSRI for depression, citalopram or escitalopram may be the safest choice; however, improvements in flushing are better with venlafaxine and desvenlafaxine, and these appear to be safe choices.

Other SSRI and SNRIs with evidence for efficacy in treating VMS include venlafaxine (37.5–150 mg daily), desvenlafaxine (100–150 mg daily), citalopram (10–20 mg daily), and escitalopram (10–20 mg daily).

15.1.5.3 Gabapentin

The mechanism of action of gabapentin in the amelioration of vasomotor symptoms is unknown, but it is thought to involve a direct effect on the hypothalamic thermoregulatory centre.

Two double-blind randomised placebo-controlled trials, examined in a meta-analysis [14], both conducted in women with breast cancer, showed a significant reduction in frequency and severity of hot flushes when taking 900 mg per day, but not when taking 300 mg per day. Titrated to 2400 mg per day continued to be superior to placebo but was not significantly different to oestrogen 0.625 mg/day. However, dizziness, unsteadiness, and fatigue were reported in the gabapentin-treated group and resulted in a higher dropout rate than in the control group.

15.1.5.4 Oxybutynin

Oxybutynin is an anticholinergic drug used as a treatment for overactive bladder symptoms. Decreased sweating is a common side effect of oxybutynin, which has led to its successful use in the treatment of generalised hyperhidrosis [19]. In a prospective, double-blind, clinical trial evaluating an extended-release formulation of oxybutynin for hot flushes, a dose of 15 mg was shown to significantly reduce the frequency and severity of HFs at 12 weeks [20] but was associated with excess toxicity and treatment discontinuation because of side effects. More recently, a dose of 2.5 or 5 mg bd has been shown to be effective with a more acceptable toxicity profile [21].

Adverse events are usually dose-dependent and most commonly include a dry mouth and urinary difficulties. Long-term use of anticholinergics may be associated with cognitive decline, particularly in older persons.

15.1.5.5 Neurokinin B Antagonists

Neurokinin B (NKB) antagonists are new nonhormonal treatments for hot flushes. Antagonising neurokinin B dampens hypersecretion of neurokinin B from the KNDy neurons onto the adjacent thermoregulatory centre in the hypothalamus, which, as described above, causes disruption of temperature control and the occurrence of reduced hot flushes.

Randomised controlled trials suggest a clinically important decrease in the number and severity of flushes [22–24].

This new treatment is an exciting novel, nonhormonal treatment for flushing, which will be a welcome addition to the options available for those who cannot, or choose not, to use HRT. As yet, Fezolinetant (Veozah®), a NKB3 antagonist, is the only licenced preparation available in the UK and the USA for the treatment of hot flushes. Phase 3 trials for a NKB1,3 antagonist are soon to be completed and may have additional benefits for sleep disturbance as well as hot flushes. Data on VMS-related mood symptoms, as well as genitourinary, sexual, cardiovascular, metabolic, and bone health, are lacking.

Elevation of hepatic enzymes has been described but was rare and resolved either during continued treatment or with treatment discontinuation.

15.1.6 Non-pharmacological Therapies

15.1.6.1 Phytoestrogens

Phytoestrogens are chemicals that resemble oestrogen and are present in most plants, vegetables, and fruits. There are three main types of phytoestrogens: soy isoflavones (the most potent), coumestans, and lignans. Soya bean and red clover are also rich in phytoestrogens. These compounds are converted into weak oestrogenic substances in the gastrointestinal tract.

Isoflavones are the most researched, and Nelson's meta-analysis included 17 RCTs. From six trials comparing Promensil (red clover isoflavone) with placebo, only one fair-quality trial found a reduction in flush frequency with Promensil, although there was no overall reduction in the meta-analysis, and no improvement in flush severity was demonstrated in any of the included trials.

Soy isoflavones were compared with placebo in the remaining 11 trials. The meta-analysis revealed an improvement in hot flushes after 12–16 weeks (4 trials) and after 6 months (2 trials), but were not significantly decreased in studies examining 4–6 weeks use.

A systematic review was also carried out by the Cochrane Collaboration [25]. They included five trials in a meta-analysis, which demonstrated no significant decrease in the frequency of hot flushes with phytoestrogens.

Thirty trials were also studied comparing phytoestrogens with control. Some of the trials found that phytoestrogens alleviated the frequency and severity of hot flushes and night sweats when compared with placebo, but many of the trials were of low quality or were underpowered. The great variability in the results of these trials may result in part from the difference in efficacy of the various types of phytoestrogens used, the exact treatment protocol, and the fraction of equol producers in the cohort. It is claimed that only 30–40% of the US population possess the gut microflora responsible for converting isoflavones to the active oestrogenic equol. It should also be noted that there was also a strong placebo response in most trials, ranging from 1% to 59%.

15.1.6.2 Black Cohosh

Black cohosh (*Actaea racemose*) is a species of flowering plant of the family Ranunculaceae. It is native to eastern North America, and it is thought to behave as a selective oestrogen receptor modulator (SERM) with mild central oestrogenic effects, although the active ingredients are unknown.

A 2012 Cochrane review [26] analysed 16 RCTS of 2027 perimenopausal and postmenopausal women. All studies used oral monopreparations of black cohosh at a median daily dose of 40 mg, for a mean duration of 23 weeks. There was no significant difference between black cohosh and placebo in the frequency of hot flushes. Evidence on the safety of black cohosh was inconclusive, owing to poor reporting, and there were insufficient data to pool results for health-related quality of life, sexuality, bone health, vulvovaginal atrophic symptoms, and night sweats.

A meta-analysis of several short-term and relatively small RCTs comparing black cohosh use with placebo "revealed a trend towards reducing vasomotor symptoms", but only in cases of mild to moderate symptoms [27]. This was particularly notable when hot flushes were associated with sleep and mood disturbances. This was confirmed in another 12-week study of 304 women in addition to improvements in mood, sleep disorders, sexual disorders, and sweating. In contrast, however, the recent Herbal Alternatives for Menopause Trial (HALT) [28] which compared black cohosh to both placebo and oestrogen replacement over 12 months suggested that black cohosh was ineffective in relieving vasomotor symptoms.

Whilst there has been no confirmation of its efficacy, many women, both cancer-free as well as breast cancer patients and survivors, will use black cohosh to relieve vasomotor symptoms since describing a drug as no more effective than placebo may mean that it may bring relief to over 30% of women. However, it is important to exercise caution as there is limited information on its potential to influence breast cancer development or progression. No effect has been seen on mammary tumour development, which would suggest that black cohosh would not influence breast cancer risk if given to women before tumour formation, but there has been an increase in the incidence of lung metastases in tumour-bearing animals when compared with mice fed with an isoflavone-free control diet. Additional studies will be needed to correlate these findings to women taking different black cohosh products at various times during breast cancer development; however, these results suggest caution for women using black cohosh, especially for extended periods of time.

Reports of possible hepatotoxicity associated with black cohosh began to appear after 2000; however, a recent critical analysis and structured causality assessment has shown no causal relationship between treatment by black cohosh and liver disease.

15.1.6.3 Dong Quai

Also known as *Angelica sinensis*, dang gui, and tang kuei; dong quai is the root of the Angelica polymorpha Maxim var. sinensis Oliv. *Angelica sinensis* grows in high altitude mountains in China, Japan, and Korea, and the yellowish-brown root of the plant had been used in traditional Chinese medicine for thousands of years. It is reputed to be oestrogenic based on reports of uterine bleeding with use and uterotropic effects in ovariectomised rats, but there is no evidence of oestrogenic activity in human studies [29].

Dong quai does not appear to be effective for hot flushes, and there may be some safety concerns, including possible photosensitisation, anticoagulation, and possible carcinogenicity [30].

15.1.6.4 Vitamin E

Three trials show varying evidence for vitamin E for treatment of vasomotor symptoms. A randomised placebo-controlled trial, in which 105 women with a history of breast cancer received placebo and vitamin E 800 IU daily for 4 weeks in a cross over design [31], demonstrated no improvement in frequency or severity of hot flushes. One hundred fifteen women were randomised to vitamin E or gabapentin in a further trial, with significant improvements in symptoms with gabapentin, and a 35% dropout rate in the vitamin E group [32]. However, in another crossover trial of

50 postmenopausal women, 4 weeks of vitamin E (400 IU) followed by placebo, or vice versa, demonstrated a small reduction in hot flushes of two flushes per day and a reduction in severity with vitamin E [33]. Care must always be taken when a toxic vitamin is ingested in excessive amounts.

15.1.6.5 Evening Primrose Oil (*Oenothera biennis*)

Oenothera biennis is a flowering plant rich in linolenic acid and ý-linolenic acid. It is a widely used product for the treatment of menopausal symptoms, although the exact mechanism of action is not fully understood. Its effectiveness has been analysed in a double-blind randomised placebo-controlled trial of 56 postmenopausal women [34]. This trial used a combination of evening primrose oil (2000 mg/day) with vitamin E (10 mg/day) versus placebo and showed a significantly greater reduction in day time flushes in the placebo group than in the treatment group. Unsurprisingly, there was a high dropout rate, only 18 women given in the EPO group and 17 in the placebo group completed the trial, due to unrelieved symptoms, and precluded reliable conclusions.

There are a number of other over-the-counter and herbal therapies that are reported to be effective in reducing vasomotor symptoms, and a comprehensive review of these can be found in the 2015 North American Menopause Society Position statement on nonhormonal management of menopause-associated vasomotor symptoms [30]. It is important to remember that herbal supplements are not as closely regulated as prescription drugs, and the amount of herbal product, quality, safety, and purity may vary between brands or even between batches of the same brand. We must make it clear to women that these therapies may also interact with prescription drugs, and as such these must be declared these to healthcare providers and may need to be stopped before any planned surgery.

15.1.6.6 CBT

Cognitive behavioural therapy (CBT), group and self-help, has been developed to help women self-manage VMS. It has been shown to be effective in reducing the impact, but not frequency, of flushing in two randomised, double-blind controlled trials, MENOS 1 [35] and MENOS 2 [36]. Improvements were maintained 26 weeks after randomisation, and there were additional benefits to quality of life, with no adverse effects.

A follow-up study [37] has revealed that beliefs about coping and control over VMS, and belief about sleep and night sweats, mediated the effect of CBT on VMS problem ratings.

NAMS has recommended CBT as an effective nonhormonal management option for vasomotor symptoms for both breast cancer survivors and menopausal women, and NICE (NG23) has recommended CBT to alleviate low mood or anxiety due to menopause.

The Update of the NICE Guideline No 23 suggests that CBT should be discussed as an alternative to HRT in the treatment of menopause symptoms. There are various options such as individual face-to-face, individual virtual, group sessions, and self-help.

The evidence review suggested an important benefit for CBT in difficulties with sleep for both people with and without a personal history of breast cancer although the evidence was considered to be low quality. Some women with breast cancer also noted an improvement in psychological symptoms and low mood [38–43].

15.1.6.7 Acupuncture
Acupuncture is a traditional component of Chinese medicine in which thin needles are inserted into the skin at key points in the body to balance the flow of energy or *chi*. Western medical acupuncture is the use of acupuncture following a medical diagnosis, and it involves stimulating sensory nerves under the skin and in the muscles of the body. This causes the production of endorphins, which may be responsible for the beneficial effects experienced.

Sham acupuncture is a placebo treatment involving needles inserted into unrelated points on the body or of special needles that do not pierce the skin.

A Cochrane review [44], and other systematic reviews [45, 46], concludes that although acupuncture is superior to no treatment, or a wait-list control, acupuncture is not superior to sham acupuncture. NAMS concluded, in their recently published position statement, that needling at acupuncture points does not appear to reduce VMS frequency or intensity independently of the superficial touch of a sham needle.

15.1.7 Alternative Treatments

15.1.7.1 Stellate Ganglion Blockade
Stellate-ganglion blocks (SGB) have been carried out safely for more than 60 years, for pain syndromes and vascular insufficiency. 0.5% bupivacaine is injected on the right side of the anterolateral aspect of the C6 vertebra under fluoroscopy and an effective block confirmed by the presence of Horner's syndrome. Adverse events, such as transient seizures, or a bleeding complication, occur rarely.

A case report published in 1985 of a 77-year old gentleman with flushing after orchidectomy for infarction his remaining testis was treated with SGB based on the belief that the flushing centre has a sympathetic outflow to the stellate ganglion. This abolished his attacks of flushing.

Four uncontrolled, open label studies [47–50] have shown that SGB reduced vasomotor symptoms, with effects ranging from a 45% to 90% reduction 6 weeks to several months after blockade. A pilot study of 13 women (age range 38–71 years), with a history of breast cancer, who suffered with severe hot flushes, demonstrated reductions in flush episodes and an improvement in sleep quality following stellate ganglion blockade [49]. A more recent study [50] revealed a benefit in only half of the 20 women in the study. The exact mechanism of action of SGB is unknown, but findings suggest that it may be an effective nonhormonal treatment for flushing. Larger trials are needed.

15.2 Vaginal Symptoms and Sexual Dysfunction

Vaginal symptoms become apparent 4–5 years after the menopause, and objective changes as well as subjective complaints are present in 25–50% of all postmenopausal women [51]. Symptoms may include vaginal dryness (75%), dyspareunia (38%), vaginal itching, burning, and pain (15%). Dyspareunia can adversely affect a postmenopausal woman's sexual quality of life or intensify pre-existing sexual disorders [52].

Vaginal oestrogens are effective in the treatment of menopause-related vulval and vaginal symptoms, and a Cochrane review reported equal efficacy across all products tested: creams, pessaries, tablets, and vaginal rings [53]. Local oestrogen therapy will lower vaginal pH, thicken the epithelium, increase blood flow, and improve vaginal lubrication.

Vaginal oestrogen is controversial in women with a history of breast cancer, in whom vulval and vaginal symptoms are common, particularly those on endocrine therapy. In a case-control study, there was no documented increase in recurrence in those women receiving endocrine therapy and use of local oestrogen compared to non-use [54]. However, in another study of breast cancer survivors, there was an initial, albeit unsustained, increase in circulating oestrogen levels [55].

Nonhormonal treatment options include lubricants and moisturisers. Lubricants are non-physiological but may reduce friction-related irritation of vaginal tissues, whilst moisturisers are hydrophilic, insoluble, cross-linked polymers which reduce vaginal pH [51]. In a trial of vaginal moisturiser compared to low-dose vaginal oestrogen, both preparations were found to be effective, but the moisturiser provided only temporary benefit [56].

Ospemifene is a non-oestrogen, tissue-selective oestrogen receptor agonist/antagonist, or selective oestrogen receptor modulator (SERM). It is approved for dyspareunia secondary to menopause-related vulvovaginal atrophy. Studies have shown improvements in vaginal pH and dryness [57, 58]; however, it should not be used in women with, or at high risk of, breast cancer.

15.3 Conclusion

Clonidine, SSRIs, and gabapentin have all shown a significant improvement in flushing, whilst vitamin E and evening primrose oil have been shown to be of no benefit. Adverse effects may limit the use of clonidine and gabapentin, but SSRIs and SNRIs have a well-established safety profile and appear to have only minor adverse effects.

The evidence surrounding the efficacy of phytoestrogens and black cohosh is contradictory. Soy isoflavones may be more effective with longer-term use than other phytoestrogens, but black cohosh, or any compound with oestrogenic properties, should be used with extreme caution in women with a history of breast cancer or any other oestrogen-dependent disease.

The effectiveness of stellate ganglion blockade for vasomotor symptoms is unconfirmed; therefore, further studies are required. It is also worth considering that the uptake of this treatment may be limited as it is costly and invasive, and the short-term side effects of Horner's syndrome may be unacceptable to some.

References

1. Annals of Internal Medicine. National Institutes of Health state-of-the-science conference statement: management of menopause-related symptoms. 2005;142(12 Pt 1):1003–13.
2. Avis NE, Crawford SL, Greendale G, Bromberger JT, Everson-Rose SA, Gold EB, et al. Duration of menopausal vasomotor symptoms over the menopause transition. JAMA Intern Med. 2015;175(4):531.
3. Freedman RR, Krell W. Reduced thermoregulatory null zone in postmenopausal women with hot flashes. Am J Obstet Gynecol. 1999;181(1):66–70.
4. Casper RF, Yen SSC, Wilkes MM. Menopausal flushes: a neuroendocrine link with pulsatile luteinizing hormone secretion. Science. 1979;205(4408):823–5.
5. Casper RF, Yen SS. Neuroendocrinology of menopausal flushes: an hypothesis of flush mechanism. Clin Endocrinol. 1985;22(3):293–312.
6. Dacks PA, Krajewski SJ, Rance NE. Activation of neurokinin 3 receptors in the median preoptic nucleus decreases core temperature in the rat. Endocrinology. 2011;152(12):4894–905.
7. Seminara SB, Messager S, Chatzidaki EE, Thresher RR, Acierno JS, Shagoury JK, et al. The GPR54 gene as a regulator of puberty. N Engl J Med. 2003;349(17):1614–27.
8. Rance NE, Young WS. Hypertrophy and increased gene expression of neurons containing neurokinin-B and substance-P messenger ribonucleic acids in the hypothalami of postmenopausal women. Endocrinology. 1991;128(5):2239–47.
9. Rance NE. Menopause and the human hypothalamus: evidence for the role of kisspeptin/neurokinin B neurons in the regulation of estrogen negative feedback. Peptides (NY). 2009;30(1):111–22.
10. Jayasena CN, Comninos AN, Stefanopoulou E, Buckley A, Narayanaswamy S, Izzi-Engbeaya C, et al. Neurokinin B administration induces hot flushes in women. Sci Rep. 2015;5(1):8466.
11. National Institute for Health and Care Excellence. Menopause: diagnosis and management of menopause. (NICE guideline).
12. Daley A, Stokes-Lampard H, MacArthur C. Exercise for vasomotor menopausal symptoms. In: Daley A, editor. Cochrane database of systematic reviews. Chichester: John Wiley & Sons, Ltd; 2007.
13. "The 2023 Nonhormone Therapy Position Statement of The North American Menopause Society" Advisory Panel. The 2023 nonhormone therapy position statement of The North American Menopause Society. Menopause. 2023;30(6):573–90.
14. Nelson HD, Vesco KK, Haney E, Fu R, Nedrow A, Miller J, et al. Nonhormonal therapies for menopausal hot flashes. JAMA. 2006;295(17):2057.
15. Rada G, Capurro D, Pantoja T, Corbalán J, Moreno G, Letelier LM, et al. Non-hormonal interventions for hot flushes in women with a history of breast cancer. Cochrane Database Syst Rev. 2010;(9):CD004923.
16. Shams T, Firwana B, Habib F, Alshahrani A, AlNouh B, Murad MH, et al. SSRIs for hot flashes: a systematic review and meta-analysis of randomized trials. J Gen Intern Med. 2014;29(1):204–13.
17. Sun Z, Hao Y, Zhang M. Efficacy and safety of desvenlafaxine treatment for hot flashes associated with menopause: a meta-analysis of randomized controlled trials. Gynecol Obstet Investig. 2013;75(4):255–62.
18. Simon JA, Portman DJ, Kaunitz AM, Mekonnen H, Kazempour K, Bhaskar S, et al. Low-dose paroxetine 7.5 mg for menopausal vasomotor symptoms. Menopause. 2013;20(10):1027–35.

19. Wolosker N, de Campos JRM, Kauffman P, Puech-Leão P. A randomized placebo-controlled trial of oxybutynin for the initial treatment of palmar and axillary hyperhidrosis. J Vasc Surg. 2012;55(6):1696–700.
20. Simon JA, Gaines T, LaGuardia KD. Extended-release oxybutynin therapy for vasomotor symptoms in women: a randomized clinical trial. Menopause. 2016;23(11):1214–21.
21. Leon-Ferre RA, Novotny PJ, Wolfe EG, Faubion SS, Ruddy KJ, Flora D, et al. Oxybutynin vs placebo for hot flashes in women with or without breast cancer: a randomized, double-blind clinical trial (ACCRU SC-1603). JNCI Cancer Spectr. 2020;4(1):pkz088.
22. Prague JK, Roberts RE, Comninos AN, Clarke S, Jayasena CN, Mohideen P, et al. Neurokinin 3 receptor antagonism rapidly improves vasomotor symptoms with sustained duration of action. Menopause. 2018;25(8):862–9.
23. Lederman S, Ottery FD, Cano A, Santoro N, Shapiro M, Stute P, et al. Fezolinetant for treatment of moderate-to-severe vasomotor symptoms associated with menopause (SKYLIGHT 1): a phase 3 randomised controlled study. Lancet. 2023;401(10382):1091–102.
24. Johnson KA, Martin N, Nappi RE, Neal-Perry G, Shapiro M, Stute P, et al. Efficacy and safety of fezolinetant in moderate to severe vasomotor symptoms associated with menopause: a phase 3 RCT. J Clin Endocrinol Metab. 2023;108(8):1981–97.
25. Lethaby A, Marjoribanks J, Kronenberg F, Roberts H, Eden J, Brown J. Phytoestrogens for vasomotor menopausal symptoms. In: Lethaby A, editor. Cochrane database of systematic reviews. Chichester: John Wiley & Sons, Ltd; 2007.
26. Leach MJ, Moore V. Black cohosh (*Cimicifuga* spp.) for menopausal symptoms. Cochrane Database Syst Rev. 2012;2012(9):CD007244.
27. Wong VCK, Lim CED, Luo X, Wong WSF. Current alternative and complementary therapies used in menopause. Gynecol Endocrinol. 2009;25(3):166–74.
28. Newton KM, Reed SD, LaCroix AZ, Grothaus LC, Ehrlich K, Guiltinan J. Treatment of vasomotor symptoms of menopause with black cohosh, multibotanicals, soy, hormone therapy, or placebo. Ann Intern Med. 2006;145(12):869.
29. Circosta C, De Pasquale R, Palumbo DR, Samperi S, Occhiuto F. Estrogenic activity of standardized extract of *Angelica sinensis*. Phytother Res. 2006;20(8):665–9.
30. Nonhormonal management of menopause-associated vasomotor symptoms. Menopause. 2015;22(11):1155–74.
31. Barton DL, Loprinzi CL, Quella SK, Sloan JA, Veeder MH, Egner JR, et al. Prospective evaluation of vitamin E for hot flashes in breast cancer survivors. J Clin Oncol. 1998;16(2):495–500.
32. Biglia N, Sgandurra P, Peano E, Marenco D, Moggio G, Bounous V, et al. Non-hormonal treatment of hot flushes in breast cancer survivors: gabapentin vs. vitamin E. Climacteric. 2009;12(4):310–8.
33. Ziaei S, Kazemnejad A, Zareai M. The effect of vitamin E on hot flashes in menopausal women. Gynecol Obstet Investig. 2007;64(4):204–7.
34. Chenoy R, Hussain S, Tayob Y, O'Brien PMS, Moss MY, Morse PF. Effect of oral gamolenic acid from evening primrose oil on menopausal flushing. BMJ. 1994;308(6927):501–3.
35. Mann E, Smith M, Hellier J, Hunter MS. A randomised controlled trial of a cognitive behavioural intervention for women who have menopausal symptoms following breast cancer treatment (MENOS 1): trial protocol. BMC Cancer. 2011;11(1):44.
36. Ayers B, Smith M, Hellier J, Mann E, Hunter MS. Effectiveness of group and self-help cognitive behavior therapy in reducing problematic menopausal hot flushes and night sweats (MENOS 2): a randomized controlled trial. Menopause. 2012;19(7):749–59.
37. Hunter MS. Letter to the Editor. Menopause. 2014;21(8):909.
38. Cheng P, Kalmbach D, Fellman-Couture C, Arnedt JT, Cuamatzi-Castelan A, Drake CL. Risk of excessive sleepiness in sleep restriction therapy and cognitive behavioral therapy for insomnia: a randomized controlled trial. J Clin Sleep Med. 2020;16(2):193–8.
39. Drake CL, Kalmbach DA, Arnedt JT, Cheng P, Tonnu CV, Cuamatzi-Castelan A, et al. Treating chronic insomnia in postmenopausal women: a randomized clinical trial comparing cognitive-behavioral therapy for insomnia, sleep restriction therapy, and sleep hygiene education. Sleep. 2019;42(2):zsy217.

40. Fenlon D, Maishman T, Day L, Nuttall J, May C, Ellis M, et al. Effectiveness of nurse-led group CBT for hot flushes and night sweats in women with breast cancer: results of the MENOS4 randomised controlled trial. Psychooncology. 2020;29(10):1514–23.
41. Green SM, Donegan E, Frey BN, Fedorkow DM, Key BL, Streiner DL, et al. Cognitive behavior therapy for menopausal symptoms (CBT-Meno). Menopause. 2019;26(9):972–80.
42. Green SM, Donegan E, McCabe RE, Fedorkow DM, Streiner DL, Frey BN. Objective and subjective vasomotor symptom outcomes in the CBT-meno randomized controlled trial. Climacteric. 2020;23(5):482–8.
43. Hardy C, Griffiths A, Norton S, Hunter MS. Self-help cognitive behavior therapy for working women with problematic hot flushes and night sweats (MENOS@Work): a multicenter randomized controlled trial. Menopause. 2018;25(5):508–19.
44. Dodin S, Blanchet C, Marc I, Ernst E, Wu T, Vaillancourt C, et al. Acupuncture for menopausal hot flushes. Cochrane Database Syst Rev. 2013;2013(7):CD007410.
45. Cho SH, Whang WW. Acupuncture for vasomotor menopausal symptoms. Menopause. 2009;16(5):1065–73.
46. Lee MS, Kim KH, Shin BC, Choi SM, Ernst E. Acupuncture for treating hot flushes in men with prostate cancer: a systematic review. Support Care Cancer. 2009;17(7):763–70.
47. Haest K, Kumar A, Van Calster B, Leunen K, Smeets A, Amant F, et al. Stellate ganglion block for the management of hot flashes and sleep disturbances in breast cancer survivors: an uncontrolled experimental study with 24 weeks of follow-up. Ann Oncol. 2012;23(6):1449–54.
48. Pachman DR, Barton D, Carns PE, Novotny PJ, Wolf S, Linquist B, et al. Pilot evaluation of a stellate ganglion block for the treatment of hot flashes. Support Care Cancer. 2011;19(7):941–7.
49. Lipov EG, Joshi JR, Xie H, Slavin KV. Updated findings on the effects of stellate-ganglion block on hot flushes and night awakenings. Lancet Oncol. 2008;9(9):819–20.
50. van Gastel P, Kallewaard JW, van der Zanden M, de Boer H. Stellate-ganglion block as a treatment for severe postmenopausal flushing. Climacteric. 2012;16(1):41–7.
51. Sturdee DW, Panay N. Recommendations for the management of postmenopausal vaginal atrophy. Climacteric. 2010;13(6):509–22.
52. Bachmann GA, Leiblum SR, Kemmann E, Colburn DW, Swartzman L, Shelden R. Sexual expression and its determinants in the post-menopausal woman. Maturitas. 1984;6(1):19–29.
53. Suckling JA, Kennedy R, Lethaby A, Roberts H. Local oestrogen for vaginal atrophy in postmenopausal women. In: Suckling JA, editor. Cochrane database of systematic reviews. Chichester: John Wiley & Sons, Ltd; 2006.
54. Le Ray I, Dell'Aniello S, Bonnetain F, Azoulay L, Suissa S. Local estrogen therapy and risk of breast cancer recurrence among hormone-treated patients: a nested case–control study. Breast Cancer Res Treat. 2012;135(2):603–9.
55. Wills S, Ravipati A, Venuturumilli P, Kresge C, Folkerd E, Dowsett M, et al. Effects of vaginal estrogens on serum estradiol levels in postmenopausal breast cancer survivors and women at risk of breast cancer taking an aromatase inhibitor or a selective estrogen receptor modulator. J Oncol Pract. 2012;8(3):144–8.
56. Biglia N, Peano E, Sgandurra P, Moggio G, Panuccio E, Migliardi M, et al. Low-dose vaginal estrogens or vaginal moisturizer in breast cancer survivors with urogenital atrophy: a preliminary study. Gynecol Endocrinol. 2010;26(6):404–12.
57. Portman DJ, Bachmann GA, Simon JA. Ospemifene, a novel selective estrogen receptor modulator for treating dyspareunia associated with postmenopausal vulvar and vaginal atrophy. Menopause. 2013;20(6):623–30.
58. Bachmann GA, Komi JO. Ospemifene effectively treats vulvovaginal atrophy in postmenopausal women. Menopause. 2010;17(3):480–6.

Complementary and Alternative Therapies for Vasomotor Symptoms During Climacteric and Beyond

Camil Castelo-Branco, Laura Ribera, and María Fernanda Garrido Oyarzún

Abstract

Complementary and alternative medicine (CAM) is more and more accepted among women to manage their menopausal complaints. Commonly, the terms "alternative" and "complementary" are often used as synonymous by health professionals and public in general, although they refer to different entities. Reasons for use of CAM range from personal beliefs to fear or individual contraindication for hormone therapy. The US National Center for Complementary and Alternative Medicine has defined this class of therapies as a group of diverse medical and health-care systems, practices, and products that are not generally considered to be part of conventional medicine.

Most complementary health approaches fall into one of two subgroups; natural products such as herbs, vitamins, minerals, and probiotics that are often sold as dietary supplements or mind and body practices including yoga, chiropractic and osteopathic manipulation, meditation, massage therapy, acupuncture, relaxation techniques, and hypnotherapy, among a huge variety of other therapies.

CAM treatments for vasomotor symptoms include a broad range of plant-based therapies such as phytoestrogens, black cohosh, Chinese herbs, and other herbs and cognitive behavioral therapies such as hypnosis, mindfulness training, paced respiration, and acupuncture.

Herein we review the characteristics, action mechanism, efficacy, and safety of CAM therapies to manage vasomotor symptoms in menopausal women.

16.1 Introduction

Vasomotor symptoms, such as hot flashes and night sweats, are very common during the menopausal transition, affecting approximately 65–76% of women in this period [1]. Although hormone therapy (HT) has traditionally been used as the most effective treatment to ameliorate these symptoms, since the publication of the Women's Health Initiative (WHI) Study in 2002 that generated concerns about the safety of this treatment, the prescription has dropped by 40–80% [2].

Nowadays, complementary and alternative medicine (CAM) has become very popular among women to treat their menopausal symptoms (up to 76% declare using at least one form of alternative therapy in a population-based survey) [3], either for personal beliefs or because they have a contraindication for HT, such as high cardiovascular risk or a personal history of hormone-dependent cancers, among others.

The US National Center for Complementary and Alternative Medicine has defined CAM as "a group of diverse medical and health care systems, practices, and products that are not generally considered to be part of conventional medicine." When describing these approaches, people often use the terms "alternative" and "complementary" interchangeably, even though they refer to different concepts. If a non-mainstream practice is used together with conventional medicine, it is considered complementary, and if a non-mainstream practice is used in place of conventional medicine, it is considered alternative [4].

Most complementary health approaches fall into one of two subgroups: natural products such as herbs, vitamins, minerals and probiotics that are often sold as dietary supplements or mind and body practices including yoga, chiropractic and osteopathic manipulation, meditation, massage therapy, acupuncture, relaxation techniques, and hypnotherapy, among a variety of other therapies [4].

CAM treatments for vasomotor symptoms include a broad range of plant-based therapies such as phytoestrogens, black cohosh, Chinese herbs, and other herbs and cognitive behavioral therapies (CBT) such as hypnosis, mindfulness training, paced respiration, and acupuncture.

This chapter will review the characteristics, action mechanism, efficacy, and safety of these CAM treatments to ameliorate vasomotor symptoms in menopausal women.

16.2 Natural Products: Plant-Based Therapies

16.2.1 Phytoestrogens

Phytoestrogens are nonsteroidal plant compounds of diverse structure that are found in many fruits, vegetables, and grains. They are categorized as isoflavones, lignans, and coumestans.

These compounds structurally resemble estradiol (E2), and, in humans, they have been suggested to act as selective estrogen receptor modulators (SERMs), exerting anti-estrogenic effects in the high estrogen environment of premenopause and estrogenic effects in the low estrogen environment of postmenopause. They act as weak agonists by stimulating estrogen receptors (ER) [5] with greater affinity for the ER beta (ERβ) than for the classical ER alpha (ERα). As a result, they preferentially express estrogenic effects in the central nervous system, blood vessels, bone, and skin without causing stimulation of the breast or uterus, mechanism by which phytoestrogens could protect against breast and endometrial cancer [6]. Thus, phytoestrogens may reduce vasomotor symptoms through their action on the vascular system without causing unwanted estrogenic effects on other body systems [7].

Nonetheless, the mode of action has other complexities such as the binding affinity of isoflavones to progesterone and androgen receptors and the capacity to induce the hepatic synthesis of sex hormone-binding globulin (SHBG), within other effects by which phytoestrogens are today considered to be endocrine disruptors [8].

All in all, phytoestrogens intake appears to cause a small and slow in onset reduction of vasomotor symptoms of menopause. Individual variations in their metabolism may account for the considerable variability in their measured effects. They also appear to improve bone mineral density and markers of cardiovascular risk (blood pressure and low-density lipoprotein cholesterol level reduction); however, there is inadequate research regarding long-term outcomes [9].

16.2.1.1 Isoflavones

Isoflavones are among the most estrogenically potent phytoestrogens, although they are much weaker than human estrogens. The most frequent source of isoflavones is soy beans (*Glycine max*) and red clover (*Trifolium pratense*). Two types of isoflavones, genistein and daidzein, are contained in the protein fraction of the soy bean, whereas formononetin and biochanin A, two precursors of genistein and daidzein, are the ones contained in red clover [10].

After their intake, phytoestrogen preparations are extensively metabolized in the gut to more or less potent metabolites by intestinal bacteria, one of them equol, the end product of the biotransformation of daidzein that possesses estrogenic activity for both ERs. However, equol is not produced in all healthy adults in response to dietary exposure to soy or daidzein. Actually, it is estimated that only 30–50% of individuals are able to produce equol, being most of them Asians or vegetarians [11]. Host genetics contribute to interindividual differences in the metabolism by determining gut microbial activity and genetic biotransformation enzyme expression. The ability to make equol is apparently the clue to the effectiveness of soy protein diets [8]. Therefore, it has been found that supplementing equol to equol nonproducers significantly lowers the incidence and/or severity of hot flashes in menopausal women [12].

A Cochrane review in 2013 evaluated the efficacy and safety of food products, extracts, and dietary supplements containing high levels of phytoestrogens (> 30 mg/d of isoflavones), to treat vasomotor menopausal symptoms in perimenopausal or postmenopausal women without a personal history of breast cancer compared with placebo and HT [7].

The Cochrane review included four trials to assess the efficacy of the treatment of menopausal hot flushes with genistein, in doses ranged from 30–60 mg/d and a duration ranging from 12 weeks to 2 years. The studies found consistent benefit with a reduction in the frequency and duration of hot flushes when compared to placebo, but in a lesser extent than HT. No severe adverse events were reported, only gastrointestinal complaints in one study. Also, no significant differences in endometrial thickness were found [7, 13–16].

Asian women have a high level of soy consumption, estimated in 50–100 mg/dL of isoflavones compared to <1 mg/dL in Western women. Although there is contradictory evidence, many studies have found a significant inverse association between the frequency of hot flushes and higher levels of soy consumption, which could explain the differences in incidence of hot flushes estimated in 14–18% in Asian woman versus 80–85% in European and American women [16, 17].

The efficacy of dietary soy was evaluated in 13 studies, with isoflavone content ranging from 42 mg/d to 134 mg/d. Of the 13 included studies, 7 indicated that no significant differences were noted between the soy intervention and control groups. The remaining six studies found a significant difference in the frequency and severity of hot flushes [18–23]. The heterogeneity of the results was not explained by the level of isoflavones in the food products and could have been caused by the ability to convert soy isoflavone to equol. Overall, no evidence suggested that a diet with high levels of soy phytoestrogens had a positive effect on hot flush frequency or severity. The most frequently reported side effects included bloating, nausea, and weight gain [24]. No evidence indicates an estrogenic stimulation of the endometrium [7].

Nine of 12 trials included in the Cochrane review that assessed the efficacy of soy extracts in capsule or tablet form, with isoflavones levels ranging from 33 mg/d to 200 mg/d, reported a positive effect on hot flush frequency or severity when compared to placebo [25–32]. An increased rate of constipation was reported in women taking soy versus placebo. No adverse event were found regarding endometrial thickness [7].

It is important to highlight the strong placebo effect noted in most trials involving soy bean, with a reduction in the frequency of hot flushes ranging from 1% to 59% [7].

The most studied red clover product is Promensil (brand name), a standardized product that contains a red clover extract. Data from five randomized trials [33–37] that assessed the effects of Promensil (40 mg/d and 80 mg/d) were combined in a metanalysis, and another four trials that assessed the effects of other red clover extracts were included in the review mentioned above. Neither reported significant differences in hot flush frequency or severity compared with placebo [7]. Neither showed an adverse effect on the endometrial thickness, and even one reported a 15% decrease in the endometrial thickness after 12 weeks of treatment with Promensil versus placebo [38].

Given the known importance of producing equol in the metabolism of daidzein to obtain the benefits from soy isoflavones and taking into account that more than one third of women are non-equol producers [16], the Cochrane review includes one trial that assessed the effect of a standardized natural S-(−) equol in the form of SE5-OH (10 mg/day) for 12 weeks in postmenopausal women with low rates of equol excretion. The study reported a significant improvement in hot flush frequency and severity when compared to placebo [39]. These results are consistent with other studies that have also shown a benefit in mood-related symptoms in perimenopausal and postmenopausal non-equol producers [40]. No serious adverse effects were reported, and no endometrial abnormalities were found, only a systemic rush in one woman [39, 40].

A recent meta-analysis including 21 randomized controlled trials (RCTs) showed that composite phytoestrogen supplementation and individual phytoestrogen interventions, such as dietary and supplemental soy isoflavones, were associated with an improvement in some menopausal symptoms, including modest reductions in hot flashes and vaginal dryness but no significant reduction in night sweats. The association between overall phytoestrogen use and menopausal symptoms by type of phytoestrogen intervention (e.g., whole foods, soy protein, and isoflavone extract supplementation groups) yielded broadly similar results. Meanwhile, the supplementation with red clover was associated with improvements in night sweats but not in the frequency of hot flashes [41].

Because of general suboptimal quality and the heterogeneous nature of the current evidence, further rigorous studies are needed to determine the association between plant-based and natural therapies with menopausal health [42].

16.2.1.2 Lignans

Lignans such as enterolactone and enterodiol are found in flaxseed, lentils, grains, fruits, and vegetables.

In the Cochrane review mentioned above, three studies compared flaxseed dietary supplement or flaxseed extract versus placebo or control and found no evidence of benefit in the frequency and intensity of hot flashes after flaxseed treatment. No serious adverse effects were reported [43–45].

16.2.1.3 Coumestans

Coumestans are another group of plant phenols that show estrogenic activity. The main coumestans with phytoestrogenic effects are coumestrol and 4′-methoxycoumestrol. Coumestans are less common in the human diet than isoflavones, yet similar to isoflavones, in that they are also found in legumes, particularly food plants such as sprouts of alfalfa and mung bean, and they are especially high in clover and soy sprouts. Coumestrol as genistein has higher binding affinities to ER than the other phytoestrogen compounds [46].

The effectiveness of coumestans in treating menopausal vasomotor symptoms has not been well studied, although it has been suggested that they could act as natural antidepressants [47].

16.2.2 Cimicifuga racemosa

The most popular and worldwide renowned herb for the treatment of menopausal symptoms is *Actaea racemosa* or *Cimicifuga racemosa* (CR), commonly known as black cohosh. It was originally used by indigenous North American Indians to treat a variety of women's diseases. Later on, it proved to be efficient to alleviate climacteric complaints [48].

CR originally grew in North America but other *Cimicifuga* species grew in Far East-Asia. In many countries where CR extracts are sold as food supplements, the preparations contain Asian CR, of which chemical constituents are quite different from North American species, and no clinical data of their effectiveness are available [48].

CR has arisen as an effective and safe treatment option for the relieving of vasomotor symptoms, even though longer study follow-ups are required. Used at the recommended dose of 40 mg/day, CR produces no significant adverse reactions [49]. A review which included 31 studies and 1839 women treated with CR provided no scientific evidence that the use of CR causes weight gain in menopausal women [50].

CR contains triterpene glycosides and phenolic acids which are identified as the possible active compounds to relieve climacteric symptoms. Ligand binding assays and cell culture experiments have indicated the presence of dopaminergic and serotoninergic compounds in CR extract (CR BNO 1055). Thus, it is possible that the proven effect of CR BNO 1055 on hot flushes is caused by dopaminergic, adrenergic, and serotoninergic compounds [51, 52].

A meta-analysis [53] on the use of black cohosh for menopausal symptoms, which included 35 clinical studies and one meta-analysis comprising 43,759 women of which 13,096 had been treated with CR, showed hormone levels remain unchanged, and therefore, estrogen-sensitive tissues (e.g., breast, endometrium) are unaffected by this treatment. The clinical data did not reveal any evidence of hepatotoxicity. Due to its good safety profile in general and at estrogen-sensitive organs, it can also be used in patients with hormone-dependent diseases who suffer from iatrogenic climacteric symptoms. This is consistent with clinical studies that reported no effect of Klimadynon (brand name of CR extract) used for 6 months in the mammary gland density determined by digitized mammography [54]. Even a case control study involving breast cancer patients demonstrated that the use of CR had a significant breast cancer protective effect [55]. However, on the other hand, CR exhibits mild inhibition of CYP2D6 that might interfere with the efficacy of concomitant chemotherapy agents or enhance their toxicity [56]. Another recent meta-analysis has corroborated previous findings regarding potentially beneficial effects of CR for relieving menopausal symptoms [57].

All in all, as benefits clearly outweigh the risks, CR at a correct dosage should be recommended as an evidence-based treatment option for climacteric symptoms.

16.2.3 Pollen Extract

A recent systematic review and meta-analysis has evaluated the efficacy of purified cytoplasm of pollen for reducing vasomotor symptoms in women [58]. It included five articles: one RCT and four observational studies ($N = 420$). Overall, pooled data suggest that vasomotor symptom improvements seen in noncontrolled studies may have been due to the placebo effect. However, its use was not associated with significant adverse effects.

16.2.4 Chinese Herbs

Traditional Chinese Medicine (TCM) is one of the most popular CAM in Eastern countries, with a history of practice exceeding 2000 years. In the last decades, it has significantly permeated a broad cross-section with western communities. Western medicine connects climacteric symptoms to a reduced function of the hypothalamic pituitary gonadal axis, while TCM frequently classifies it as a "kidney deficiency" and imbalance of Yin and Yang [59].

Traditionally, drugs in Chinese herbal medicine (CHM) are not given as single substances. They are combined in complex individualized prescriptions for each patient and their disease and are then modified at different stages of the patient's recovery or illness [60].

Traditionally, prescriptions are prepared as decoction (raw materials are cooked over a longer period), but, over the last decades, several additional forms of application have been proposed and investigated such as pills, liniments, plasters, and ointments that concentrate powder and liquid extracts prepared with modern pharmaceutical procedures. The routes of administration also differ and can be either oral, topical, intravenous, or injections into specific acupuncture points [59, 60].

More than 185 herbs and 73 classic formulae have been used to treat menopausal complaints. Some herbs such as Ren Shen (Radix Panax ginseng) and Dang Gui have been linked with an estrogen-like effect, while in other formulae no estrogenic action has been detected, remaining the mechanisms of action still unknown [59].

A Cochrane review in 2016 included 22 RCTs to assess the effectiveness of CHM. The review found that CHM was no better than placebo for vasomotor symptoms in terms of frequency and severity. It also did not find any benefit in relation to quality of life (QoL). No serious adverse events were reported, only mild to moderate symptoms such as diarrhea, breast tenderness, and gastric discomfort, among others, which were solved once the CHM was terminated [59].

However, a recent systematic review and meta-analysis evaluating TCM in the treatment of menopause-like syndrome for breast cancer survivors, which included 42 studies involving 3112 female patients, showed that TCM can effectively improve these symptoms in this collective [61]. In the TCM group, the scores of hot flashes and night sweats were significantly decreased (95% CI [− 1.1- -0.27]). Follicle-stimulating hormone (FSH) and estradiol (E_2) had no significant difference compared with the control group, meaning that the use of TCM does not negatively affect endocrine therapy and may even have a synergistic effect.

Nevertheless, there are few randomized, double-blind, placebo-controlled studies on TCM treatment of menopausal syndrome, and future studies should be undertaken to confirm its merits [62].

16.3 Mind and Body Practices

16.3.1 Acupuncture

Acupuncture is among the most popular forms of complementary medicine with an estimated prevalence of acupuncture use by mid-life women ranging from 1% to 10.4% [63].

Acupuncture is defined as the practice of inserting a needle or needles into certain points in the body for therapeutic purposes. The most used types of acupuncture include traditional Chinese acupuncture (TCA) that involves the insertion of needles; electroacupuncture that involves passing small electric currents through the inserted acupuncture needles; acupressure, a technique that involves manual pressure on the acupoints; and ear acupuncture that uses acupuncture needles, seeds, or magnetic pearls to stimulate the acupoints located on the ear and scalp acupuncture that involves the use of acupuncture needles along the surface of the head. Sham acupuncture (SA), also called placebo, consists in light touches of the skin that are performed off the acupuncture points established by TCA [63, 64].

It has been suggested that acupuncture may have the potential to reduce hot flush frequency and severity in the menopause and also during the menopausal transition [65], but the mechanism by which it might affect health or menopausal symptoms is not completely understood. It has been proposed that TCA may affect the release of serotonin and beta-endorphins in the central nervous system, therefore influencing and stabilizing the thermoregulatory center, normalizing body temperature, and reducing hot flashes and sweating [63, 64].

In the Eastern view of acupuncture, which is based on Chinese medical philosophy, acupuncture tries to reestablish the energy balance in order to treat disease through the stimulation of specific points. When acupuncture is specifically used for menopausal symptoms, it is designed to correct a condition known as deficient heat [63, 64].

A Cochrane meta-analysis of 16 RCTs [64] was performed in 2013 to assess the effectiveness and safety of acupuncture to reduce hot flushes and improve the QoL of menopausal women. When acupuncture was compared with SA, no differences were found in hot flashes frequency, but there was a benefit in terms of their severity. No differences were found when compared with relaxation and electroacupuncture in any outcome. More frequent hot flashes were reported in the TCA group comparing with the HT group, but TCA proved to be significantly more effective than no intervention regarding hot flashes frequency and severity and in terms of QoL. No serious adverse events were reported.

Another meta-analysis of 12 RCT in 2015 [66] was designed to investigate the effects of acupuncture on menopause-related symptoms and QoL in women experiencing natural menopause. Acupuncture compared with no intervention significantly reduced the frequency and severity of hot flashes with long-term effects remaining up to 3 months. Regarding QoL, acupuncture improved QoL in the vasomotor domain of the Menopause-Specific Quality of Life questionnaire but not in the psychiatric, physical, or sexual domains. However, SA showed comparable treatment effects with TCA. This could be explained by a limbic response induced by the touch of the skin of the SA, resulting in emotional and hormonal reactions such as the endorphins release that could reduce hot flashes.

These results are consistent with a RCT [67] performed in multiple health centers in Australia. This study showed that an 8-week course of standardized TCA did not reduce menopausal hot flashes more than SA. Hot flashes decreased in both groups by approximately 40% with an effect sustained for 6 months. No effects were found over QoL for neither acupuncture type.

Patients with cancer often show interest in complementary and integrative modalities because HT is contraindicated for these women. Several clinical trials have suggested a role for acupuncture in managing moderate to severe hot flashes in women with breast cancer. However, the superiority of acupuncture has not been demonstrated when using SA as a control or nonoptimal acupuncture intervention in women with mixed menopausal symptoms.

One RCT [68] involving 190 women with breast cancer compared acupuncture (85 women received 10 TCA sessions involving needling of predefined acupoints) plus enhanced self-care with enhanced self-care alone (105 women received a booklet with information about climacteric syndrome and its management). The study showed that women with breast cancer treated with acupuncture plus enhanced self-care for 12 weeks experienced fewer vasomotor symptoms than women who received self-care alone. Acupuncture was associated with improvements in all health-related QoL outcomes except for the sexual dimension, suggesting a specific effect of acupuncture. These effects persisted for at least 6 months after the end of the treatment and were not associated with significant adverse events during the study period.

A systematic review [69] including a total of 943 patients from 13 RCTs aimed to evaluate how long the effect of acupuncture on breast cancer-related hot flashes and menopause symptoms last showed, however, a significant 3-month maintenance effect of ameliorating menopause symptoms after treatment ended. No adverse events were reported and the improvement did not persist any longer. Therefore, the authors suggested additional acupuncture at 3 months after the initial treatment course could be considered.

Nevertheless, provided, in the end, an individual improvement is sought, an effort to identify genetic predictors to acupuncture response for hot flashes in breast cancer survivors has been performed. A randomized controlled trial [70] which included 57 women receiving electroacupuncture or SA analyzed single nucleotide polymorphisms in genes involved in neurotransmission, thermoregulation, and inflammation. It identified six genotypes, which were associated with response (70.3% in carriers vs 37.5% in noncarriers), defined as a 50% reduction in the hot flash composite score of the participants at the end of the treatment.

A review [64] that included 5 RCT showed a slight superiority of TCA compared with SA for reducing the frequency and intensity of hot flashes in 3 studies, while two other studies suggested that both interventions, TCA and SA, are beneficial for the treatment of hot flashes because they reduced their symptoms, even though there were no significant differences between the two intervention methods.

The similarity between the results of TCA and SA may arise because the patient's expectations regarding the intervention influence its effects and could also be related to the different administration protocols and the limbic effect induced by SA as was mentioned above. This is a crucial aspect of clinical research that requires rigorous evaluation.

16.3.2 Mind–Body Therapies

Cognitive-behavioral, behavioral, and mindfulness-based therapies have been used to deal with menopausal symptoms, mainly depression, though evidence is limited.

Mind–body techniques including yoga, meditation, hypnosis, and tai chi have been tested for pain and other chronic medical conditions in several clinical trials, but the paucity of data regarding vasomotor symptoms has not proven any beneficial effect so far. Nevertheless, tai chi was associated with a positive effect on bone density and balance, as well as a reduction in the frequency of falls in elderly women [71]. Yoga practitioners have shown better anthropometric and biochemical variables regarding carbohydrates and lipid metabolism when compared to sedentary women, with no clinical effect on vasomotor symptoms [72]. Similar results regarding body composition have been found with the practice of other meditative movement [73]. The psychological and emotional symptoms of menopause can also be dealt with music therapy [74]. Paced respiration has also been tried as an intervention for hot flashes. However, its efficacy has not been demonstrated [75].

A Cochrane review concluded that there is no evidence indicating that relaxation techniques could reduce the number of hot flashes per 24 h or their severity, although evidence is insufficient in this field [76].

16.3.3 Exercise and Lifestyle Modifications

There is evidence that body mass index, smoking, alcohol consumption, and sedentary lifestyle are associated with reports of vasomotor symptoms. However, there are few papers addressing the direct effect of lifestyle modifications on flushes [77].

A Cochrane review examined the effectiveness of any type of exercise intervention in the management of vasomotor symptoms in symptomatic perimenopausal and postmenopausal women. The evidence of 5 RCTs (733 women) was insufficient to show whether exercise is an effective treatment for vasomotor menopausal symptoms when compared with no active treatment, or with yoga [76]. A more recent meta-analysis [78] including 9 RCTs in which any type of exercise was compared with no active treatment, also found no evidence for the effects of exercise on vasomotor symptoms, although positive effects on physical and psychological QoL scores were found.

References

1. Randolph JF Jr, Sowers M, Bondarenko I, Gold EB, Greendale GA, Bromberger JT, et al. The relationship of longitudinal change in reproductive hormones and vasomotor symptoms during the menopausal transition. J Clin Endocrinol Metab. 2005;90(11):6106–12.
2. Burger HG, MacLennan AH, Huang KE, Castelo-Branco C. Evidence-based assessment of the impact of the WHI on women's health. Climacteric. 2012;15(3):281–7.
3. Newton KM, Buist DS, Keenan NL, Anderson LA, LaCroix AZ. Use of alternative therapies for menopause symptoms: results of a population-based survey. Obstet Gynecol. 2002;100(1):18–25.
4. Complementary, Alternative, or Integrative Health: What's In a Name? NCCAM;2016. https://nccih.nih.gov/health/integrative-health.
5. Seibel MM. Treating hot flushes without hormone replacement therapy. J Fam Pract. 2003;52(4):291–6.
6. Kuiper GG, Carlsson B, Grandien K, Enmark E, Häggblad J, Nilsson S, et al. Comparison of the ligand binding specificity and transcript tissue distribution of estrogen receptors alpha and beta. Endocrinology. 1997;138(3):863–70.
7. Lethaby A, Marjoribanks J, Kronenberg F, Roberts H, Eden J, Brown J. Phytoestrogens for menopausal vasomotor symptoms. Cochrane Database Syst Rev. 2013;12:CD001395.
8. Villaseca P. Non-estrogen conventional and phytochemical treatments for vasomotor symptoms: what needs to be known for practice. Climacteric. 2012;15(2):115–24.
9. Rowe IJ, Baber RJ. The effects of phytoestrogens on postmenopausal health. Climacteric. 2021;24(1):57–63.
10. Booth NL, Overk CR, Yao P, Burdette JE, Nikolic D, Chen SN, et al. The chemical and biologic profile of a red clover (Trifolium pratense L.) phase II clinical extract. J Altern Complement Med. 2006;12(2):133–9.
11. Setchell KD, Brown NM, Lydeking-Olsen E. The clinical importance of the metabolite equol-a clue to the effectiveness of soy and its isoflavones. J Nutr. 2002;132(12):3577–84.
12. Daily JW, Ko BS, Ryuk J, Liu M, Zhang W, Park S. Equol decreases hot flashes in postmenopausal women: a systematic review and meta-analysis of randomized clinical trials. J Med Food. 2019;22(2):127–39.
13. Crisafulli A, Marini H, Bitto A, Altavilla D, Squadrito G, Romeo A, et al. Effects of genistein on hot flushes in early postmenopausal women: a randomized, double-blind EPT and placebo—controlled study. Menopause. 2004;11:400–4.
14. D'Anna R, Cannata ML, Atteritano M, Cancellieri F, Corrado F, Baviera G, et al. Effects of the phytoestrogen genistein on hot flushes, endometrium, and vaginal epithelium in postmenopausal women: a 1-year randomized, double-blind, placebo-controlled study. Menopause. 2007;14(4):648–55.
15. Evans M, Elliott JG, Sharma P, Berman R, Guthrie N. The effect of synthetic genistein on menopause symptom management in healthy postmenopausal women: a multi-center, randomized, placebo-controlled study. Maturitas. 2011;68(2):189–96.
16. Thomas AJ, Ismail R, Taylor-Swanson L, Cray L, Schnall JG, Mitchell ES, et al. Effects of isoflavones and amino acid therapies for hot flashes and co-occurring symptoms during the menopausal transition and early postmenopause: a systematic review. Maturitas. 2014;78(4):263–76.
17. Nagata C, Takatsuka N, Kawakami N, Shimizu H. Soy product intake and hot flashes in Japanese women: results from a community-based prospective study. Am J Epidemiol. 2001;153(8):790–3.
18. Carmigiani LO, Pedro AO, Cost-Paiva LH, Pinto-Neto AM. The effect of dietary soy supplementation compared to estrogen and placebo on menopausal symptoms: a randomised controlled trial. Maturitas. 2010;67:262–9.
19. Albertazzi P, Pansini F, Bonaccorsi G, Zanotti L, Forini E, De Aloysio D. The effect of dietary soy supplementation on hot flushes. Obstet Gynecol. 1998;91(1):6–11.

20. Brzezinski A, Adlercreutz H, Shaoul R, Rosler A, Shmueli A, Tanos V, et al. Short-term effects of phytoestrogen rich diet on postmenopausal women. Menopause. 1997;4(2):89–94.
21. Radhakrishnan G, Agarwal N, Vaid N. Evaluation of isoflavone rich soy protein supplementation for postmenopausal therapy. Pak J Nutr. 2009;8(7):1009–17.
22. Cheng G, Wilczek B, Warner M, Gustafsson J-A, Landgren B-L. Isoflavone treatment for acute menopausal symptoms. Menopause. 2007;14(3, Part 1):468–73.
23. Hanachi P, Golkho S. Assessment of soy phytoestrogens and exercise on lipid profiles and menopause symptoms in menopausal women. J Biol Sci. 2008;8(4):789–93.
24. Knight DC, Howes JB, Eden JA, Howes LG. Effects on menopausal symptoms and acceptability of isoflavone containing soy powder dietary supplementation. Climacteric. 2001;4:13–8.
25. Bicca ML de O, Horta BL, Lethaby AE. Double-blind randomized clinical trial to assess the effectiveness of soy isoflavones in the relief of climacteric symptoms. (unpublished data only).
26. Faure ED, Chantre P, Mares P. Effects of a standardised soy extract on hot flushes: a multicentre, double-blind, randomised placebo-controlled study. Menopause. 2002;9(5):329–34.
27. Khaodhiar L, Ricciotti HA, Li L, Pan W, Schickel M, Zhou J, et al. Daidzein-rich isoflavone-aglycones are effective in reducing hot flashes in menopausal women. Menopause. 2008;15(1):125–32.
28. Nahas E, Nahas-Neto J, Orsatti F, Carvalho E, Oliveira M, Dias R. Efficacy and safety of a soy isoflavone extract in postmenopausal women: a randomized double-blind, and placebo controlled study. Maturitas. 2007;58(3):249–58.
29. Ye Y-B, Wang Z-L, Zhuo S-Y, Lu W, Liao H-F, Verbruggen MA, et al. Soy germ isoflavones improve menopausal symptoms but have no effect on blood lipids in early postmenopausal Chinese women: a randomised placebo controlled trial. Menopause. 2012;19(7):791–8.
30. Han KK, Soares JM, Haidar MA, de Lima GR, Baracat EC. Benefits of soy isoflavone therapeutic regimen on menopausal symptoms. Obstet Gynecol. 2002;99(3):389–94.
31. Jou H-J, Wu S-C, Chang F-W, Ling P-Y, Chu KS, Wu WH. Effect of intestinal production of equol on menopausal symptoms in women treated with soy isoflavones. Int J Gynaecol Obstet. 2008;102(1):44–9.
32. Upmalis DH, Lobo R, Bradley L, Warren M, Cone FL, Lamia CA. Vasomotor symptom relief by soy isoflavone extract tablets in postmenopausal women: a multicenter double-blind randomized placebo-controlled study. Menopause. 2000;7(4):236–42.
33. Baber RJ, Templeman C, Morton T, Kelly GE, West L. Randomized placebo-controlled trial of an isoflavone supplement and menopausal symptoms in women. Climacteric. 1999;2(2):85–92.
34. Jeri A. The use of an isoflavone supplement to relieve hot flushes. Female Patient. 2002;27:47–9.
35. Knight DC, Howes JB, Eden JA. The effect of Promensil, an isoflavone extract, on menopausal symptoms. Climacteric. 1999;2(2):79–84.
36. Tice JA, Ettinger B, Ensrud K, Wallace R, Blackwell T, Cummings SR. Phytoestrogen supplements for the treatment of hot flashes: the Isoflavone clover extract (ICE) study: a randomized controlled trial. JAMA. 2003;290(2):207–14.
37. van de Weijer PH, Barentsen R. Isoflavones from red clover (Promensil) significantly reduce menopausal hot flush symptoms compared with placebo. Maturitas. 2002;42(3):187–93.
38. Imhof M, Gocan A, Reithmayr F, Lipovac M, Schimitzek C, Chedraui P, et al. Effects of a red clover extract (MF11RCE) on endometrium and sex hormones in postmenopausal women. Maturitas. 2006;55(1):76–81.
39. Aso T, Uchiyama S, Matsumura Y, Taguchi M, Nozaki M, Takamatsu K, et al. A natural S-equol supplement alleviates hot flushes and other menopausal symptoms in equol nonproducing postmenopausal Japanese women. J Womens Health (Larchmt). 2012;21(1):92–100.
40. Ishiwata N, Melby MK, Mizuno S, Watanabe S. New equol supplement for relieving menopausal symptoms: randomized, placebo-controlled trial of Japanese women. Menopause. 2009;16(1):141–8.
41. Franco OH, Chowdhury R, Troup J, Voortman T, Kunutsor S, Kavousi M, et al. Use of plant-based therapies and menopausal symptoms: a systematic review and meta-analysis. JAMA. 2016;315(23):2554–63.

42. Kang I, Rim CH, Yang HS, Choe JS, Kim JY, Lee M. Effect of isoflavone supplementation on menopausal symptoms: a systematic review and meta-analysis of randomized controlled trials. Nutr Res Pract. 2022;16(Suppl 1):S147–59.
43. Colli MC, Bracht A, Soares AA, de Oliveira AL, Bôer CG, de Souza CG, et al. Evaluation of the efficacy of flaxseed meal and flaxseed extract in reducing menopausal symptoms. J Med Food. 2012;15(9):840–5.
44. Dalais FS, Rice GE, Wahlqvist ML, Grehan M, Murkies AL, Medley G, et al. Effects of dietary phytoestrogens in postmenopausal women. Climacteric. 1998;1(2):124–9.
45. Lewis JE, Nickell LA, Thompson LU, Szalai JP, Kiss A, Hilditch JR. A randomized controlled trial of the effect of dietary soy and flaxseed muffins on quality of life and hot flashes during menopause. Menopause. 2006;13(4):631–42.
46. Ososki AL, Kennelly EJ. Phytoestrogens: a review of the present state of research. Phytother Res. 2003;17(8):845–69.
47. Patra S, Gorai S, Pal S, Ghosh K, Pradhan S, Chakrabarti S. A review on phytoestrogens: current status and future direction. Phytother Res. 2023;37(7):3097–120.
48. Wuttke W, Jarry H, Haunschild J, Stecher G, Schuh M, Seidlova-Wuttke D. The non-estrogenic alternative for the treatment of climacteric complaints: black cohosh (Cimicifuga or Actaea racemosa). J Steroid Biochem Mol Biol. 2014;139:302–10.
49. Castelo-Branco C, Navarro C, Beltrán E, Losa F, Camacho M. On the behalf of the natural products study Group of the Spanish Menopause Society. Black cohosh efficacy and safety for menopausal symptoms. The Spanish menopause society statement. Gynecol Endocrinol. 2022;38(5):379–84.
50. Naser B, Castelo-Branco C, Meden H, Minkin MJ, Rachoń D, Beer AM, Pickartz S. Weight gain in menopause: systematic review of adverse events in women treated with black cohosh. Climacteric. 2022;25(3):220–7.
51. Beer AM, Osmers R, Schnitker J, Bai W, Mueck AO, Meden H. Efficacy of black cohosh (Cimicifuga racemosa) medicines for treatment of menopausal symptoms—comments on major statements of the Cochrane collaboration report 2012 "black cohosh (Cimicifuga spp.) for menopausal symptoms (review)". Gynecol Endocrinol. 2013;29(12):1022–5.
52. Powell SL, Gödecke T, Nikolic D, Chen SN, Ahn S, Dietz B, Farnsworth NR, et al. In vitro serotonergic activity of black cohosh and identification of N(omega)-methylserotonin as a potential active constituent. J Agric Food Chem. 2008;56(24):11718–26.
53. Castelo-Branco C, Gambacciani M, Cano A, Minkin MJ, Rachoń D, Ruan X, Beer AM, Schnitker J, Henneicke-von Zepelin HH, Pickartz S. Review & meta-analysis: isopropanolic black cohosh extract iCR for menopausal symptoms—an update on the evidence. Climacteric. 2021;24(2):109–19.
54. Lundström E, Hirschberg AL, Söderqvist G. Digitized assessment of mammographic breast density—effects of continuous combined hormone therapy, tibolone and black cohosh compared to placebo. Maturitas. 2011;70(4):361–4.
55. Rebbeck TR, Troxel AB, Norman S, Bunin GR, De Michele A, Baumgarten M, et al. A retrospective case-control study of the use of hormone-related supplements and association with breast cancer. Int J Cancer. 2007;120(7):1523–8.
56. Nikander E, Kilkkinen A, Metsä-Heikkilä M, Adlercreutz H, Pietinen P, Tiitinen A, et al. A randomized placebo-controlled crossover trial with phytoestrogens in treatment of menopause in breast cancer patients. Obstet Gynecol. 2003;101(6):1213–20.
57. Sadahiro R, Matsuoka LN, Zeng BS, Chen KH, Zeng BY, Wang HY, Chu CS, Stubbs B, Su KP, Tu YK, Wu YC, Lin PY, Chen TY, Chen YW, Suen MW, Hopwood M, Yang WC, Sun CK, Cheng YS, Shiue YL, Hung CM, Matsuoka YJ, Tseng PT. Black cohosh extracts in women with menopausal symptoms: an updated pairwise meta-analysis. Menopause. 2023;30(7):766–73.
58. Acquarulo EL, Hernandez EC, Kodzodziku F, Nemec EC. The efficacy of purified pollen extract for reducing vasomotor symptoms in women: a systematic review and meta-analysis. Menopause. 2024;31(2):154–9.
59. Zhu X, Liew Y, Liu ZL. Chinese herbal medicine for menopausal symptoms. Cochrane Database Syst Rev. 2016;3:CD009023.

60. Eisenhardt S, Fleckenstein J. Traditional Chinese medicine valuably augments therapeutic options in the treatment of climacteric syndrome. Arch Gynecol Obstet. 2016;294(1):193–200.
61. Wang R, Wang Y, Fang L, Xie Y, Yang S, Liu S, Fang Y, Zhang Y. Efficacy and safety of traditional Chinese medicine in the treatment of menopause-like syndrome for breast cancer survivors: a systematic review and meta-analysis. BMC Cancer. 2024;24(1):42.
62. Wang YP, Yu Q. The treatment of menopausal symptoms by traditional Chinese medicine in Asian countries. Climacteric. 2021;24(1):64–7.
63. Dodin S, Blanchet C, Marc I, Ernst E, Wu T, Vaillancourt C, et al. Acupuncture for menopausal hot flushes. Cochrane Database Syst Rev. 2013;7:CD007410.
64. Lopes-Júnior CL, Cruz LA, Leopoldo VC, Campos FR, Almeida AM, Silveira RC. Effectiveness of traditional Chinese acupuncture versus sham acupuncture: a systematic review. Rev Lat Am Enfermagem. 2016;24:e2762.
65. Soares JM Jr, Branco-de-Luca AC, da Fonseca AM, Carvalho-Lopes CM, Arruda-Veiga EC, Roa CL, Bagnoli VR, Baracat EC. Acupuncture ameliorated vasomotor symptoms during menopausal transition: single-blind, placebo-controlled, randomized trial to test treatment efficacy. Menopause. 2020;28(1):80–5.
66. Chiu HY, Pan CH, Shyu YK, Han BC, Tsai PS. Effects of acupuncture on menopause-related symptoms and quality of life in women in natural menopause: a meta-analysis of randomized controlled trials. Menopause. 2015;22(2):234–44.
67. Ee C, Xue C, Chondros P, Myers SP, French SD, Teede H, et al. Acupuncture for menopausal hot flashes: a randomized trial. Ann Intern Med. 2016;164(3):146–54.
68. Lesi G, Razzini G, Musti MA, Stivanello E, Petrucci C, Benedetti B, et al. Acupuncture as an integrative approach for the treatment of hot flashes in women with breast cancer: a prospective multicenter randomized controlled trial (AcCliMaT). J Clin Oncol. 2016;34(15):1795–802.
69. Chien TJ, Liu CY, Fang CJ, Kuo CY. The maintenance effect of acupuncture on breast cancer-related menopause symptoms: a systematic review. Climacteric. 2020;23(2):130–9.
70. Romero SAD, Li QS, Orlow I, Gonen M, Su HI, Mao JJ. Genetic predictors to acupuncture response for hot flashes: an exploratory study of breast cancer survivors. Menopause. 2020;27(8):913–7.
71. Reid R, Abramson B, Blake J, Desindes S, Dodin S, Johnston S, et al. Managing menopause. Chapter 9: Complementary and alternative medicine (CAM). J Obstet Gynaecol Can. 2014;36(9):830–3.
72. Souza LACE, Lima AA. Anthropometric, biochemical and clinical parameters in climacteric yoga practitioners. Climacteric. 2022;25(3):293–9.
73. James DL, Larkey LK, Evans B, Sebren A, Goldsmith K, Ahlich E, Hawley NA, Kechter A, Sears DD. Mechanisms of improved body composition among perimenopausal women practicing meditative movement: a proposed biobehavioral model. Menopause. 2023;30(11):1114–23.
74. Kim S, Kim SM, Hwang H, Kim MK, Kim HJ, Park S, Han DH. The effects of music therapy on the psychological status of women with perimenopause syndrome. Menopause. 2023;30(10):1045–52.
75. Mintziori G, Lambrinoudaki I, Goulis DG, Ceausu I, Depypere H, Erel CT, et al. EMAS position statement: non-hormonal management of menopausal vasomotor symptoms. Maturitas. 2015;81(3):410–3.
76. Saensak S, Vutyavanich T, Somboonporn W, Srisurapanont M. Relaxation for perimenopausal and postmenopausal symptoms. Cochrane Database Syst Rev. 2014;7:CD008582.
77. Sassarini J, Lumsden MA. Non-hormonal management of vasomotor symptoms. Climacteric. 2013;16(Suppl 1):31–6.
78. Nguyen TM, Do TTT, Tran TN, Kim JH. Exercise and quality of life in women with menopausal symptoms: a systematic review and meta-analysis of randomized controlled trials. Int J Environ Res Public Health. 2020;17(19):7049.

Lifestyle: Physical Activity

17

Nicolás Mendoza Ladrón de Guevara,
Carlos de Teresa Galván, and Débora Godoy Izquierdo

Abstract

Physical activity (PA) is a promoter of health in general. Its benefits include maintaining proper weight, providing stress relief, increasing muscle strength, improving balance and coordination, increasing bone strength, and increasing mental focus. In addition, PA improves the evolution of diseases such as hypertension, diabetes, osteoporosis, and dementia. We can infer that PA is more than a lifestyle; it constitutes a form of therapy in itself.

The aim of this chapter is to analyse the impact of healthy PA during peri- and postmenopause, to determine the PA-associated improvements in the symptoms and processes that emerge during this period, and to identify the optimal PA recommendations for those purposes.

17.1 Introduction

PA is related to protecting and promoting physical and mental health, increasing quality of life (QoL), and preventing premature death from any cause for people of any age, sex, or health status. In contrast, sedentary behaviour can triple the risk of

---

N. M. L. de Guevara (✉)
Department of Obstetrics and Gynaecology, University of Granada, Granada, Spain
e-mail: nicomendoza@ugr.es

C. de Teresa Galván
Centro Andaluz de Medicina del Deporte, Granada, Granada, Spain
e-mail: cdeteresa@ugr.es

D. Godoy Izquierdo
Instituto Universitario de Investigación de Estudios de las Mujeres y de Género,
Department of Personality, Psychological Assessment and Treatment,
University of Granada, Granada, Spain
e-mail: debora@ugr.es

© The Author(s), under exclusive license to Springer Nature Switzerland AG 2025
A. Cano (ed.), *Menopause*, https://doi.org/10.1007/978-3-031-83979-5_17

disease and exacerbates the risks associated with such health hazards as smoking, obesity, and hypertension [1].

Sedentary behaviour not only endangers peri- and postmenopausal women health but also increases the problems associated with this life stage. In this sense, there is abundant evidence linking PA practice with improvements in many health indicators and QoL and the prevention or treatment of various ailments that emerge during and after menopause. We can infer that PA is more than a lifestyle; rather, it constitutes a form of therapy in itself [2].

There is an increasing demand by women for interventions to improve that has influenced the demand for therapies to improve signs and symptoms of ageing and allow them to reach old age with the best possible QoL. PA is a promoter of health and well-being in general. Its benefits include proper weight maintenance, stress relief, increased muscle strength, improved balance and coordination, increased bone strength, and increased mental focus [3]. In addition, PA improves the evolution of diseases such as hypertension, diabetes, osteoporosis, and dementia. The aim of this chapter is to analyse the impact of PA and to determine its benefits, requirements, and the optimal types of PA for postmenopausal women.

17.2 Risks of Sedentary Behaviour

Menopause is a transition period influenced by a multitude of physiological and psychological changes. It is not a disease, but it sometimes affects QoL and general health: it is accompanied by vasomotor symptoms and changes in body composition. These changes amplify those caused by a sedentary lifestyle; they can lead to real pathologies such as metabolic syndrome and cardiovascular diseases (CVD) and can increase the intensity and frequency of hot flashes.

Sedentary habits have been installed in modern societies, and new technologies continue to reduce the effort required to perform physical tasks jobs. Sedentary behaviour could be considered a risk factor (RF) or trigger for multiple diseases [3]:

- Overweight-obesity and excess abdominal fat are RFs for diabetes and CVD.
- Diabetes mellitus is a metabolic disease caused by insulin resistance produced mainly by high sugar intake but also sedentary habits and overweight.
- PA has been linked to improved HDL and LDL, while the sedentary lifestyle has an inverse effect on the lipid profile, increasing the risk of CVD.
- Fibromyalgia is a disease that causes marked functional and social limitations because of chronic pain in the joints and muscles. A sedentary lifestyle lowers the pain threshold and favours the development of this ailment.
- A sedentary lifestyle has been linked to many types of cancers, such as breast, colon, and pancreas cancer.

17.3 Cardiometabolic Benefits

It has been shown that PA alone reduces the risk of cardiometabolic mortality regardless of age, sex, or weight. Consequently, PA reduces the risk of cardiovascular mortality in postmenopausal women, and it falls within the prevention recommendations for CVD. PA has a dose-dependent benefit; that is, the level of physical fitness is inversely related to mortality [4].

PA reduces the risk of cardiovascular mortality by reducing its main RFs (e.g. hypertension, dyslipidaemia, and diabetes). Improvements of hypertension have been observed with the practice of various forms of training [5].

In postmenopausal women, PA decreases hypertension by mitigating arterial ageing, causing functional and structural vascular adaptations that help to maintain or normalize arterial pressure levels. It has been observed that individuals who exercise more frequently exhibit less arterial stiffness than sedentary individuals and that when sedentary individuals engage in PA, arterial stiffness decreases. This seems to result from the release of a vasodilator (nitrous oxide), which improves the per-O2 supply to the cells of the endothelium (the intima of the blood vessels), preventing deterioration and death [6]. PA also increases the sensitivity of the beta-adrenergic receptors and reduces the release of catecholamines [7].

Along with chronic systemic inflammation, oxidative stress, abdominal visceral adipose tissue, and dyslipidaemia, a sedentary lifestyle is an RF associated with metabolic syndrome in postmenopausal women. Aerobic PA (running, cycling) and muscle training with resistance (weightlifting) have been associated with general health improvements, including normalizing the lipid profile, anti-inflammatory responses, and antioxidant enzyme expression and reducing adipose tissue [8].

Aerobic PA has been shown to decrease weight and increase insulin sensitivity, which are important mechanisms for preventing diabetes and metabolic syndrome. Diabetes is also associated with overweight and increased visceral adipose tissue level. Additionally, postmenopausal hypoestrogenism results in fat redistribution (male-type obesity), which is an important cardiometabolic RF.

There is a direct relationship between PA and weight reduction: the more PA is performed, the more fat mass is eliminated. However, after a PA session, the appetite increases and the individual tends to eat more; therefore, during the first few weeks of a PA programme, weight loss is not very evident, and weight even tends to increase. Additionally, PA increases muscle mass. Therefore, PA should be a consistent part in an individual's routine, along with a healthy diet. Although few studies have evaluated the effectiveness of PA in postmenopausal women, it appears that PA is more effective when it is more intense [9–11]. A systematic review found that in postmenopausal overweight/obese women, PA plus a hypocaloric diet for 54 weeks reduced BMI and abdominal fat [12].

17.4 Bone Benefits

In postmenopausal women, PA has been shown to have a beneficial effect on bone metabolism, both by preventing the loss of bone mass and by improving balance and reducing the risk of falls. A meta-analysis of 22 cohort studies with a total of 14,843 fractures showed a reduced risk of fractures in 29% of subjects [13]. Other meta-analyses found similar results and suggested that the fracture prevention benefits from PA result from the reduced risk of falls [14, 15].

Some studies have examined the most appropriate type of PA considering such factors as intensity, duration, and permanency. The most effective types of PA were those that combine resistance exercises (squats and push-ups), direct impact on the lower limbs (such as jumping and running), and light loads (weights) and possibly mechanical vibration. However, a recent meta-analysis found that only combined resistance exercise protocols had protective effects on bone mineral density (BMD) in postmenopausal women, whereas resistance-alone protocols produced a nonsignificant positive effect. Combined resistance training protocols were defined as the combination of resistance training and high-impact or weight-bearing exercise [16].

In comparison, PA such as swimming and cycling is performed under microgravity conditions. Studies have shown that the BMD of subjects who perform these types of PA is similar to that of a sedentary population and inferior to that achieved with PA that includes impact [17, 18]. In addition, walking, which is likely the PA that most menopausal women prefer, has shown an insufficient protective effect on BMD, even in the long term [19].

17.5 Sarcopenia

Sarcopenia is the progressive and generalized loss of muscle mass and strength. It is very common in older people, especially in postmenopausal women, and is related to the loss of oestrogen and testosterone. Recent studies have found that sarcopenia is closely related to osteoporosis and balance disturbances and that it increases the risk of falls and bone fractures. Sarcopenia is also secondary to inadequate protein intake or physical inactivity after dieting. Although it is a sign of ageing, sarcopenia by itself increases the risk of physical disability, decreases physical function, and results in a poor QoL.

PA is probably the best strategy for preventing and treating sarcopenia and balance disturbances. PA that combines strength and balance (e.g., Pilates) can improve postural muscle mass and tone. Other activities, such as Tai-chi, have also been shown to be effective for increasing muscle mass and improving strength.

It is estimated that the prevalence of sarcopenia in postmenopausal women is 10–40% [20], and although it can result from other causes, one of the principal factors in sarcopenia is hypoestrogenism [21]. During menopause, women experience a deterioration of balance that is related to android-type fat distribution, low BMD, and falls [22].

In addition to its effects on bone health, PA is a principal strategy for preventing and treating sarcopenia. Progressive resistance exercise (PRE) training programmes increase muscle mass and function; improve flexibility, balance, and physical function; and correct disability [23, 24]. Although it has not shown clear effects as the only strategy for improving balance and reducing the risk of falls, PA is successful when combined with balance-training programmes or aerobic exercise [25].

Exercise programmes based on virtual reality, which are alternatives to conventional activities, have been associated with improved postural control in older individuals [26].

Other recently popularized types of PA (e.g., Pilates) also show benefits for improving balance and preventing falls [27]. Step training and whole-body vibration training can improve function and restore balance, but not strength, in older individuals [28]. Recently, exercises that incorporate electrical muscle stimulation, increased muscle mass, and maximal isometric strength have also shown this benefit [29].

17.6 Quality of Life

Health-related QoL is defined as the perception of aspects of life that are most likely affected by changes in health status. It covers aspects such as health, physical, and emotional functioning and limitations in performing different roles in everyday life and social functioning. A variety of instruments and scales have been used to assess QoL, although not all of them are applicable to specific populations (female sex, menopause status) and personal characteristics. Therefore, specific tools are needed for each condition, and in addition to being sensitive to physical changes, they must also evaluate psychological, social, and sexual well-being. The Spanish Menopause Society recommends and prioritizes the use of the Cervantes Scale [30].

The main complaints of postmenopausal women are vasomotor symptoms, especially hot flashes. Although there is disparity in results when only changes in hot flashes are rated, PA can affect hot flashes if other symptoms are reduced and the QoL is improved.

Insomnia is another symptom experienced by postmenopausal women. PA increases the production of melatonin, a hormone associated with wakefulness-sleep, thus allowing a better night's sleep. Menopause also affects mood because it is a new stage with many changes that are not always welcome; PA releases endorphins, which improve mood. Within the psychosocial sphere, PA improves anxiety, depression, and sleep quality [31, 32].

PA reduces weight and the consequences of obesity (aesthetic, medical, mental) associated with menopausal symptoms. In addition, PA improves the pain of fibromyalgia, joint diseases, and even some cancers, such as breast cancer. In breast cancer patients, PA improves pain, QoL, and mood, allowing the patient to face the disease with greater hope, which results in improved adherence to treatment. In addition to being an RF for other diseases, weight gain worsens the QoL of postmenopausal women; however, it is unclear whether this is because of the weight gain alone or the existence of comorbidities (hot flashes, urinary incontinence, anxiety, and depressed mood) [33] or social pressures to meet the feminine-body cultural beauty cannons.

17.7 Cognitive and Neurodegeneration Protection

PA is inversely related to the risk of dementia, and it improves cognitive functioning to a higher degree in middle-aged women than in men of the same age. A systematic review describes a reduction in the risk of developing Alzheimer's disease when PA is continuous and intense [34]. In addition, beneficial effects have been reported in patients with neurodegeneration and dementia with respect to anxiety, depression, sleep quality, and general well-being [35].

17.8 Pain During Menopause

There are many diseases that cause pain, and pain becomes more pronounced with age and is more common in women (e.g., osteoarticular pain and fibromyalgia). PA plus weight loss improves pain along with other health indicators and associated symptoms. In women with fibromyalgia, PA improves general health, physical status, and the perception of pain [36]. PA did not reduce pain in breast cancer patients who underwent surgery, but it did improve the well-being of these patients by reducing fatigue, depression, mobility, and postsurgical lymphoedema. Furthermore, exercise alleviates joint pain derived from the use of aromatase inhibitors [37, 38].

PA also improves gynaecological pain. For example, the combination of pelvic floor exercises and local oestrogen was associated with a reduction in dyspareunia [39]. Nevertheless, PA was not sufficient for treating vaginismus, which required desensitization techniques and cognitive-behavioural therapy to achieve relief [40].

17.9 Requirements

Generally, everyone should include PA in their daily activities. However, although it could be considered a form of therapy because of its multiple benefits, there are contraindications for its implementation. In postmenopausal women, the requirements for practicing PA do not differ from those for other healthy adults of the same age and either sex. In any case, before starting PA, cardiovascular RFs should be evaluated, along with personal and family antecedents of cardiorespiratory and metabolic diseases. The type of PA prescribed will depend on the individual's general status of health and level of physical fitness. Regardless, a medical history must be completed that indicates the presence of RFs (smoking, hypercholesterolemia, diabetes, sedentary lifestyle, and arterial hypertension) and existing symptoms (dizziness, syncope, chest pain, dyspnoea, palpitations) [41].

The PA level in daily life can be used to classify women into distinct groups (sedentary, insufficiently active, active and very active) and permits stratification by variables that predict performance and mortality; such classifications will determine the prescription and monitoring of PA to ensure that the woman can perform it safely.

Other tests may be necessary to determine the appropriate type of PA for an individual. We recommend following the indications of the Spanish Society of Cardiology and the American Heart Association (AHA) [42, 43]:

- For mild-moderate PA, no special proof is required, unless some of the above factors are present; if they are, a medical assessment will be necessary.
- For intense PA, more specific studies are needed (a baseline ECG for women over 50 years old and a stress test) to prevent serious complications, such as sudden death during exercise. In these cases, the medical history should emphasize the symptoms that occurred during previous PA (such as syncope or angina) [44]. The most frequently used test to assess the cardiovascular risks associated with PA in postmenopausal women is the ergometer or stress test. It is sensitive as a diagnostic test because of the higher prevalence of silent ischaemic cardiopathy in women than in men of the same age [45].

Notwithstanding the above, recommended levels of PA and exercise for peri- and postmenopausal women are similar to international guidelines for adults [46]. Although any type of PA is welcome for postmenopausal women, the most highly recommended type of PA at this stage is probably a combination of HIIT with short recovery periods and exercises that promote the improvement of balance, such as Pilates [47–49]. These activities yield fat loss and muscle gain in less time than conventional PA practiced alone (running, swimming, cycling). They have the benefit of closely resembling daily activities and may have better adherence among users. Other types of PA, such as Tai-chi and yoga, have also been proven to be helpful, although not all of them provide all the benefits of HIIT [50–52].

Additionally, as initiation and maintenance of health-related lifestyle changes are challenging, and most adults find it extremely difficult to be adherent to recommended healthy behaviours after clinicians' advice, alliances between healthcare providers such as gynaecologists and exercise and sports experts including sport medicine professionals and behavioural sciences experts particularly health psychologists may improve a woman's skills for self-regulation and lifestyle modifications success [53]. By identifying behavioural determinants of health and well-being, such as adopting an active lifestyle, and the psychosocial processes involved in health-related behavioural changes and long-term adherence, effective interventions can be developed involving the most successful behavioural modification theories and behaviour change techniques to increase health, quality of life, and longevity. This collaborative work can address the main factors affecting middle-aged women's active behaviour at each stage of the change process, including perceived barriers, expected benefits, motivation, self-confidence, and self-regulation resources, among others. This approach should also consider the interactive influences of psychosocial, sociocultural, and biomedical factors and processes that influence the initiation and adherence to active behaviour. Thus, health psychologists can effectively support women in self-managing the entire behavioural change process. These interventions can also be tailored to be sensitive to the unique experiences, needs, desires, and opportunities of women during this life stage, enabling them to navigate the behaviour change process more successfully while empowering their sense of agency over their behaviour, identity, well-being, and ageing [54].

Below, we summarize the recommendations of the Spanish Menopause Society on benefits of PA in postmenopausal women:

- PA produces cardiovascular and metabolic benefits in postmenopausal women. These benefits are manifested in the early months of practice. To maintain the benefits of PA, it must be continued and adapted to the individual's physical condition, medication use, and other lifestyle factors. PA should always be supervised and should be varied to improve adherence.
- PA has proven to be beneficial for preventing and treating osteoporosis, sarcopenia, and balance disorders and reducing the risk of falls and their complications.
- Although exercise does not seem to lead to a significant reduction in vasomotor symptoms, the evidence does indicate that it improves quality of life, especially when associated with other psychosocial interventions.
- PA has a moderate efficacy for reducing pain postmenopausal women, but its effectiveness increases if it is associated with education, nutrition, and physical therapy.
- The recommendations regarding the practice of PA should be extended to all postmenopausal women in any condition. If moderate- or high-intensity PA is prescribed, cardiovascular, metabolic, and bone RFs should be determined using anthropometric, bone, ECG, and stress tests.
- PA that combines HIIT and Pilates seems to be the most appropriate type for postmenopausal women.

17.10 Conclusions

In general, PA is recommended for health promotion for any woman, regardless of her age and condition, and has shown benefits at many levels (cardiovascular, bone, muscular, metabolic, QoL, mental well-being, etc.). In addition, adherence to PA is an excellent way to treat some of the ailments that become more prevalent in postmenopausal women.

Acknowledgements This chapter has been translated and edited by American Journal Experts.

References

1. Lin X, Zhang X, Guo J, Roberts CK, McKenzie S, Wu WC, Liu X, Song Y. Effects of exercise training on cardiorespiratory fitness and biomarkers of cardiometabolic health: a systematic review and meta-analysis of randomized controlled trials. J Am Heart Assoc. 2015;4:e002014.
2. Pedersen BK, Saltin B. Exercise as medicine—evidence for prescribing exercise as therapy in 26 different chronic diseases. Scand J Med Sci Sports. 2015;25(Suppl 3):1–72.
3. Spanish Association for the Study of Menopause (AEEM). Menoguía: physical exercise in postmenopausal [Internet]. Madrid: AEEM; 2021 [cited 2024 Jun 17]. https://www.aeem.es/menoguia-physical exercise in postmenopausal women.
4. Grindler NM, Santoro NF. Menopause and exercise. Menopause. 2015;22:1351–8.
5. Klonizakis M, Moss J, Gilbert S, Broom D, Foster J, Tew GA. Low-volume high-intensity interval training rapidly improves cardiopulmonary function in postmenopausal women. Menopause. 2014;21:1099–05.
6. Matsubara T, Miyaki A, Akazawa N, Choi Y, Ra SG, Tanahashi K, Kumagai H, Oikawa S, Maeda S. Aerobic exercise training increases plasma klotho levels and reduces arterial stiffness in postmenopausal women. Am J Physiol Heart Circ Physiol. 2014;306:H348–55.
7. Tanahashi K, Akazawa N, Miyaki A, Choi Y, Ra SG, Matsubara T, Kumagai H, Oikawa S, Maeda S. Aerobic exercise training decreases plasma asymmetric dimethylarginine concentrations with increase in arterial compliance in post-menopausal women. Am J Hypertens. 2014;27(3):415–21.
8. Glouzon BK, Barsalani R, Lagacé JC, Dionne IJ. Muscle mass and insulin sensitivity in postmenopausal women after 6-month exercise training. Climacteric. 2015;18:846–51.
9. Zhang J, Chen G, Lu W, et al. The effect of physical exercise on health-related quality of life and blood lipids in perimenopausal women: a randomized, placebo-controlled trial. Menopause. 2014;21(12):1269–76.
10. Moreau KL, Deane KD, Meditz AL, Kohrt WM. Tumor necrosis factor-α inhibition improves endothelial function and decreases arterial stiffness in estrogen-deficient postmenopausal women. Atherosclerosis. 2013;230(2):390–6.
11. Walker AE, Kaplon RE, Pierce GL, Nowlan MJ, Seals DR. Prevention of age-related endothelial dysfunction by habitual aerobic exercise in healthy humans: possible role of nuclear factor-κB. Clin Sci (Lond). 2014;127(11):645–54.
12. Jull J, Stacey D, Beach S, Dumas A, Strychar I, Ufholz LA, Prince S, Abdulnour J, Prud'homme D. Lifestyle interventions targeting body weight changes during the menopause transition: a systematic review. J Obes. 2014;2014:824310.
13. Qu X, Zhang X, Zhai Z, Li H, Liu X, Li H, Liu G, Zhu Z, Hao Y, Dai K. Association between physical activity and risk of fracture. J Bone Miner Res. 2014;29:202–11.
14. Kemmler W, Häberle L, von Stengel S. Effects of exercise on fracture reduction in older adults: a systematic review and meta-analysis. Osteoporos Int. 2013;24:1937–50.
15. Silva RB, Eslick GD, Duque G. Exercise for falls and fracture prevention in long-term care facilities: a systematic review and meta-analysis. J Am Med Dir Assoc. 2013;14:685–9.
16. Zhao R, Zhao M, Xu Z. The effects of differing resistance training modes on the preservation of bone mineral density in postmenopausal women: a meta-analysis. Osteoporos Int. 2015;26:1605–18.
17. Okubo Y, Schoene D, Lord SR. Step training improves reaction time, gait and balance and reduces falls in older people: a systematic review and meta-analysis. Br J Sports Med. 2017;51(7):586–93.
18. Abrahin O, Rodrigues RP, Marçal AC, Alves EAC, Figueiredo RC, Sousa ECD. Swimming and cycling do not cause positive effects on bone mineral density: a systematic review. Rev Bras Reumatol. 2016;56:345–51.

19. Sydora BC, Turner C, Malley A, Davenport M, Yuksel N, Shandro T, Ross S. Can walking exercise programs improve health for women in menopause transition and postmenopausal? Findings from a scoping review. Menopause. 2020;27(8):952–63.
20. Yuan S, Larsson SC. Epidemiology of sarcopenia: prevalence, risk factors, and consequences. Metabolism. 2023;144:155533.
21. Smith-Ryan AE, Hirsch KR, Cabre HE, Gould LM, Gordon AN, Ferrando AA. Menopause transition-a cross-sectional evaluation on muscle size and quality. Med Sci Sports Exerc. 2023;55(7):1258–64.
22. Hita-Contreras F, Martínez-Amat A, Lomas-Vega R, Álvarez P, Mendoza N, Romero-Franco N, Aránega A. Relationship of body mass index and body fat distribution with postural balance and risk of falls in Spanish postmenopausal women. Menopause. 2013;20:202–8.
23. Sá KMM, da Silva GR, Martins UK, Colovati MES, Crizol GR, Riera R, et al. Resistance training for postmenopausal women: systematic review and meta-analysis. Menopause. 2023;30(1):108–16.
24. Forte R, De Vito G. Comparison of neuromotor and progressive resistance exercise training to improve mobility and fitness in community-dwelling older women. J Sci Sport Exerc. 2019;1:124–31.
25. Anek A, Bunyaratavej N. Effects of circuit aerobic step exercise program on musculoskeletal for prevention of falling and enhancement of postural balance in postmenopausal women. J Med Assoc Thail. 2015;98(Suppl 8):S88–94.
26. Laufer Y, Dar G, Kodesh E. Does a Wii-based exercise program enhance balance control of independently functioning older adults? A systematic review. Clin Interv Aging. 2014;23(9):1803–13.
27. Cruz-Díaz D, Martínez-Amat A, De la Torre-Cruz MJ, Casuso RA, de Guevara NM, Hita-Contreras F. Effects of a six-week Pilates intervention on balance and fear of falling in women aged over 65 with chronic low-back pain: a randomized controlled trial. Maturitas. 2015;82(4):371–6.
28. Marin-Cascales E, Alcaraz PE, Ramos-Campo DJ, Martinez-Rodriguez A, Chung LH, Rubio-Arias JA. Whole-body vibration training and bone health in postmenopausal women: a systematic review and meta-analysis. Medicine. 2018;97(34):e11918.
29. Kemmler W, Bebenek M, Engelke K, von Stengel S. Impact of whole-body electromyostimulation on body composition in elderly women at risk for sarcopenia: the training and ElectroStimulation trial (TEST-III). Age (Dordr). 2014;36:395–406.
30. Coronado PJ, Sánchez-Borrego R, Ruiz MA, Baquedano L, Sánchez S, Argudo C, Fernández-Abellán M, González S, Iglesias E, Calleja J, Presa J, Duque A, Ruiz F, Otero B, Rejas J. Psychometric attributes of the Cervantes short-form questionnaire for measuring health-related quality of life in menopausal women. Maturitas. 2016;84:55–62.
31. Fausto DY, Leitão AE, Silveira J, Martins JB, Dominski FH, Guimarães AC. An umbrella systematic review of the effect of physical exercise on mental health of women in menopause. Menopause. 2023;30(2):225–34.
32. Zhang Z, Zhao M. Comparison of physical exercise and psychological intervention in the healthcare of menopausal women. Int J Healthc Inf Syst Inform. 2023;18(1):1–9.
33. Blümel JE, Chedraui P, Aedo S. Obesity and its relation to depressive symptoms and sedentary lifestyle in middle-aged women. Maturitas. 2015;80:100–5.
34. Marques-Aleixo I, Beleza J, Sampaio A, Stevanović J, Coxito P, Gonçalves I, Ascensão A, Magalhães J. Preventive and therapeutic potential of physical exercise in neurodegenerative diseases. Antioxid Redox Signal. 2021;34(8):674–93.
35. Demurtas J, Schoene D, Torbahn G, Marengoni A, Grande G, Zou L, et al. Physical activity and exercise in mild cognitive impairment and dementia: an umbrella review of intervention and observational studies. J Am Med Dir Assoc. 2020;21(10):1415–22.
36. Sañudo B, Carrasco L, de Hoyo M, Figueroa A, Saxton JM. Vagal modulation and symptomatology following a 6-month aerobic exercise program for women with fibromyalgia. Clin Exp Rheumatol. 2015;33(1 Suppl 88):S41–5.

37. De Groef A, Van Kampen M, Dieltjens E, Christiaens MR, Neven P, Geraerts I, Devoogdt N. Effectiveness of postoperative physical therapy for upper-limb impairments after breast cancer treatment: a systematic review. Arch Phys Med Rehabil. 2015;96:1140–53.
38. Irwin ML, Cartmel B, Gross CP, Ercolano E, Li F, Yao X, Fiellin M, Capozza S, Rothbard M, Zhou Y, Harrigan M, Sanft T, Schmitz K, Neogi T, Hershman D, Ligibel J. Randomized exercise trial of aromatase inhibitor-induced arthralgia in breast cancer survivors. J Clin Oncol. 2015;33:1104–11.
39. Fausto DY, Martins JBB, Moratelli JA, Lima AG, Guimarães ACDA. The effect of body practices and physical exercise on sexual function of menopausal women. A systematic review with meta-analysis. Int J Sex Health. 2023;35(3):414–26.
40. Goldfinger C, Pukall CF, Thibault-Gagnon S, McLean L, Chamberlain S. Effectiveness of cognitive-behavioral therapy and physical therapy for provoked vestibulodynia: a randomized pilot study. J Sex Med. 2016;13:88–94.
41. Kohli P, Gulati M. Exercise stress testing in women: going back to the basics. Circulation. 2010;122:2570–80.
42. Barbat-Artigas S, Filion ME, Dupontgand S, Karelis AD, Aubertin-Leheudre M. Effects of tai chi training in dynapenic and nondynapenic postmenopausal women. Menopause. 2011;18:974–9.
43. Soria-Gila MA, Chirosa IJ, Bautista IJ, Baena S, Chirosa LJ. Effects of variable resistance training on maximal strength: a meta-analysis. J Strength Cond Res. 2015;29:3260–70.
44. Rikkonen T, Sund R, Koivumaa-Honkanen H, Sirola J, Honkanen R, Kröger H. Effectiveness of exercise on fall prevention in community-dwelling older adults: a 2-year randomized controlled study of 914 women. Age Ageing. 2023;52(4):afad059. https://doi.org/10.1093/ageing/afad059.
45. Troiano RP, Stamatakis E, Bull FC. How can global physical activity surveillance adapt to evolving physical activity guidelines? Needs, challenges and future directions. Br J Sports Med. 2020;54(24):1468–73.
46. Dupuit M, Maillard F, Pereira B, Marquezi ML, Lancha AH Jr, Boisseau N. Effect of high intensity interval training on body composition in women before and after menopause: a meta-analysis. Exp Physiol. 2020;105(9):1470–90.
47. Lindner R, Raj IS, Yang AWH, Zaman S, Larsen B, Denham J. Moderate to vigorous-intensity continuous training versus high-intensity interval training for improving VO2max in women: a systematic review and meta-analysis. Int J Sports Med. 2023;44(7):484–95.
48. de Sousa AG, Júnior EDLC, da Costa NF, de Araújo RJ, Ribeiro APL, Filgueiras LA. The influence of the Pilates method on postmenopausal women: literature review. Health Biosci. 2022;3(1):44–58.
49. Parveen A, Kalra S, Jain S. Effects of Pilates on health and Well-being of women: a systematic review. Bull Fac Phys Ther. 2023;28(1):1–12.
50. Shepherd-Banigan M, Goldstein KM, Coeytaux RR, McDuffie JR, Goode AP, Kosinski AS, Van Noord MG, Befus D, Adam S, Masilamani V, Nagi A, Williams JW Jr. Improving vasomotor symptoms; psychological symptoms; and health-related quality of life in peri-or post-menopausal women through yoga: an umbrella systematic review and meta-analysis. Complement Ther Med. 2017;34:156–64.
51. Sharifi N, Afshari F, Bahri N. The effects of yoga on quality of life among postmenopausal women: a systematic review study. Post Reprod Health. 2021;27(4):215–21.
52. Wang Y, Shan W, Li Q, Yang N, Shan W. Tai chi exercise for the quality of life in a perimenopausal women organization: a systematic review. Worldviews Evid-Based Nurs. 2017;14(4):294–305.
53. Liu F, Wang S. Effect of tai chi on bone mineral density in postmenopausal women: a systematic review and meta-analysis of randomized control trials. J Chin Med Assoc. 2017;80(12):790–5.
54. Godoy-Izquierdo D, de Teresa C, Mendoza N. Exercise for peri-and postmenopausal women: some recommendations from synergistic alliances of Women's medicine and Health Psychology for the promotion of an active lifestyle. Maturitas. 2024;185:107924.

Nutritional Management of Menopausal Women

18

Annamaria Colao and Roberta Scairati

Abstract

The term "menopause" comes from the ancient Greek words "meno" (month) and "pause" (stop), and thus, it indicates literally the date of last menstrual bleeding due to decreased estrogen levels and loss of ovulation. Natural menopause is defined by the absence of menses for 12 consecutive months, typically occurring between the late 30 s and late 50 s, with most women entering this phase between ages 48 and 55 years (Wylie-Rosett J., Am J Clin Nutr 81:1223S–31S, 2005). The most common symptoms of menopause are hot flashes or flushes, night sweats, and sleep disturbances reported by 60%, 48%, and 41% of the women, respectively (Keenan et al., Menopause 10:507–15, 2003). Women undergoing hysterectomy and ovariectomy experience surgical menopause often associated with rapid onset of vasomotor symptoms. Chemotherapy and radiation for cancer can also induce a rapid onset of menopausal symptoms: approximately 30% of women under 35 years of age experience ovarian failure after chemotherapy with increase in the proportion of ovarian failure related to the age of chemotherapy up to 75–90% for women over 40 years of age (Overlie et al., Maturitas 41:69–77, 2002). Indeed, the risk of premature menopause is strongly influenced by both age at the time of chemotherapy and the cumulative dose administered. Treatment of menopausal symptoms in this group is a more difficult complex because of concomitant treatments for cancer and the associated risk related to cancer as well as the abrupt onset of symptoms. Nutrition plays an essential role in menopausal women both in limiting clinical complaints, such as vasomotor symptoms and hair loss, and in preventing more serious diseases such osteoporosis (discussed in other chapters of this book) and overweight/obesity.

A. Colao (✉) · R. Scairati
Department of Clinical Medicine and Surgery, Unit of Endocrinology, Diabetology, Andrology and Nutrition; "Federico II" University of Naples, Naples, Italy
e-mail: colao@unina.it

18.1 Introduction

The term "menopause" comes from the ancient Greek words "meno" (month) and "pause" (stop), and thus, it indicates literally the date of last menstrual bleeding due to decreased estrogen levels and loss of ovulation. Natural menopause is defined by the absence of menses for 12 consecutive months, typically occurring between the late 30 s and late 50 s, with most women entering this phase between ages 48 and 55 years [1]. The most common symptoms of menopause are hot flashes or flushes, night sweats, and sleep disturbances as reported by 60%, 48%, and 41% of women, respectively [2]. Women undergoing hysterectomy and ovariectomy experience surgical menopause often associated with quick onset of vasomotor symptoms. Chemotherapy and radiation for cancer can also induce a rapid onset of menopausal symptoms due to ovarian failure, defined either as the absence of regular menses in premenopausal women or as FSH levels increased (> 40 IU/L) [3]. Approximately 30% of women under 35 years of age experience ovarian failure after chemotherapy with increase in the proportion of ovarian failure related to the age of chemotherapy up to 75–90% for women over 40 years of age [4]. Indeed, the risk of premature menopause is strongly influenced by both age at the time of chemotherapy and the cumulative dose administered. Treatment of menopausal symptoms in this group is a more difficult complex because of concomitant treatments for cancer and the associated risk related to cancer as well as the abrupt onset of symptoms.

Together with the specific symptoms of ovarian failure, there are relevant changes in body composition evolving naturally with aging. As reported by Munro [4] in a men-only population, the muscle mass of a 20 years of age was 50% greater than fat mass; in 40 s, muscle mass was virtually identical to fat mass, while in 60 s and over, data of muscle and fat mass was virtually the opposite of the values recorded in 20 years of age. In woman population, aging causes similar changes in the body composition particularly at the time of menopause: body weight and total body fat increase, with a concurrent decrease in fat-free mass [5].

The reported changes in the body composition have relevant clinical consequences.

The Study of Women's Health Across the Nation (SWAN) has significantly added to our understanding of changes in women's bone health over the menopause transition [6]. Among the most important effects which substantially vary across race/ethnicity groups, the progressive decrease in bone mass produces loss of height, changes in posture, and osteoporotic fractures [7]. Low-trauma fractures of the hip, the major cause of physical disability, and early mortality are more common in White women than in Asian, Black, and Hispanic women.

Modifications of the spine cause alteration of the chest cage such as restriction and distortion, compromising pulmonary vital capacity and maximal breathing capacity [8]. Since overall skeletal mobility is impaired, all basic daily movements are limited; thus, daily energy expenditure is reduced. Moreover, the progressive loss of muscle mass and increase in fat tissue produce a progressive decrease of caloric requirements for weight maintenance with aging.

The decrease in metabolic rate with aging is largely attributable to these changes in body composition [9]. However, some other alterations also contribute to a fall in energy expenditure. The thyroid function also falls with aging [10]: thyroid-stimulating hormone and free triiodothyronine levels tend to reduce in elderly persons, even healthy elderly. This decline might contribute to the reduction in metabolic rate with aging, even if the magnitude hormonal decrement is probably too small to have a major effect on metabolic rate. The decrease in resting metabolic rate of aged subjects may be partly due also to a decrease in energy expenditure that occurs progressively throughout adult life from 20 to 100 years of age [11].

A body of evidence now clearly shows that reduced life expectancy in elderly individuals is associated with either major weight gain or major weight loss. In fact, many studies reported that mortality rates are a function of weight changes, exhibiting a U-shaped relation [12]: stable obesity across adulthood, weight gain from young to middle adulthood, and weight loss from middle to late adulthood were associated with increased risks of mortality. As known, obesity has a striking effect on mortality and morbidity by inducing diabetes, hypertension, cardiovascular disease, and certain forms of cancer among adults with a mean age of 60 years [13].

On the other hand, it is increasingly appreciated that losing weight is not necessarily indicative of gaining good health [14]. Elderly individuals may be losing weight because of progressive or preexisting disease. In fact, before death, many elderly persons tend to lose weight, and weight loss may be related to frailty rather than of good health, and so it greatly increases the risk of osteoporosis and fracture [15].

This chapter focuses on the nutritional management of menopause symptoms and on management of overweight/obesity that are considered the major problems of postmenopausal women. We do not consider the nutritional management of osteoporosis, that is, object of other chapter of this book.

18.2   Nutrition and Menopausal Symptoms

Considered as the most evident and complained symptom of menopause, hot flashes are caused by dysfunction of the central thermoregulatory system when estrogen concentration is decreased. The central pathways of norepinephrine and serotonin likely lower the set point for the thermoregulatory nucleus, which allows heat loss to be regulated by a subtle change in core temperature [1]. Endorphins and catechol estrogen, derivatives of estrogen, and other sex hormones are considered to contraregulate the elevation in core temperature induced by norepinephrine and serotonin. Micronutrients, phytochemicals, and herbal supplements commonly used to treat menopausal symptoms include vitamin E, black cohosh (*Actaea racemosa*), and soy (and other phytoestrogens), which are used to treat the vasomotor symptoms; ginkgo biloba, ginseng, and St. John's wort (*Hypericum perforatum*), which are used for mood-related symptoms; and valerian which has been used for sleep disturbances associated with menopause. Interpretation of study findings using these compounds is hampered by the small sample size, variability in the product tested (especially

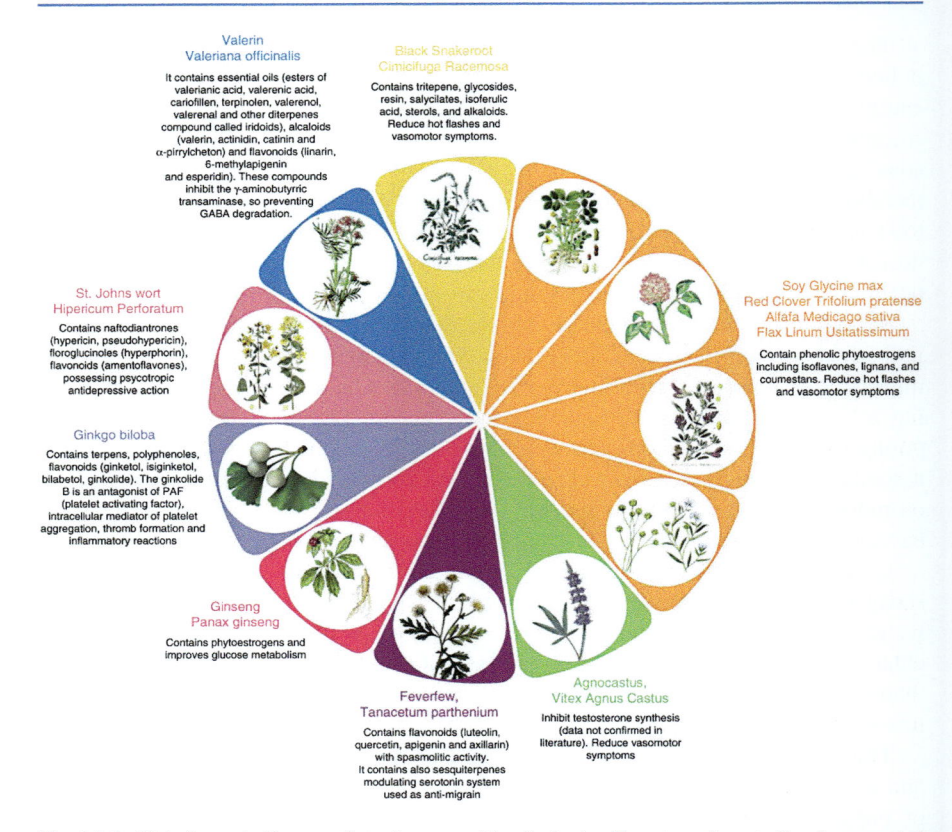

Fig. 18.1 This figure indicates a list of women-friendly herbs. To note, a few studies documented the detailed effects in postmenopausal women, while many herbal integrations come from an ancient tradition in many different population

for the soy), and wide variability in the clinical characteristics of the study population. A list of women-friendly herbs is illustrated in Fig. 18.1. Research that focuses on micronutrient and related treatments is likely to increase to provide an evidence-based document to address questions posed by menopausal women and their care providers.

18.2.1 Vitamin E

Although vitamin E is widely used for treating hot flashes, the research database is extremely limited [16]. Barton et al. [17] in a randomized crossover trial (4 weeks per treatment condition) conducted in 120 women treated for breast cancer found that vitamin E (800 IU) resulted only in 1 fewer hot flash per day than the placebo. Whether these findings can be generalized to women undergoing naturally occurring or surgical menopause remains to be determined. A randomized controlled trial carried out on 52 postmenopausal women aged 40–65 compared the effect of a vitamin E vaginal suppository with that of conjugated estrogen vaginal cream on genitourinary syndrome of menopause. The improvement in Abbreviated Sexual Function Questionnaire (ASFQ) scores after the 12th week showed that vitamin E vaginal suppository could be an alternative to vaginal estrogen to relieve symptoms of vaginal atrophy in postmenopausal women, especially if hormonal therapy is contraindicated [18]. A recent systematic review including 16 quality studies aimed to investigate the role of vitamin E in relieving hot flashes, vascular modulation, plasma lipid profile levels, and vaginal health. Compared to vitamin E, estrogen administration leads to better clinical effects, but further controlled studies are needed to draw firm conclusions [19].

Controlled studies are needed to assess the effects of vitamin E on symptoms using one of the standardized menopausal symptom questionnaires and on hormones affected by menopause. Research also needs to specifically address how vitamin E affects the metabolic pathways involved in the hot flash reaction. Vitamin E concentration is high in fresh virgin olive oil.

18.2.2 Black Cohosh (*Cimicifuga racemosa*, Black Snakeroot)

Black cohosh, botanically a member of the buttercup family, has been widely used by Native Americans as therapy for a variety of problems including dysmenorrhea, labor pains, and menopausal symptoms [1]. It has been difficult to discern the effects of black cohosh despite the availability of a standardized formulation and reported findings from 3 of 4 randomized trials indicating a reduction in menopausal symptoms [20, 21]. Black cohosh contains a number of compounds with potential bioactivity including triterpene, glycosides, resin, salicylates, isoferulic acid, sterols, and alkaloids. The analysis of black cohosh from various woodlands in the Eastern USA and Remifemin did not find any formononetin inside, the phytoestrogen thought to account for the reported reduction in menopausal symptoms [20, 21], and thus the mechanism of action of black cohosh in reducing hot flashes is still not completely understood. Black cohosh does not modify the hormonal pattern associated with menopause, low estrogen accompanied by elevated luteinizing hormone and follicle-stimulating hormone. Additional rigorously controlled studies are needed to ascertain the true effects of black cohosh on menopausal symptoms and to make an evidenced-based decision regarding who may benefit and for whom its use the risks are likely to outweigh any potential benefits [21].

18.2.3 Phytoestrogens from Soy, Red Clover, and Flax

The phytoestrogens that have been isolated from a variety of plant food are phenolic (rather than steroidal) compounds, structurally or functionally similar to estradiol (E2); the major categories of phytoestrogens include isoflavones, lignans, and coumestans [22]. Phytoestrogens function as selective estrogen receptor modulators

(SERMs) as they bind to receptors for estrogen metabolites. SERMs may function as estrogen metabolites in some tissues but not in others. SERMs developed in laboratory are widely used to treat women with estrogen receptor-positive cancers, while SERM function of phytoestrogens is much less understood. Soy, other beans, red clover (*Trifolium pratense*), and alfalfa (*Medicago sativa*) contain isoflavone precursors, which are converted to genistein, daidzein, and equol by intestinal bacteria. Flax seeds (*Linum usitatissimum*), other seeds, legumes, whole grains, and some fruits and vegetables (essential part of the Mediterranean diet) contain lignan precursors that can be converted to enterolactone and enterodiol by intestinal bacteria. The phytoestrogens can have estrogenic activity as potential dietary-derived modulators with endocrine function.

Unfortunately to date the studies addressing the use of phytoestrogens to improve vasomotor symptoms of menopause are small and lack of statistical power, and aggregation is not possible due to differences in their methodologies. In the systematic review by Kronenberg and Fugh-Berman [20], only 3 of the 12 randomized controlled trials found that soy phytoestrogen supplements or soy products reduced the frequency or severity of hot flashes. In one of the studies, the decrease in hot flashes was accompanied by increases in 17β-estradiol and decreases in total and LDL cholesterol [20]. Flax seeds have been reported to have estrogenic, antiestrogenic, and steroid-like activity [23].

Red clover contains the phytoestrogen formononetin, biochanin A, daidzein, and genistein, but the overall finding of research to date reports that red clover and its related supplements are not superior than placebo in controlling hot flashes.

The control of other symptoms of menopause from other micronutrients, phytochemicals, and herbal compounds is not supported by sufficient data. In a recent systematic review, Izzo et al. [24] reported preliminary or satisfactory clinical evidence for agno-castus (*Vitex agnus-castus*) for premenstrual complaints, flax seed for hypertension, feverfew (*Tanacetum parthenium*) for migraine prevention, ginseng (*Panax ginseng*) for improving fasting glucose levels, as well as phytoestrogens and St John's wort for the relief of some symptoms in menopause, but firm conclusions of efficacy cannot be generally drawn. In another cross-section of ethnically diverse women 40–55 years of age (35.5% African American, 60.2% Caucasian), Dailey et al. [25] documented that herbal product users reported more menopause symptoms than nonusers and 68% of the users said that the herbs improved their symptoms. Lastly, in a German revision of 22 studies by Aiselsburger et al. [26], high doses of isolated genistein were shown to reduce the frequency/intensity of hot flashes, while low doses of genistein show no significant effect. Furthermore, intake of isoflavone extract such as genistein, daidzein, and glycitein in various combinations did not have an effect on improvement of cognitive function or vaginal dryness [26]. The effect of black cohosh and hop extract for menopausal complaints cannot be determined since results are heterogenous [26]. The combination of isoflavone, black cohosh, agno-castus, valerian, and vitamin E had a positive effect on menopause symptoms. To date, the 2023 nonhormone therapy position statement from North American Menopause Society addressed alternatives to estrogen therapy [27]. The specific recommendations pointed first to lifestyle changes, while the administration of dietary supplements is complex and challenging because there is little data from randomized clinical trials from which to evaluate supplements and a lack of regulation to ensure their purity and safety. For moderate to severe menopause-related hot flashes, SSRIs and SNRIs, gabapentin, and fezolinetant can be used [27].

18.3 Nutrition and Hair Loss

Hair loss during the period of premenopause is physiological and is mainly due to estrogen reduction together with increase in androgen levels: hair loss appears as a spread thinning of hair mainly in the central and forehead part and sometimes also in the parietal and occipital part [28]. Nutrition is essential in keeping hair strength and density in menopausal age, through the following nutrients: standard value proteins containing sulfur amino acids, vitamin C, group B and A vitamins, and minerals such as Zn, Fe, Cu, Se, Si, Mg, and Ca [29].

18.3.1 Macronutrients: Proteins, Fat, and Carbohydrates

Fundamental elements of any diet for hair building include proteins containing sulfur amino acids such as cysteine and methionine which are precursors to keratin. Protein malnutrition impairs hair synthesis (hair fragility and brittleness) and strength (hair are in the form of lanugo) and causes hair loss [30]. Cysteine, as a keratin ingredient, occurs in hair in the highest amount (10–17%), and its synthesis depends on methionine presence. The hair growth rate, diameter, and keratin synthesis are related to cysteine concentration. The active form of pyridoxal phosphate (vitamin B6) increases L-cysteine incorporation to keratin, but other essential amino acids like L-lysine, mainly present in the inner part of hair root, are responsible for hair shape and volume. L-lysine has also a significant impact on zinc and iron absorption [31, 32].

Proteins should make 10–15% of energy value of the diet in the amount of 0.9 g/kg of body mass per day: the source of cysteine and L-lysine in diets is represented by cheese, yoghurt, fish, meat, poultry, legumes, seeds, nuts, grain products, and eggs.

Fats that participate in steroid hormones synthesis (from cholesterol) thus have influence on keeping hair in skin integument, but saturated fatty acids increase sebum secretion. The protective layer for skin integument and its products are ceramides, sterols, and phospholipids and also free fatty acids: thus, deficiency of these compounds in a women's body causes decrease in hair hydration, even to their loss as a result of improper state of the hair bulbs. In a diet, reduced amount of linoleic and linolenic acids and long-chain polyunsaturated fatty acids causes hair loss. Fatty acids from the omega-3 polyunsaturated fatty acids (EPA and DHA) family are found mainly in fish, flax seeds, walnuts, and wheat sprouts [29]. Omega-6 polyunsaturated fatty acids, present in plant oils, are also needed for a proper hair building, but their excess might lead to inflammation states, which in turn might cause hair asthenia and their loss [33]. Fats should constitute 25–35% energy value of the diet, and their source should be fish, poultry, eggs, olive oil, and rapeseed oil.

Carbohydrates also influence the state of hair: consumption of simple sugars stimulates sebum secretion by sebaceous glands, and sebum excess becomes food for microorganisms found on the skin, which cause decomposition of triacylglycerols contained inside [34]. Furthermore, excessive intake of simple sugars implies hyperglycemia and hyperinsulinemia, which contributes directly to increase synthesis of ovarian androgens and indirectly through suppression of sex hormone binding globulin synthesis in the liver and insulin-like growth factor 1. In hair follicles, insulin has a direct impact on hair growth, on increase of DHT concentration which leads to miniaturization [22], and also on local microcirculation nourishing the scalp, thus leading to local hypoxia which contributes to hair loss [35]. On this basis, a healthy diet should contain products rich in complex carbohydrates, with low glycemic index and load containing fiber-regulating carbohydrate-lipid metabolism of the body, as beautifully indicated in the scheme of the Mediterranean diet [36]. Carbohydrates should form 50–70% energy value of the diet from full grain breads, grits, rice, whole meal pasta, vegetables, and fruit with low glycemic load.

18.3.2 Micronutrients: Vitamins and Minerals

Vitamins have relevant impact on the state of hair, in particular, vitamins of group B, vitamin C, vitamin A, and vitamin D (Table 18.1).

Folates contribute to red blood cells and hemoglobin production and in oxygen transport to all organs and also to tissues building hair. The dietary source of folates is constituted by green vegetables and some fishes like halibut and cod but also in small amounts consumed eggs and poultry liver. The recommended dietary allowance of food folate is 400 μg daily for adults, which is supported by required fortification of some foods in the USA [45]. Pantothenic acid (vitamin B5) prevents early hair graying and can also restore their natural color, has anti-inflammatory properties, protects, has moisturizing abilities, regulates functioning of sebum glands, and accelerates melanin creating [29]. Products rich in B5 vitamin that is a mixture of pantothenic acid, pantein, panthenol, and coenzyme A are mushrooms, cauliflower, liver, soya, hen eggs, and baking yeast, whole grains, beans, milk, and green leafy vegetables [29]. Biotin (vitamin B7, vitamin H) is a vitamin taking part in fat and protein metabolism, and its deficiency might lead to hair loss; biotin deficiency induces increase in palmitic acid concentration in the liver and hypercholesterolemia, leading to erythematous and seborrheic skin inflammation (conjunctivitis, greasy hair, hair loss, and nails brittleness) [46]. Biotin can be found in cereal germs, milk and vegetables (free form), meat, liver, egg yolk, yeast, and some nuts (bound form). An adequate intake of biotin for adults is 30 μg/day in US populations [47]. Niacin (vitamin PP) detoxifies skin, and its main source is meat, whole wheat grains, legume vegetables, seeds, milk, green leafy vegetables, fish, peanuts, shellfish, and yeast.

Table 18.1 The vitamins helpful for hair and skin health in menopause

Tocopherol—Vitamin E

α-Tocopherol is the main source in the European diet (olive and sunflower oils), while γ-tocopherol is the main source in the American diet (soybean and corn oil). The recommended daily amount (RDA) is 15 mg/day. Low-fat diets can reduce its levels. Vitamin E is widely used as an inexpensive [37, 38] antioxidant in cosmetics and foods. It reduces vasomotor symptoms

Pantothenic acid—Vitamin B5

Vitamin B5 is found in whole unprocessed foods, in meat such as Turkey, tuna, liver, legumes (pulses or beans), whole grains, mushrooms, cauliflower, soya, and hen eggs. It is involved in the oxidation of fatty acids and carbohydrates. Coenzyme A, synthesized from pantothenic acid, is involved in the synthesis of amino acids, fatty acids, ketones, cholesterol, phospholipids, steroid hormones, neurotransmitters (such as acetylcholine), and antibodies [39]. It prevents early hair graying and can also restore their natural color, has anti-inflammatory properties, and regulates functioning of sebum glands and accelerates melanin creating. Its deficiency results in acne and paresthesia

Biotin—Vitamin B7

Biotin is found in cereal germs, milk, and vegetables (free form) and in meat, liver, egg yolk, yeast, and some nuts (bound form). It plays a key role in lipids, proteins, and carbohydrates metabolism. It is a critical coenzyme of four carboxylases: Acetyl CoA carboxylase, which is involved in the synthesis of fatty acids from acetate; pyruvate CoA carboxylase, involved in gluconeogenesis; β-methylcrotonyl CoA carboxylase, involved in the metabolism of leucine; and propionyl CoA carboxylase, which is involved in the metabolism of energy, amino acids, and cholesterol [40]. Biotin deficiency induces increase in palmitic acid concentration in liver and hypercholesterolemia, leading to erythematous and seborrheic skin inflammation (conjunctivitis, greasy hair, hair loss, and nails brittleness)

(continued)

Table 18.1 (continued)

Folic acid—Vitamin B9

The dietary source of folate is constituted by green vegetables and some fishes like halibut and cod but also in small amounts consumed eggs and poultry liver. Folic acid acts as a coenzyme in the form of tetrahydrofolate (THF), involved in pyrimidine nucleotide synthesis, so is needed for normal cell division, especially during pregnancy and infancy, which are times of rapid growth. Folate also contributes to production of red blood cells [41] and so in oxygen transport to all organs and also to tissues building hair

Nicotinamide—niacin—Vitamin PP

Vitamin PP is found in meat, whole wheat grains, legume vegetables, seeds, milk, green leafy vegetables, fish, peanuts, shellfish, and yeast. Nicotinamide in the form of a cream is used as a treatment for acne: It has anti-inflammatory actions and thus may be beneficial to people with inflammatory skin conditions. Nicotinamide increases the biosynthesis of ceramides in human keratinocytes in vitro and improves the epidermal permeability barrier in vivo. There is tentative evidence that it may reduce the risk of skin cancer and bullous pemphigoid [42]

Ascorbic acid—L-ascorbic acid—Vitamin C

Ascorbate and ascorbic acid are both naturally present in the body that increase absorption of non-heme iron, originating from plant products, and are found in vegetables (green parsley leaves, kale, horseradish, peppers, Brussels sprouts, broccoli, cauliflower, spinach, and savoy) and fruit (black currants, strawberries, wild strawberries, kiwi, red currants, and citrus fruit). Vitamin C is a cofactor of at least eight enzymatic reactions, including several collagen syntheses. Ascorbate also acts as an antioxidant, protecting against oxidative stress. Insufficient supply of vitamin C in diet influences the creation of the hair shaft and might be an indirect cause of telogenic baldness

Retinol–retinal–retinoic acid—Vitamin A

Retinol, the vitamin A form from animal food sources, is a yellow, fat-soluble substance. The carotenes alpha-carotene, beta-carotene, and gamma-carotene and the xanthophyll beta-cryptoxanthin serve as provitamin A in herbivore and omnivore animals, which possess the enzyme beta-carotene 15,15′-dioxygenase for cleaving beta-carotene in the intestinal mucosa and converting it into retinol. Vitamin A is found in many foods: High amount are present in cod liver oil, liver Turkey, beef, pork, and chicken and less in some vegetables such as red capsicum, sweet potatoes, carrots, broccoli, spinach, pumpkin, and cantaloupe melon. Vitamin A plays a role in a variety of functions throughout the body [43] such as vision, gene transcription, immune function, embryonic development and reproduction, and hematopoiesis. For menopausal women, vitamin A is relevant for bone metabolism, skin, and cellular health, and it is responsible for moisturizing and protecting hair, giving them resistance from being fragile, and thus its deficiency may cause decrease in cycle speed of cell regeneration

Calcitriol—Vitamin D

Vitamin D refers to a group of fat-soluble secosteroids involved in intestinal absorption of calcium, iron, magnesium, phosphate, and zinc. Vitamin D is present in very few foods such as fat fish (marcel, salmon, and sardines), whale, or tuna liver oil and in lower amounts in meat, poultry, eggs, and full fat diary. Consumption of mushrooms and yeast will additionally supply body in D2 (ergocalciferol). Vitamin D synthesis (specifically cholecalciferol) is in the skin. Dermal synthesis of vitamin D from cholesterol is dependent on sun exposure (specifically UVB radiation). In humans, the most important compounds in this group are vitamin D3 (also known as cholecalciferol) and vitamin D2 (ergocalciferol). Cholecalciferol and ergocalciferol can be ingested from the diet and from supplements. In the liver, cholecalciferol (vitamin D3) is converted to calcifediol. Ergocalciferol (vitamin D2)—Abbreviated 25(OH)D2). Part of the calcifediol is converted by the kidneys to calcitriol, the biologically active form of vitamin D. Calcitriol circulates as a hormone in the blood [44], regulating the concentration of calcium and phosphate in the bloodstream and promoting the healthy growth and remodeling of bone. Calcitriol also affects neuromuscular and immune function. Vitamin D promotes hair follicle differentiation, without affecting proliferation

Insufficient supply of vitamin C in diet influences the creation of the hair shaft and might be an indirect cause of telogenic baldness. However, no randomized controlled data correlated vitamin C levels and hair loss. Vitamin C increases absorption of non-heme iron, originating from plant products, and it is present in vegetables (green parsley leaves, kale, horseradish, peppers, Brussels sprouts, broccoli, cauliflower, spinach, and savoy) and fruit (black currants, strawberries, wild strawberries, kiwi, red currants, and citrus fruit).

Vitamin A is responsible for moisturizing and protects hair giving them resistance from being fragile, and thus its deficiency may cause decrease in cycle speed of cell regeneration. However, excess in vitamin A, coming from animal products cumulated in the liver, can also be a cause of hair loss, so a good source is its form derived from carotenoids present in vegetables and fruit [29]. The recommended dietary allowance of vitamin A for adults aged ≥19 years is 1300 µg/day (4300 IU) for US populations [48]. Finally, vitamin D promotes hair follicle differentiation, without affecting proliferation. Endogenous vitamin D synthesis starts in the skin (mainly in the prickle layer of epidermis) with 7-dehydrocholesterol under the influence of UVB (290–315 nm), subsequently undergoing two hydroxylations in the liver and in the kidney. The best source of D3 vitamin in women's diet should be fat fish (marcel, salmon, and sardines), whale or tuna liver oil, and also products containing lower amounts such as meat, poultry, eggs, and full fat diary. Consumption of mushrooms and yeast will additionally supply body in D2 (ergocalciferol). Overweight and obese women have low serum levels of calcitriol (the active form of vitamin D), and after the age of 70 s, it is reported a low synthesis of vitamin D from sun exposure [49]. In animal studies, the activation of VDR receptor was shown to play a significant role in the hair follicle cycle, especially in anagen initiation, and is independent of calcium and phosphorus content in diet [50].

Many minerals influence hair growth, namely, Zn, Fe, Cu, Se, Si, Mg, and Ca. Zinc takes part in carbohydrates, proteins, and fats metabolism and at the same time influences hair follicles and hair growth. Zinc also influences vitamin A keratinizing hair. Its deficiency in diet suppresses hair growth and can lead to telogen effluvium, thin white, and brittle hair and cause hair fall, especially in women using diuretic drugs [31]. Iron deficiency has been associated with hair loss as in alopecia areata, androgenetic alopecia, and telogen effluvium [50]. The best iron sources are animal products containing better assimilated heme iron (beef and pork, poultry, pork and lamb liver, and fish), but valuable diet variety are plant products such as soya, white beans, pasticcio nuts, green parsley leaves, dried apricots, and figs [29]. Copper is crucial for aminoxidases required for oxidation of thiol groups to dithio- cross-links and is essential for keratin fiber strength, has a stimulating effect on the proliferation of keratinocytes and fibroblasts in monolayers, has a vital role in the activation of key enzyme systems specific to tissue formation and repair, and participates in the cross-linking and maturation of collagen in healing wounds [51]. Copper is present in the same products as iron. Selenium is an essential component for antioxidant defense, formation of thyroid hormones, DNA synthesis, fertility, and reproduction, and it is a component of at least 35 proteins many of which are enzymes and with its deficiency in the body hair loss with pseudo albinism occurs [29]. Although much less common than selenium deficiency, selenium toxicity can affect individuals as a result of oversupplementation, which results in hair loss. The main food groups providing selenium in the diet are bread and cereals, meat, liver, fish (cod, canned tuna), eggs, and milk/dairy products. Fruit and vegetables typically contain relatively small amounts of selenium [52]. Calcium is also an element playing significant role in keeping hair in proper state, and in hair, calcium concentration exceeds by 200 times that in blood serum and erythrocytes. Women, in particular, in the perimenopause period, are exposed to its deficiency, and so they should be supplemented. Calcium in diet is present in all dairy products containing lactose facilitating its absorption and also soya, parsley green leaves, hazelnuts, white beans, kale, walnuts, fish, and cabbages. Magnesium, taking part in protein transformation, is responsible for division, growth, and maturation processes of cells, taking into consideration its role in immunological reactions, protecting, and alleviating inflammation states, and thus its deficiency directly or indirectly contributes to hair fall. The sources of magnesium in women's diet are cocoa, grits, whole grain breads, nuts, and legumes.

18.3.3 Liquids

Water influences the hydration degree and state of hydrolipid layer on its surface. Physiologically, the amount of water in the skin represents 20% of the total [53]. That is why mineral and spring waters containing minerals are a very good source of water and minerals. Liquids should be consumed in the amount 30–35 mL/kg of body mass/day including 1.5 L in the form of water (boiled, mineral) best between meals.

In summary, to prevent hair loss, diet should include large amount of fresh vegetable and grains, with a proper intake of proteins and fat, and the best scheme is represented by the Mediterranean diet [54]. External supplementation of micronutrients might be indicated after medical consultation.

18.4 Nutritional Management of Overweight and Obesity

Worldwide, obesity prevalence has nearly tripled since 1975. In 2016, more than 1.9 billion adults, 18 years and older, were overweight. Of these over 650 million were obese [55]. In 2013, the report of the 53 WHO European Region Member States (2013) shows overweight in men ranging from 31% in Tajikistan to 72% in Czech Republic, while in women it ranged from 31% of Tajikistan to 64% of Turkey. In Italy, overweight is present in 32.6% of the adult population and 10.4% is frankly obese [56]. There is a gap between North and South in Italy, with the southern regions presenting the higher prevalence of obesity (Basilicata 13.3% and Molise 15.3%) or overweight (Campania 38.2% and Puglia 38.1%) than the northern (Valle d'Aosta 3 and 16.1%, respectively). The prevalence of overweight and obesity increases with aging up to a maximum at the age of 75 years, then it lowers slightly.

Similar data are reported in Canada where 58% of the women aged 40–59 years are considered overweight or obese [57].

Poor eating habits and physical inactivity contribute to the increasing prevalence of overweight and obese individuals.

As stated before in this chapter, during the menopause transition body composition changes by increasing in abdominal fat mass as well as associated alterations in cardio-metabolic risk due to hormone-related decreases in energy expenditure and fat oxidation [54, 55].

Lifestyle interventions to minimize gains in fat mass and changes in body composition and body fat distribution predominantly include exercise and healthy nutrition. Current guidelines recommend (a) assessing factors contributing to overweight (body mass index (BMI) 25–29.9 kg m^2) and obesity (BMI $\geq$ 30 kg m^2) in adults and (b) intervening with counseling and treatment of obesity [56].

Jull et al. [57] systematically reviewed the effectiveness of exercise and/or nutrition interventions on mitigating changes in body weight, body composition, and body fat distribution in women specifically in menopause transition stage. They reported that only one study was appropriate for this aim [57], and this study included women exposed to a program of combined exercise and caloric restriction dietary interventions for 54 weeks. Using this combined program, women had improved body weight, and reduced abdominal adiposity and significant reductions in waist circumference and body fat were maintained beyond 4 years [57]. In other studies with less stringent study design, exercise or both exercise and caloric reduction interventions were able to limit the process and patterns of weight gain and change in body fat distribution during the menopause transition stage [58, 59].

These findings are consistent with guidelines on the prevention and management of obesity that recommend lifestyle intervention as the first approach for preventing or treating obesity.

Evidence points towards a role of the Mediterranean diet in preventing obesity [60–62]. It covers most nutritional recommendations, like low content of refined carbohydrates, high fiber content, moderate fat content—mostly unsaturated—and moderate-to-high content of vegetable proteins and energy expenditure via a daily physical exercise (Fig. 18.2). The Mediterranean diet also appears as a safe strategy to treat metabolic syndrome and to reduce associated cardiovascular risk [60], to combat obesity, and to reduce low-grade inflammation, thus limiting the onset of many of the modern noncommunicable diseases.

18.4.1 Chrononutrition

The study of biological rhythms and circadian cycles of living organisms and how they adapt to external changes is known as chronobiology [63]. These circadian rhythms have a significant impact on hormones (e.g., insulin, glucagon, cortisol, and growth hormone), influencing many patterns as sleep/wake rhythms and nutrition/fasting. The mammalian circadian system consists of three key components: the input, the 24-h oscillator, and the outputs. The central and most crucial circadian

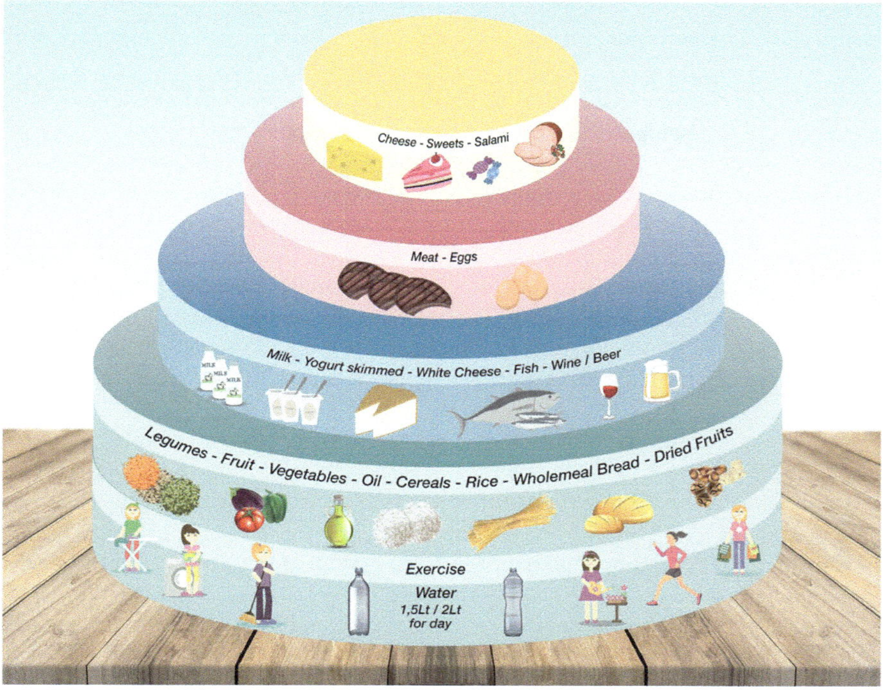

Fig. 18.2 The pyramid of Mediterranean diet redrafted for women. The first step includes the required daily activities and food to be consumed. The second step includes food to be used only three times per week (wine and beer are alternatives). The third step includes food to be used only one time per week, and the top step includes food to be seldom used in the month

oscillator resides in the suprachiasmatic nucleus (SCN) of the hypothalamus. This central pacemaker system governs circadian rhythmicity in various regions of the brain and peripheral tissues by transmitting them both neural and humoral signals. While most peripheral tissues and organs typically operate under the guidance of the SCN, certain conditions, such as restricted nutrition, jet-lag, and shift work, can lead to a loss of synchronization between these peripheral oscillators and the SCN [63]. Furthermore, external factors such as an individual's chronotype, meal timing and frequency, and food choices can also profoundly influence this complex system, ultimately playing a role in the development of obesity and metabolic diseases [64]. Notably, metabolic enzymes and transport systems related to cholesterol, glucose, and lipid metabolism are also influenced by the circadian system, and disruptions in these cycles can lead to conditions like obesity, type 2 diabetes, dyslipidemias, and hypertension [65]. Indeed, dietary fat consumption may impact circadian rhythm-related gene expression, and the timing of food intake may influence personal response to weight loss treatments; some studies indicate a link between obesity and the timing of food consumption, particularly late lunch and late dinner consumption [66–68]. Disruptions in circadian rhythms can be caused by various factors, such as constant light exposure or altered feeding behaviors, and have negative effects on metabolism, energy expenditure, and overall health. Light exposure and shift work can lead to an increased risk of metabolic disorders, emphasizing the importance of maintaining a regular circadian rhythm [69]. Practical nutritional guidance is supported by the following evidence-based recommendations:

- Do not skip breakfast, as it can help prevent metabolic syndrome and obesity.
- Balance breakfast and lunch with a mix of carbohydrates, fiber, proteins, and a moderate amount of fat.
- Take adequate protein intake, especially from sources like whey proteins.
- Most daily carbohydrates should be consumed during the first half of the day.
- Calorie and carbohydrate intake should be reduced in the evening.
- Foods rich in tryptophan (e.g., meat, poultry, fish, and milk) can aid muscle growth and sleep.
- Foods that contain melatonin (e.g., cherries, strawberries, and kiwis) can promote sleep.
- Limit fat consumption and opt for foods rich in polyunsaturated fats, like fish and seeds.
- Consider incorporating polyphenol-rich foods such as tea, grapes, red fruits, and dark chocolate.
- Avoid excessive consumption of coffee, alcohol, and high-fat foods, as they can disrupt circadian rhythms [70].

18.5 Conclusion

Nutrition plays an essential role in the well-being of menopausal women both in limiting clinical complaints, such as vasomotor symptoms and hair loss, and in preventing more serious diseases such osteoporosis (discussed in other chapters of this book) and overweight/obesity. A recommended daily dietary regimen for menopausal women is reported in Fig. 18.3: this together with constant physical exercise will produce lifelong sustained benefits.

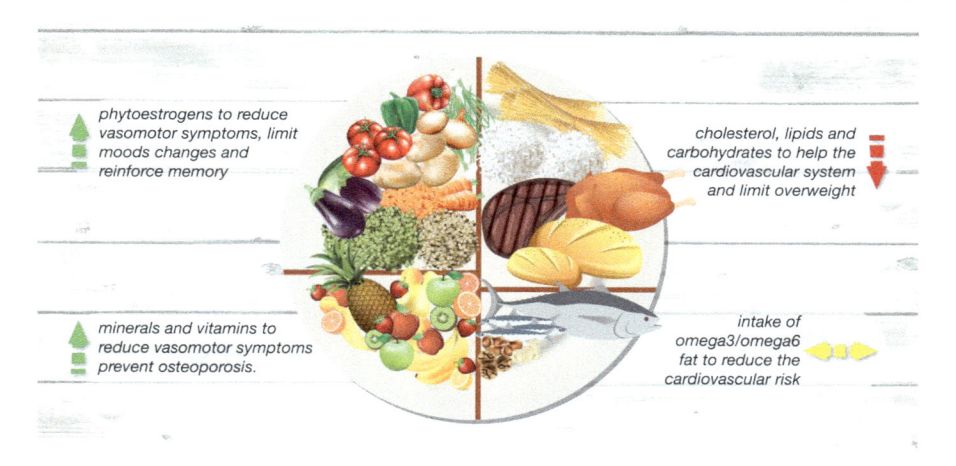

Fig. 18.3 This is the perfect plate to eat everyday. More fibers, vegetables, and integral pasta or rice, little portion of fish, and some fruit ensure a perfect balance of minerals, vitamins, and good proteins, carbohydrates, and fat for limiting the appearance of chronic comorbidities

References

1. Wylie-Rosett J. Menopause, micronutrients, and hormone therapy. Am J Clin Nutr. 2005;81(5):1223S–31S.
2. Keenan NL, Mark S, Fugh-Berman A, Browne D, Laczmarczyk J, Hunter C. Severity of menopausal symptoms and use of both conventional and complementary alternatives. Menopause. 2003;10:507–15.
3. Overlie I, Moen MH, Holte A, Finset A. Androgens and estrogens in relation to flushes during the menopause transition. Maturitas. 2002;41:69–77.
4. Munro HN. Aging. In: Kinney JM, Jeejeebhoy KN, Hill GL, Owen OE, editors. Nutrition and metabolism in patient care. Philadelphia: WB Saunders; 1988. p. 145–66.
5. Guo SS, Zeller C, Chumlea WC, et al. Aging, body composition, and lifestyle: the Fels longitudinal study. Am J Clin Nutr. 1999;70:405–11.
6. Greendale GA, Sowers M, Han W, Huang MH, Finkelstein JS, Crandall CJ, Lee JS, Karlamangla AS. Bone mineral density loss in relation to the final menstrual period in a multiethnic cohort: results from the Study of Women's Health Across the Nation (SWAN). J Bone Miner Res. 2012;27(1):111–8.
7. Culhan EG, Jimenez HA, King CE. Thoracic kyphosis, rib mobility, and lung volumes in normal women and women with osteoporosis. Spine. 1994;19:1250–5.
8. Melton LJ III. Adverse outcomes of osteoporotic fractures in the general population. J Bone Miner Res. 2003;18:1139–41.
9. Roubenoff R. The pathophysiology of wasting in the elderly. J Nutr. 1999;129(suppl):256S–9S.
10. Weissel M. Disturbances of thyroid function in the elderly. Wien Klin Wochenschr. 2006;118:16–20.
11. Roberts SB, Dallal GE. Energy requirements and aging. Public Health Nutr. 2005;8:1028–36.
12. Troiano RP, Frongillo EA, Sobol J, Levitsky DA. The relationship between body weight and mortality: a quantitative analysis of combined information from existing studies. Int J Obes Relat Metab Disord. 1996;20:63–75.
13. McTigue KM, Hess R, Ziouras J. Obesity in older adults: a systematic review of the evidence for diagnosis and treatment. Obesity. 2006;14:1485–97.

14. Rivlin RS. Keeping the young-elderly healthy: is it too late to improve our health through nutrition? Am J Clin Nutr. 2007;86:1572S–6S.
15. Flegal KM, Graubard BI, Williamson DF, Gail MH. Excess deaths associated with underweight, overweight and obesity. JAMA. 2005;293:1861–7.
16. Philp HA. Hot flashes—a review of the literature on alternative and complementary treatment approaches. Altern Med Rev. 2003;8:284–302.
17. Barton DL, Loprinzi CL, Quella SK, et al. Prospective evaluation of vitamin E for hot flashes in breast cancer survivors. J Clin Oncol. 1998;16:495–500.
18. Golmakani N, Parnan Emamverdikhan A, Zarifian A, Sajadi Tabassi SA, Hassanzadeh M. Vitamin E as alternative local treatment in genitourinary syndrome of menopause: a randomized controlled trial. Int Urogynecol J. 2019;30(5):831–7.
19. Feduniw S, Korczyńska L, Górski K, Zgliczyńska M, Bączkowska M, Byrczak M, Kociuba J, Ali M, Ciebiera M. The effect of Vitamin E supplementation in postmenopausal women-a systematic review. Nutrients. 2022;15(1):160.
20. Kronenberg F, Fugh-Berman A. Complementary and alternative medicine for menopausal symptoms: a review of randomized controlled, trials. Ann Intern Med. 2002;137:805–13.
21. Blumenthal M. The use of black cohosh to treat symptoms of menopause. Sex Reprod Menopause. 2004;2:27–34.
22. Nabaie L, Kavand S, Robati N, et al. Androgenic alopecia and insulin resistance: are they realy related? Clin Exp Dermatol. 2009;34:694–7.
23. Huntley AL, Ernst E. A systematic review of herbal medicine products for the treatment of menopausal symptoms. Menopause. 2003;10:465–76.
24. Izzo AA, Hoon-Kim S, Radhakrishnan R, Williamson EM. A critical approach to evaluating clinical efficacy, adverse events and drug interactions of herbal remedies. Phytother Res. 2016;30:691–700.
25. Dailey RK, Neale AV, Northrup J, West P, Schwartz KL. Herbal product use and menopause symptom relief in primary care patients: a MetroNet study. J Womens Health (Larchmt). 2003;12:633–41.
26. Aidelsburger P, Schauer S, Grabein K, Wasem J. Alternative methods for the treatment of postmenopausal troubles. GMS. Health Technol Assess. 2012;8:Doc03.
27. The 2023 Nonhormone Therapy Position Statement of The North American Menopause Society Advisory Panel. The 2023 nonhormone therapy position statement of The North American Menopause Society. Menopause. 2023;30(6):573–90.
28. Herskovitz I, Tosti A. Female pattern hair loss. Int J Endocrinol Metab. 2013;11:e9860.
29. Goluch-Koniuszy ZS. Nutrition of women with hair loss problem during the period of menopause. Prz Menopauzalny. 2016;15(1):56–61.
30. Jen M, Yan AC. Syndromes associated with nutritional deficiency and excess. Clin Dermatol. 2010;28:669–85.
31. D'Agostini F, Fiallo P, Pennisi TM, De Flora S. Chemoprevention of smoke-induced alopecia in mice by oral administration of L-cystine and vitamin B6. J Dermatol Sci. 2007;46:189–98.
32. Rushton DH, Norris MJ, Dover R, Busuttil N. Causes of hair loss and the developments in hair rejuvenation. Int J Cosmet Sci. 2002;24:17–23.
33. Pappas A. Epidermal surface lipids. Dermatoendocrinol. 2009;1:72–6.
34. James MJ, Gibson RA, Cleland LG. Dietary polyunsaturated fatty acids and inflammatory mediator production. Am J Clin Nutr. 2000;71(1 suppl):343S–8S.
35. Matilainen V, Laakso M, Hirsso P, et al. Hair loss, insulin resistance, and heredity in middle-aged women. A population-based study. J Cardiovasc Risk. 2003;10:227–31.
36. Saulle R, Semyonov L, La Torre G. Cost and cost-effectiveness of the Mediterranean diet: results of a systematic review. Forum Nutr. 2013;5:4566–86.
37. Wagner K-H, Kamal-Eldin A, Elmadfa I. Gamma-tocopherol—an underestimated vitamin? Ann Nutr Metab. 2004;48(3):169–88.
38. Jiang Q, Christen S, Shigenaga MK, Ames BN. Gamma-tocopherol, the major form of vitamin E in the US diet, deserves more attention. Am J Clin Nutr. 2001;74(6):714–22. PMID 11722951.

39. Gropper S, Smith J. Advanced nutrition and human metabolism. Belmont: Cengage Learning; 2009.
40. University of Bristol. Biotin. 2012. Accessed 17 Sep 2012.
41. National Academy of Sciences, Institute of Medicine, Food and Nutrition Board. Folate. In: Dietary reference intakes for thiamine, riboflavin, niacin, vitamin B6, folate, vitamin B12, pantothenic acid, biotin and choline. Washington, DC: National Academy Press; 1998.
42. Chen AC, Damian DL. Nicotinamide and the skin. Aust J Dermatol. 2014;55(3):169–75.
43. Vitamin A. MedlinePlus, National Library of medicine, US National Institutes of Health. Accessed 2 Dec 2016.
44. Norman AW. From vitamin D to hormone D: fundamentals of the vitamin D endocrine system essential for good health. Am J Clin Nutr. 2008;88(2):491S–9S.
45. Institute of Medicine, Food and Nutrition Board. Dietary reference intakes: thiamin, riboflavin, niacin, vitamin b6, folate, vitamin b12, pantothenic acid, biotin, and choline. Washington, DC: National Academy Press; 1998.
46. Said HM. Cell and molecular aspects of human intestinal biotin absorption. J Nutr. 2009;139:158–62.
47. Almohanna HM, Ahmed AA, Tsatalis JP, Tosti A. The role of vitamins and minerals in hair loss: a review. Dermatol Ther (Heidelb). 2019;9(1):51–70.
48. Muscogiuri G, Mitri J, Mathieu C, Badenhoop K, Tamer G, Orio F, Mezza T, Vieth R, Colao A, Pittas A. Mechanisms in endocrinology: vitamin D as a potential contributor in endocrine health and disease. Eur J Endocrinol. 2014;171:R101–10.
49. Bolland MJ, Ames RW, Grey AB, et al. Does degree of baldness influence vitamin D status? Med J Aust. 2008;189:674–5.
50. Trost LB, Bergfeld WF, Calogeras E, et al. The diagnosis and treatment of iron deficiency and its potential relationship to hair loss. J Am Acad Dermatol. 2006;54:824–44.
51. Driscoll MS, Kwon EK, Skupsky H, et al. Nutrition and the deleterious side effects of nutritional supplements. Clin Dermatol. 2010;28:371–9.
52. Fairweather-Tait SJ, Bao Y, Broadley MR, et al. Selenium in human health and disease. Antioxid Redox Signal. 2011;14:1337–83.
53. Kacalak-Rzepka A, Bielecka-Grzela S, Klimowicz A, et al. Dry skin as a dermatological and cosmetic problem. Ann Acad Med Stetin. 2008;54:54–7.
54. Barrea L, Balato N, Di Somma C, Macchia PE, Napolitano M, Savanelli MC, Esposito K, Colao A, Savastano S. Nutrition and psoriasis: is there any association between the severity of the disease and adherence to the Mediterranean diet? J Transl Med. 2015;13:18.
55. WHO Country profiles on nutrition, physical activity and obesity in the 53 WHO European Region Member States. 2013. http://www.euro.who.int/en/health-topics/noncommunicable-diseases/obesity/publications/2013/country-profiles-on-nutrition,-physical-activity-and-obesity-in-the-53-who-european-region-member-states.-methodology-and-summary-2013.
56. ISS Osservasalute. 2013. http://www.epicentro.iss.it.
57. Jull J, Stacey D, Beach S, Dumas A, et al. Lifestyle interventions targeting body weight changes during the menopause transition: a systematic review. J Obes. 2014;2014:824310.
58. Ogwumike OO, Arowojolu AO, Sanya AO. Effects of a 12-week endurance program on adiposity and flexibility of Nigerian perimenopausal and postmenopausal women. Niger J Physiol Sci. 2011;26:199–206.
59. Hagner W, Hagner-Derengowska M, Wiacek M, Zubrzycki IZ. Changes in level of VO2max, blood lipids, and waist circumference in the response to moderate endurance training as a function of ovarian aging. Menopause. 2009;16:1009–13.
60. Giugliano D, Esposito K. Mediterranean diet and metabolic diseases. Curr Opin Lipidol. 2008;19:63–8.
61. Méndez MA, Popkin BM, Jakszyn P, Berenguer A, Tormo MJ, Sánchez MJ, et al. Adherence to a Mediterranean diet is associated with reduced 3-year incidence of obesity. J Nutr. 2006;136(11):2934–8.

62. Goulet J, Lapointe A, Lamarche B, Lemieux S. Effect of a nutritional intervention promoting the Mediterranean food pattern on anthropometric profile in healthy women from the Québec city metropolitan area. Eur J Clin Nutr. 2007;61(11):1293–300.
63. McKenna H, van der Horst GTJ, Reiss I, Martin D. Clinical chronobiology: a timely consideration in critical care medicine. Crit Care. 2018;22(1):124.
64. Asher G, Sassone-Corsi P. Time for food: the intimate interplay between nutrition, metabolism, and the circadian clock. Cell. 2015;161(1):84–92.
65. Mi SJ, Kelly NR, Brychta RJ, Grammer AC, Jaramillo M, Chen KY, et al. Associations of sleep patterns with metabolic syndrome indices, body composition, and energy intake in children and adolescents. Pediatr Obes. 2019;14(6):e12507.
66. Eckel-Mahan KL, Patel VR, De Mateo S, Orozco-Solis R, Ceglia NJ, Sahar S. Reprogramming of the circadian clock by nutritional challenge. Cell. 2013;155(7):1464–78.
67. Lopez-Minguez J, Dashti HS, Madrid-Valero JJ, Madrid JA, Saxena R, Scheer FAJL. Heritability of the timing of food intake. Clin Nutr. 2019;38(2):767–73.
68. Lucassen EA, Zhao X, Rother KI, Mattingly MS, Courville AB, de Jonge L, et al. Evening Chronotype is associated with changes in eating behavior, more sleep apnea, and increased stress hormones in short sleeping obese individuals. PLoS One. 2013;8(3):e56519.
69. Barrea L, Frias-Toral E, Aprano S, Castellucci B, Pugliese G, Rodriguez-Veintimilla D, Vitale G, Gentilini D, Colao A, Savastano S, Muscogiuri G. The clock diet: a practical nutritional guide to manage obesity through chrononutrition. Minerva Med. 2022;113(1):172–88.
70. Bone mineral density loss in relation to the final menstrual period in a multiethnic cohort: Results from the Study of Women's Health Across the Nation (SWAN) Abstract Journal of Bone and Mineral Research (2012) (2012) (2011);27(1):111–118. https://doi.org/10.1002/jbmr.534.

Part V
Menopause in the Context of Healthy Ageing

Frailty and Comorbidities: Frailty in Women

19

Esperanza Navarro-Pardo, Patricia Villacampa-Fernández, Ruth E. Hubbard, Emily Gordon, and Antonio Cano

Abstract

Frailty is a dynamic and multidimensional clinical condition characterized by the depletion of system reserves, resulting in a loss of redundancy and increased vulnerability to any stressful event. This loss of resilience implies not only a poorer and more difficult recovery from baseline homeostasis but a disproportionate increase in harmful health outcomes from even minor insults. There are two models of frailty that have received the most attention within the community: the frailty phenotype and the frailty index. Frailty and comorbidity represent two distinct, but related, clinical concepts. The term comorbidity designates the co-occurrence of different noncommunicable diseases (NCDs) in the same individual. Comorbidity, however, does not only represent the sum of different NCDs, but a clinical condition in itself. In fact, it is conceived as a synergy of the different NCDs associated with worse health outcomes and a more complex clinical management than the simple sum of the individual NCDs. Evidence

---

E. Navarro-Pardo (✉) · P. Villacampa-Fernández
Department of Developmental and Educational Psychology, University of Valencia, Valencia, Spain
e-mail: esperanza.navarro@uv.es; patricia.villacampa@uv.es

R. E. Hubbard
PA Southside Clinical Unit, Centre for Research in Geriatric Medicine,
Translational Research Institute, The University of Queensland, Brisbane, Australia
e-mail: r.hubbard1@uq.edu.au

E. Gordon
Geriatric Medicine, Princess Alexandra Hospital, School of Medicine and Centre for Research in Geriatric Medicine, The University of Queensland, Woolloongabba, Australia
e-mail: e.gordon@uq.edu.au

A. Cano
Full Professor of Obstetrics and Gynecology, Salus Vitae Women's Health Clinical Center, Valencia, Spain
e-mail: Antonio.cano@uv.es

© The Author(s), under exclusive license to Springer Nature Switzerland AG 2025
A. Cano (ed.), *Menopause*, https://doi.org/10.1007/978-3-031-83979-5_19

supports the role of frailty and comorbidity as mutual risk factors. Women have been found to acquire slightly more general comorbidities than men, but paradoxically enjoy a longer life expectancy. Women also experience poorer health which has, at least in part, been attributed to psychosocial differences. It is unclear why women live longer despite suffering higher levels of frailty. This may be due to the distinctive profile of NCDs, which may not be life-threatening in women, a lower physiological reserve in men, or other reasons.

19.1 Introduction

"Frailty, thy name is woman!"

Hamlet, Act 1 Scene II.In the past, "frailty" was associated with the female sex. Before reproductive biology was understood, women's recurring menstrual cycles were considered to render them unstable and imperfect. Aristotle argued that menstruation was a sign of women's inferiority, a direct cause of their physical weakness. Victorians expanded on this hypothesis, proposing the uterus as the weakest part of the female body (since it failed to hold its contents) through which emotional problems could both originate and manifest. Locating physical and psychological weakness in the womb excluded men from such faults.

It is now accepted that frailty may be seen in both sexes, but it is not identical. Men and women tend to age in different ways. Women experience more disability, dependency, and chronic disease yet have a longer life expectancy. Compared to their age-matched male peers, women could be considered both *more* frail (because they have poorer health) and *less* frail (because they are less vulnerable to the adverse outcome of death).

In this chapter, we explore the frailty concept by reviewing its definition and different approaches to its measurement. The link between frailty and chronic disease is reviewed before considering how frailty in older women differs to that of older men.

19.2 Frailty

To a contemporary layperson, frailty is a derogatory term, identifying multiple losses: of strength, social engagement, levels of activity, and even moral stature [1]. In gerontological research, on the other hand, frailty represents a dynamic and multidimensional clinical condition characterized by depletion of the system's reserve that translates into a loss of redundancy and increased vulnerability when facing any stressor event. This loss of resilience implies not only a poorer and harder recovery of baseline homeostasis but also a disproportionate increment in deleterious health outcomes when facing even minor insults.

Regarding the factors involved in the triggering of frailty, it appears that the losses and cumulative damage imposed by aging, the impact of acute or chronic disease, the psychosocial resources and coping strategies, and the individual's own genetic endowment may be at play [2, 3]. However, a holistic and definite knowledge of the aetiology of frailty remains yet to be accomplished. Clegg and colleagues [2] identified the nervous, endocrine, immune, and musculoskeletal as the main systems in which the development of frailty has been best investigated and provided a very illustrative description of the role each systems plays in the so-called spiral of physiological decline.

The concept of frailty may be understood as what Schefer [4] calls a *foreseeing tipping point*, namely, as a broad and comprehensive indicator that determines whether the complex biopsychosocial system is on the brink of a dramatic shift or collapse due to the loss of its redundancy. In order to facilitate a better understanding of the frailty concept, a visual representation of the increased vulnerability to stressors due to the system's redundancy depletion linked to its loss of reserve is displayed in Fig. 19.1.

19.2.1 Frailty Paradigms

Consensus has not yet been achieved among the scientific and practitioner experts of the field for a definitive operational definition of frailty [5, 6]. There are, even so, two main paradigms that have received most of the attention within the community: the frailty phenotype [7] and the frailty index [8]. Both approaches consider frailty

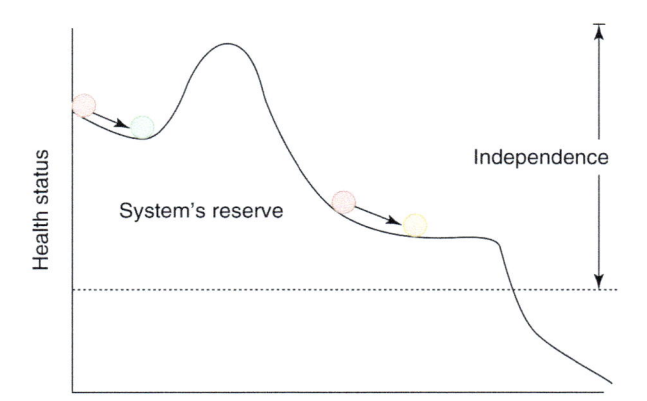

Fig. 19.1 Increased vulnerability to stressors of frail individuals due to the system's reserve depletion. The *green circle* represents a robust elder person, while the *orange circle* represents a frail one. *Red circles* represent a certain minor insult. The *horizontal dashed line* represents the cutoff between dependency and independency regarding functional capacity. Due to the depletion in the system's reserve and loss of redundancy, when facing the same minor stressor event, the frail individual presents a higher risk of adverse health outcomes, loss of functional capacity, and difficulty to recover baseline homeostasis. On the contrary, the preservation of the system's reserve and redundancy buffers the strain repercussions for the robust individual, making it more resilient by preventing a disproportionate impairment of health status and allowing a quick and easy recovery of homeostasis. (*Note*: For the elaboration of this figure, inspiration was drawn from the visual representation of tipping points and leading indicators provided by Schefer [4] as well as from the diagram of vulnerability of frail elderly people provided by Clegg and colleagues [2])

as an age-related, dynamic, stochastic, multidimensional, and nonlinear depletion of systems that leads to a loss of physiological reserve and redundancy where even minor stressors can lead to adverse health outcomes and complications due to the inability of the system to recover homeostasis [7–13]. Notwithstanding, they differ in their conceptual framework, naming them differently: a cycle of frailty versus a model of fitness and frailty. Based on the differences regarding their conceptualization of frailty, each operationalization has generated a distinct assessment tool (see Table 19.1).

- The *frailty phenotype* recognizes frailty as a clinical syndrome identified by the presence of three or more of the following components: sarcopenia (weight loss), weakness (grip strength), exhaustion (poor endurance and energy), slowness (gait speed), and sedentary lifestyle (low physical activity) [7]. This operationalization considers as intermediate, or prefrail, people with one or two of those characteristics present and as robust all those free of any of those features. The most consistent critic to this conceptualization is the omission of important dimensions, like cognitive and other psychosocial components [6, 8, 14–16].
- The *frailty index*, also known as cumulative deficit model, is a mathematical model that identifies frailty as an accumulation of health deficits [8]. It can be based on Comprehensive Geriatric Assessment (CGA), and the principle is to count health deficits in a whole range of areas from purely physical to more psychosocial. These health deficits should be age-related yet not too early saturated and would include symptoms, signs, diseases, disabilities, or laboratory, radiographic, or electrocardiographic abnormalities [17]. Frailty, then, is operationalized as the ratio between the number of deficits present in an individual and the

Table 19.1 The dominant frailty paradigms

	Elements	Interpretation
Frailty phenotype [7]	*Sarcopenia*: Unintentional weight loss *Weakness*: Low grip strength *Exhaustion*: Poor endurance and energy *Slowness*: Low gait speed *Sedentary lifestyle*: Low physical activity	None present: Robust 1–2 present: Pre-frail 3 or more present: Frail
Frailty index [17]	Accounts for the *accumulation of health deficits*: Symptoms, signs, diseases, disabilities Computes a *ratio* between the health deficits counted in the list and the ones present in the individual assessed. *Criteria* for the elaboration: – Deficits must be associated to health status (e.g., gray hair cannot be considered) – Deficits must be age-related – Deficits must not saturate too early (e.g., impaired vision cannot be considered) – It must cover a wide range of systems from purely physical to psychosocial – For longitudinal assessments, the deficits list must remain unaltered	Frail: (approximately) ≥ 0.20 The higher the ratio, the frailer the individual Upper limit: (approximately) 0.7

total number of deficits counted [8, 10, 17–19]. It is important to note that, although the theoretical maximum of the frailty index by definition is 1, the 99% upper limit has consistently been proven to be less than 0.722 [9].

Existing evidence supports the ability of both operationalizations to predict health status impairment with its consequent decay in functional capacity and mortality [11]. Up to now, most of the interest within the community has been captured by the frailty phenotype. A great part of its success resides in the categorical nature of the approach [12]. The discretization of the individuals in categories (i.e., robust, pre-frail, or frail), rather than providing a certain ratio, increases the assessment outcome intuitiveness and ease of interpretation for general practitioners. Even so, the frailty index is the preferred operationalization for policymakers and the majority of the researchers, as its continuous character turns it more sensitive to changes plus a better and more sensitive predictor of deleterious health outcomes [6, 8, 15, 16].

19.3 Frailty and Comorbidities

The clinical conditions of frailty, comorbidity, and disability have traditionally been used interchangeably as they are highly interrelated and overlapping in a considerable amount of people [20]. However, they represent three distinct clinical concepts [7, 21]. The differentiation between disability and comorbidity and frailty is quite apparent due to the former representing a clear impairment in functional status. Nonetheless, to disentangle frailty and comorbidity is a more complex task [5].

19.3.1 Comorbidities

The term comorbidity designates the co-occurrence of different noncommunicable diseases (NCDs) in the same individual, that is, the presence of two or more chronic diseases in the same person [22–24]. Some authors have proposed a distinction between comorbidity and multimorbidity, but this conceptual differentiation goes beyond the scope of the present chapter, where both terms are used interchangeably (see Fig. 19.2). Chronic diseases are those diseases that are permanent, caused by nonreversible pathological alteration, and/or require rehabilitation or a long period of care. The traditional concept of chronic diseases has been integrated in the more recent and increasingly popular denomination of NCDs [25]. The cluster of cardiovascular diseases accounts for most of the deaths related to NCDs, followed by cancer, chronic obstructive pulmonary disease, and diabetes mellitus. These four clusters of diseases account for the majority of the NCD-related mortality. Other common NCDs are painful conditions, depression, anxiety, heart failure, stroke/transient ischemic attack, atrial fibrillation, and dementia [22].

It is worth noting, however, that comorbidity does not just represent the sum of different NCDs but a clinical condition itself [25]. Indeed, it is envisaged as a

```
┌─────────────────────────────────────────┐
│                 NCDs                     │
│ Most incidents:                          │
│   • Cardiovascular diseases              │
│   • Cancer                               │
│   • Chronic Obstructive Pulmonary Disease│
│   • Diabetes mellitus                    │
│                                          │
│ Other common ones:                       │
│ Painful condition, depression, anxiety,  │
│ heart failure, stroke/transient ischemic │
│ attack, atrial fibrillation, dementia,...│
└─────────────────────────────────────────┘
                    ──when 2 or more──▶ ┌──────────────┐
                        are present     │ Co-morbidity │
                                        └──────────────┘
```

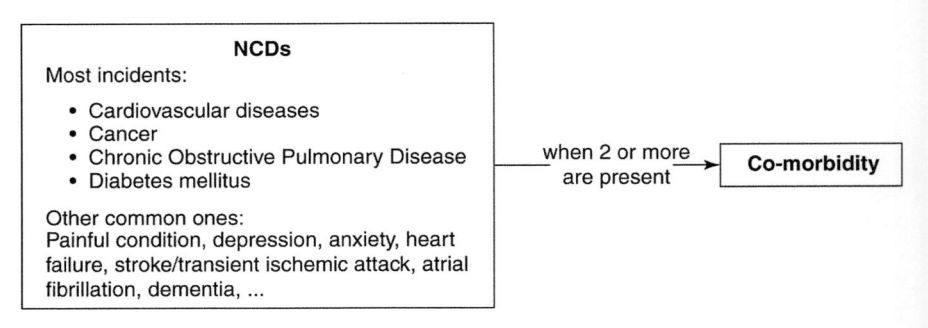

Fig. 19.2 Noncommunicable diseases and comorbidity

synergy of the different NCDs associated with worse health outcomes and a more complex clinical management than the simple addition of the single NCDs [26] (see Fig. 19.2). Low socioeconomic status and female gender have been confirmed as social risk factors for comorbidity [27, 28], while a large social network appears to be a protective factor [24]. Like frailty, comorbidity is age related, for its prevalence rates increase substantially with aging, ranging from 55% to 98% in people aged 65 years or older [22, 24, 26]. Comorbidity prevalence rates, however, are strongly affected by the operationalization of the condition, that is, the cutoff point taken for the number of diagnoses and the range of health conditions that is contemplated. Most researchers usually take a conservative approach establishing the presence of three (instead of two) or more NCDs as a cutoff point for the presence comorbidity in order to prevent the disproportionate prevalence rates associated to a lower cutoff point. The prevalence rates variations between studies, nonetheless, are possibly due also to methodological biases, or other reasons.

As a way to find consensus among the wide variety of operationalizations for comorbidity, the European General Practice Research Network [28] proposed a comprehensive definition of the concept as:

> Any combination of chronic disease with at least one other disease (acute or chronic) or biopsychosocial factor (associated or not) or somatic risk factor. Any biopsychosocial factor, any risk factor, the social network, the burden of diseases, the health care consumption, and the patient's coping strategies may function as modifiers (of the effects of multimorbidity).

19.3.2 Frailty–Comorbidity Connection

Existing evidence supports the role of frailty and comorbidity as risk factors for each other, as well as to be both predictors of diminished quality of life, of health and well-being, of disability, and of mortality [15, 17, 19, 22, 24, 27, 29].

As proposed by Villacampa-Fernández and colleagues [21], both comorbidity and frailty are crucial clinical conditions in the system failure process of an aging

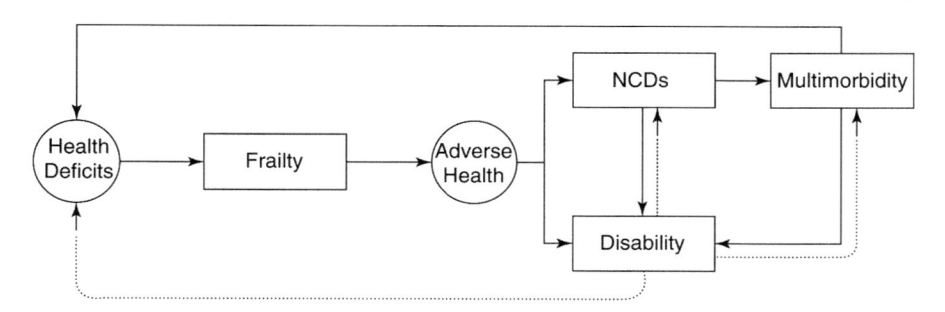

Fig. 19.3 Flowchart of the aging system failure process. *Notes*: *Circles* represent inputs/outputs, *rectangles* represent clinical conditions, *continuous lines* represent direct effects, *dotted lines* represent indirect or secondary effects, *NCDs* represent noncommunicable diseases. (*Source*: Villacampa-Fernández et al. [21]. With permission of Elsevier from Villacampa-Fernández et al. Maturitas 2017; 95:31. Permission conveyed through Copyright Clearance Center, Inc.)

individual (see Fig. 19.3 for the graphical representation). Comorbidities, as already discussed above, are major predictors for an increase in health deficits. This accumulation of health deficits triggers a depletion of the system's reserve and redundancy, leading to a higher vulnerability to stressors known as frailty. Frailty, in turns, leads to a highly increased probability of adverse health outcomes when facing minor insults. By adverse health outcomes, a range of possible diseases and/or impairments is included, with institutionalization and mortality as the worst scenarios. Within the wide range of diseases and/or impairments that trigger the adverse health outcomes related to frailty status, the already discussed NCDs and their consequent comorbidities, in conjunction with disability, stand out for their deleterious effects on the individual. Disability is proposed to indirectly trigger NCDs and comorbidity, along with frailty through the increase in health deficits.

19.3.3 Sex Differences in Comorbidities

While older males and females acquire new comorbidities with age, females have been found to acquire slightly more overall [30]. In addition, the types of diseases commonly acquired by females, such as osteoarthritis, depression, and anxiety, appear to be more likely to impact negatively on function and quality of life [31–35]. While males and females differ in terms of their approach to defining and assessing well-being, the number and nature of chronic illnesses has been found to be a significant confounding factor for sex differences in self-rated health [31]. Women also report (and experience) more disability than men [30, 32, 34–36]. The high prevalence of functional limitation experienced by women may be due to a higher incidence (in the setting of low physical activity and "disabling" chronic conditions) and/or lower recovery rates [37, 38].

19.4 The Sex–Frailty Paradox

Women tend to live longer lives than men. The sex differential in longevity is seen in most countries across the developed and developing world [39]. At a global level, the gap between the sexes has remained stable (at approximately 4.5 years) over the last 25 years [40]. Historical data suggests that this is not a recent phenomenon [41, 42]. Yet, as we have discussed, older women experience more chronic disease and disability. So while increasing frailty is associated with worse mortality for both sexes, women seem to be able to tolerate a higher level of frailty. This so-called sex–frailty paradox [43, 44] is one of several fundamental paradoxes of aging that remain unexplained.

19.4.1 Why Do Women Have Poorer Health?

Psychosocial factors have been identified as potential mediators of the sex–morbidity gap. In studies using self-report data, conclusions regarding sex differences in comorbidity, disability, and self-rated health depend to some degree upon whether males and females assess and report health in the same way. Even though it has been hypothesized (and sometimes assumed) that sex differences in disease incidence reflect a female tendency to overreport and a male tendency to underreport health problems, the literature is far from conclusive [36, 45, 46]. Females have been shown to access healthcare services more often than males (even after removing reproduction-related presentations) [46]. While this might contribute to higher female incidence of self-reported medical diagnoses, it is not clear whether this is due to real sex differences in morbidity prevalence or sex differences in health–illness perception or help-seeking behavior.

Sex differences in biological factors, such as inflammatory cytokines and sarcopenia, are emerging in the literature and likely underpin sex differences in comorbidity, functional decline, and, ultimately, frailty [47, 48]. Abdominal adiposity, which accumulates to a greater extent in older women than men, may play a particularly important role in the chronic inflammatory state thought to be at the crux of frailty [48].

While sex differences in pathophysiology may develop in middle to late age, it is also possible that differences stem from divergent physiological investment during reproductive years. The "disposable soma" theory proposes a trade-off between somatic maintenance and reproduction, which would manifest as an inverse dose–response relationship between parity and life expectancy [49, 50]. Arguably, a relationship between parity and frailty may be expected to emerge first, but this has not been examined in the literature to date. In keeping with this theory, there is some evidence that pregnancy and childbirth are associated with chronic medical conditions, poor functional performance, and self-rated health, as well as late-life mortality, in older women [51–54]. However, the fact that nulliparous women have not demonstrated superior longevity and the life expectancies of fathers were not insensitive to increasing parity oppose this theory and emphasize that other (probably psychosocial) factors are relevant [50, 51]. The impact of reproduction on the late-life health of women remains a focus of contemporary research.

19.4.2 Why Do Women Live Longer Lives?

Multiple factors contribute to sex differences in longevity. Certainly, there are biological factors, such as sex differences in immunocompetence and hormonal modulation of inflammation, that may contribute to mortality rates [46]. In particular, the favorable impact of estrogen on lipid profiles with subsequent delays to the onset of cardiovascular disease after menopause has been frequently cited in the literature [55]. Longevity benefits associated with the presence of two X-chromosomes has also been speculated [44, 55]. Risk-related activities, such as smoking and alcohol intake, have also been identified as contributing to higher male mortality rates, possibly through their contribution to increased incidence of "lethal" comorbidities [31, 34, 44, 46]. Sex differences in healthcare utilization, particularly in terms of access to early intervention and preventative medicine [44, 46], also probably contribute to the male–female mortality gap.

19.4.3 Why Do Women Tolerate a Greater Frailty Burden?

These health and longevity factors, however, do not explain the "male–female health–survival paradox"—why or how do females live longer despite greater frailty? It has been proposed that the paradox is an artefact of female longevity. That is, females have more time to acquire a greater number of health problems, which they then have for a longer period of time. However, the frailty differential emerges in middle age and, as a result, cannot be solely attributed to longer life span [44].

Perhaps the sex paradox is underpinned by sex differences in the "nature" of chronic medical illnesses. There is some evidence to suggest that females experience chronic conditions that are typically "non-life-threatening" or "disabling," resulting in high morbidity and low mortality, whereas males experience more "life-threatening" chronic conditions, resulting in high mortality [30–32, 56, 57].

The sex paradox may also transpire because males have lower physiological reserve than females. Studies using the cumulative deficit model of frailty have determined sex differences in frailty limits (i.e., the frailty score at which survival approaches zero) [35, 58]. In particular, the frailty limit was found to be significantly lower for males than females and males reached the frailty limit at a younger age [35].

Hubbard and Rockwood [44] proposed that there are evolutionary drivers for sex differences in physiological reserve. In males, optimal physical function in youth may be achieved at the expense of longevity. In evolutionary terms, this fitness-frailty pleiotropy is advantageous to the species as it maximizes progeny. However, the consequence is lower physiological reserve with early system failure (relatively to females). In females, on the other hand, pregnancy and childbirth may be key drivers. Reproduction is physiologically demanding and may lead to early decrements in system reserve. Thus, in order to maximize fecundity, there would need to be an evolutionary increase in female physiological reserve. This fertility–frailty pleiotropy would mean that even though females acquire damage during their reproductive lives and are more likely to enter middle and late age with frailty, the sexes would have a similar life expectancy. The mortality gap between the sexes, therefore, might be indicative of the contemporary trend towards limiting parity, whereby females enter their post-reproductive years with less system damage.

An alternative, or complementary, theory is that the benefits of the post-reproductive female life may drive an evolutionary increase in physiological reserve. The "mother effect" emphasizes the advantage of women living for some years after the birth of their last child to ensure that their children achieve sexual and economic maturity [59]. The presence of grandmothers may also convey a survival advantage by supporting offspring to successfully produce their own progeny [59]. However, it may be argued that the "grandmother effect" does not drive biological evolution of female systems; rather the advantage may lie in supporting daughters to cope with increased frailty during and after reproduction.

It has been hypothesized that females tolerate frailty better than males because they have increased social supports [60]. However, higher levels of social support for females have not been consistently demonstrated, particularly when marital status and cultural background have been taken into account [34, 61–63]. Socioeconomic factors have been independently associated with frailty and mortality [63–67], and there is some evidence that the size and direction of the impact differs between the sexes [62, 64, 68]. Overall, it is unclear how social factors may impact the male–female health–survival paradox.

19.5 Conclusions

Frailty is a construct for examining health status and risk of adverse outcomes in the aging population. It is related to, but distinct from, comorbidity. Even though consensus regarding the best way to diagnose frailty has not been reached, it is generally agreed that at the crux of this condition is the increased vulnerability to stressors in the setting of reduced system's reserve and redundancy.

Frailty affects both sexes. However, the relationship between sex and frailty is not straightforward. Consistent with the observation that women tend to have more health problems than men in old age, women are more frail. However, women also appear to be more resilient to the deleterious effects of frailty. This paradox, well cited in the literature, remains controversial but highlights future directions for aging research.

The ultimate aim of frailty research is to identify targets for intervention in the hope that frailty can be delayed or slowed, thereby improving the health and quality of life of older adults. Although it is tempting to focus on untangling the weaknesses that contribute to frailty in women and mortality in men, it is equally important to explore resilience in older, frail women. Interventions targeting modifiable behavioral risk factors for frailty and comorbidity, such as physical activity, nutrition, responsible consumption of drugs, and education, are likely to be highly beneficial and cost-effective. From a health policy point of view, greater understanding of the balance between vulnerability and resilience in aging may help to shift care of the elderly from a traditional disease-centered paradigm to a preventive, multidisciplinary approach that promotes functionality and independence.

References

1. Warmoth K, Lang IA, Phoenix C, Abraham C, Andrew MK, Hubbard RE, Tarrant M. 'Thinking you're old and frail': a qualitative study of frailty in older adults. Ageing Soc. 2015;36:1–8.
2. Clegg A, Young J, Iliffe S, Rikkert MO, Rockwood K. Frailty in elderly people. Lancet. 2013;381:752–62.
3. Xue QL. The frailty syndrome: definition and natural history. Clin Geriatr Med. 2011;27:1–15.
4. Scheffer M. Foreseeing tipping points. Nature. 2010;467:411–2.
5. Rodríguez-Mañas L, Féart C, Mann G, Viña J, Chatterji S, Chodzko-Zajko W, Harmand MG, Bergman H, Carcaillon L, Nicholson C, Scuteri A. Searching for an operational definition of frailty: a delphi method based consensus statement. The frailty operative definition-consensus conference project. J Gerontol A Biol Sci Med Sci. 2013;68:62–7.
6. Sternberg SA, Wershof Schwartz A, Karunananthan S, Bergman H, Clarfield AM. The identification of frailty: a systematic literature review. J Am Geriatr Soc. 2011;59:2129–38.
7. Fried LP, Tangen CM, Walston J, Newman AB, Hirsch C, Gottdiener J, Seeman T, Tracy R, Kop WJ, Burke G, McBurnie MA. Frailty in older adults: evidence for a phenotype. J Gerontol A Biol Sci Med Sci. 2001;56:808–13.
8. Rockwood K, Song X, MacKnight C, Bergman H, Hogan DB, McDowell I, Mitnitski A. A global clinical measure of fitness and frailty in elderly people. Can Med Assoc J. 2005;173:489–95.
9. Rockwood K, Mitnitski A. Limits to deficit accumulation in elderly people. Mech Ageing Dev. 2006;127:494–6.
10. Rockwood K, Mitnitski A. Frailty in relation to the accumulation of deficits. J Gerontol A Biol Sci Med Sci. 2007;62A:722–7.
11. Woo J, Leung J. Multi-morbidity, dependency, and frailty singly or in combination have different impact on health outcomes. Age. 2014;36:923–31.
12. Bandeen-Roche K, Xue Q-L, Ferrucci L, Walston J, Guralnik JM, Chaves P, Zeger SL, Fried LP. Phenotype of frailty: characterization in the women's health and aging studies. J Gerontol A Biol Sci Med Sci. 2006;61:262–6.
13. Fried LP, Xue QL, Cappola AR, Ferrucci L, Chaves P, Varadhan R, Guralnik JM, Leng SX, Semba RD, Walston JD, Blaum CS. Nonlinear multisystem physiological dysregulation associated with frailty in older women: implications for etiology and treatment. J Gerontol A Biol Sci Med Sci. 2009;64:1049–57.
14. Cano A. Cognitive frailty, a new target for healthy ageing. Maturitas. 2015;82:139–40.
15. Rockwood K, Andrew M, Mitnitski A. A comparison of two approaches to measuring frailty in elderly people. J Gerontol A Biol Sci Med Sci. 2007;62:738–43.
16. Collard RM, Boter H, Schoevers RA, Oude Voshaar RC. Prevalence of frailty in community-dwelling older persons: a systematic review. J Am Geriatr Soc. 2012;60:1487–92.
17. Searle SD, Mitnitski A, Gahbauer EA, Gill TM, Rockwood K. A standard procedure for creating a frailty index. BMC Geriatr. 2008;8:24.
18. Rockwood K, Mitnitski A. How might deficit accumulation give rise to frailty? J Frailty Aging. 2012;1:8–12.
19. Rockwood K, Mitnitski A. Frailty defined by deficit accumulation and geriatric medicine defined by frailty. Clin Geriatr Med. 2011;27:17–26.

20. Fried LP, Ferrucci L, Darer J, Williamson JD, Anderson G. Untangling the concepts of disability, frailty, and comorbidity: implications for improved targeting and care. J Gerontol A Biol Sci Med Sci. 2004;59:M255–63.
21. Villacampa-Fernández P, Navarro-Pardo E, Tarín JJ, Cano A. Frailty and multimorbidity: two related yet different concepts. Maturitas. 2017;95:31–5.
22. Barnett K, Mercer SW, Norbury M, Watt G, Wyke S, Guthrie B. Epidemiology of multimorbidity and implications for health care, research, and medical education: a cross-sectional study. Lancet. 2012;380:37–43.
23. Salisbury C. Multimorbidity: redesigning health care for people who use it. Lancet. 2012;380:7–9.
24. Marengoni A, Angleman S, Melis R, Mangialasche F, Karp A, Garmen A, et al. Aging with multimorbidity: a systematic review of the literature. Ageing Res Rev. 2011;10:430–9.
25. Hunter DJ, Reddy KS. Noncommunicable diseases. N Engl J Med. 2013;369:1336–43.
26. Starfield B. Threads and yarns: weaving the tapestry of comorbidity. Ann Fam Med. 2006;4:101–3.
27. Fortin M, Stewart M, Poitras M, Almirall J, Maddocks H. A systematic review of prevalence studies on multimorbidity: toward a more uniform methodology. Ann Fam Med. 2012;10:142–51.
28. Le Reste JY, Nabbe P, Manceau B, Lygidakis C, Doerr C, Lingner H, et al. The European general practice research network presents a comprehensive definition of multimorbidity in family medicine and long term care, following a systematic review of relevant literature. J Am Med Dir Assoc. 2013;14:319–25.
29. Gijsen R, Hoeymans N, Schellevis FG, Ruwaard D, Satariano WA, Van Den Bos GAM. Causes and consequences of comorbidity: a review. J Clin Epidemiol. 2001;54:661–74.
30. Avendano M, Mackenbach J. Changes in physical health among older Europeans. In: Health and health care; 2008. p. 116.
31. Case A, Paxson C. Sex differences in morbidity and mortality. Demography. 2005;42:189–214.
32. Crimmins EM, Kim JK, Solé-Auró A. Gender differences in health: results from SHARE, ELSA and HRS. Eur J Pub Health. 2010;21:81–91.
33. Ferrucci L, Turchi A, Fumagalli S, Di Bari M, Silvestrini G, Zacchei S, Nesti A, Magherini L, Tarantini F, Pini R, Antonini E. Sex-related differences in the length of disability prior to death in older persons. Aging Clin Exp Res. 2003;15:310–4.
34. Gorman BK, Read JN. Gender disparities in adult health: an examination of three measures of morbidity. J Health Soc Behav. 2006;47:95–110.
35. Shi J, Yang Z, Song X, Yu P, Fang X, Tang Z, Peng D, Mitnitski A, Rockwood K. Sex differences in the limit to deficit accumulation in late middle-aged and older Chinese people: results from the Beijing longitudinal study of aging. J Gerontol A Biol Sci Med Sci. 2014;69:702–9.
36. Merrill SS, Seeman TE, Kasl SV, Berkman LF. Gender differences in the comparison of self-reported disability and performance measures. J Gerontol A Biol Sci Med Sci. 1997;52:M19–26.
37. Hardy SE, Allore HG, Guo Z, Gill TM. Explaining the effect of gender on functional transitions in older persons. Gerontology. 2008;54:79–86.
38. Oman D, Reed D, Ferrara A. Do elderly women have more physical disability than men do? Am J Epidemiol. 1999;150:834–42.
39. Leon DA. Trends in European life expectancy: a salutary view. Int J Epidemiol. 2011;40:271–7.
40. World Health Organization. World health statistics. Monitoring health for the SDGs. Geneva: WHO; 2016.
41. Austad SN. Why women live longer than men: sex differences in longevity. Gend Med. 2006;3:79–92.
42. Gage TB. Are modern environments really bad for us?: revisiting the demographic and epidemiologic transitions. Am J Phys Anthropol. 2005;48:96–117.
43. Hubbard RE. Sex differences in frailty. Interdiscip Top Gerontol Geriatr. 2015;41:41–53.
44. Hubbard RE, Rockwood K. Frailty in older women. Maturitas. 2011;69:203–7.

45. Macintyre S, Ford G, Hunt K. Do women 'over-report' morbidity? Men's and women's responses to structured prompting on a standard question on long standing illness. Soc Sci Med. 1999;48:89–98.
46. Oksuzyan A, Juel K, Vaupel JW, Christensen K. Men: good health and high mortality. Sex differences in health and aging. Aging Clin Exp Res. 2008;20:91–102.
47. Canon ME, Crimmins EM. Sex differences in the association between muscle quality, inflammatory markers, and cognitive decline. J Nutr Health Aging. 2011;15:695–8.
48. Hubbard RE, Lang IA, Llewellyn DJ, Rockwood K. Frailty, body mass index, and abdominal obesity in older people. J Gerontol A Biol Sci Med Sci. 2010;65A:377–81.
49. Westendorp RG, Kirkwood TB. Human longevity at the cost of reproductive success. Nature. 1998;396:743–6.
50. Zeng Y, Ni ZM, Liu SY, Gu X, Huang Q, Liu JA, Wang Q. Parity and all-cause mortality in women and men: a dose-response meta-analysis of cohort studies. Sci Rep. 2016;6:19351.
51. Barclay K, Keenan K, Grundy E, Kolk M, Myrskylä M. Reproductive history and post-reproductive mortality: a sibling comparison analysis using Swedish register data. Soc Sci Med. 2016;155:82–92.
52. Díaz-Venegas CA, Sáenz JL, Wong R. Family size and old-age wellbeing: effects of the fertility transition in Mexico. Ageing Soc. 2016;37:495.
53. Engelman M, Agree EM, Yount KM, Bishai D. Parity and parents' health in later life: the gendered case of Ismailia. Popul Stud (Camb). 2010;64:165–78.
54. Read S, Grundy E, Wolf DA. Fertility history, health, and health changes in later life: a panel study of British women and men born 1923–49. Popul Stud. 2011;65:201–15.
55. Eskes T, Haanen C. Why do women live longer than men? Eur J Obstet Gynecol Reprod Biol. 2007;133:126–33.
56. Newman A, Brach J. Gender gap in longevity and disability in older persons. Epidemiol Rev. 2001;23:343–53.
57. Verburgge L. Gender and health: an update on hypotheses and evidence. J Health Soc Behav. 1985;26:156–82.
58. Garcia-Gonzalez J, Garcia-Pena C, Franco-Marina F, Gutierrez-Robeldo L. A frailty index to predict mortality risk in a population of senior Mexican adults. BMC Geriatr. 2005;48:96–117.
59. Lachmann PJ. The grandmother effect. Gerontology. 2011;57:375–7.
60. Berges IM, Graham JE, Ostir GV, Markides KS, Ottenbacher KJ. Sex differenes in mortality among older frail Mexican Americans. J Womens Health (Larchmt). 2009;18:1475–51.
61. Andrew M, Mitnitski A, Rockwood K. Social vulnerability, frailty and mortality in elderly people. PLoS One. 2008;3(5):e2232. https://doi.org/10.1371/journal.pone.0002232.
62. Gu D, Dupre ME, Sautter J, Zhu H, Liu Y, Yi Z. Frailty and mortality among Chinese at advanced ages. J Gerontol B Psychol Sci Soc Sci. 2009;64B:279–89.
63. Woo J, Goggins W, Sham A, Ho S. Social determinants of frailty. Gerontology. 2005;51:402–8.
64. Bassuk S, Berkman L, Amick B. Socioeconomic status and mortality among elderly: findings from four US communities. Am J Epidemiol. 2001;155:520–33.
65. Lang I, Hubbard RE, Andrew M, Llewellyn D, Melzer D, Rockwood K. Neighborhood deprivation, individual socioeconomic status, and frailty in older adults. J Am Geriatr Soc. 2009;57:1776–80.
66. Romero-Ortuno R. Frailty index in Europeans: association with determinants of health. Geriatr Gerontol Int. 2014;14(2):420–9.
67. Szanton SL, Seplaki CL, Thorpe RJ Jr, Allen JK, Fried LP. Socioeconomic status is associated with frailty: the Women's health and ageing studies. J Epidemiol Community Health. 2010;64:63–7.
68. Major J, Doubeni C, Freedman N, Park Y, Lian M, Hollenbeck A, Schatzkin A, Graubard B, Sinha R. Neighborhood socioeconomic deprivation and mortality: NIH-AARP diet and health study. PLoS One. 2010;5(11):e15538. https://doi.org/10.1371/journal.pone.0015538.

20. Muscle Strength, Dynapenia, and Sarcopenia During Female Midlife and Beyond

Faustino R. Pérez-López, Pascual García-Alfaro, and Ignacio Rodríguez

Abstract

Muscle-skeletal symptoms are highly prevalent among peri- and postmenopausal women and more frequently display in women than in men of similar age. They are unrelated to other causes of dynapenia or sarcopenia. The handgrip strength is a simple screening test for dynapenia. In healthy postmenopausal women living in Spain, age less than 65 years, with normal vitamin D levels and normal body mass index, the handgrip strength is 24.10 ± 3.88 Kg. Some gene variations of the vitamin D receptor are associated with reduced handgrip strength and the dynapenia risk. Women with early menopause have increased risk of reduced appendicular muscle mass and no difference of handgrip strength. Ethnicity, environment, lifestyle, and nutrition may influence muscle strength and the risk of dynapenia. Subclinical chronic inflammation and increased fat mass may contribute to handgrip strength reduction and fracture risk in older women.

20.1 Introduction

Muscle-skeletal symptoms are more prevalent in peri- and postmenopausal women than the typical vasomotor complaints, persisting long after these symptoms disappear or become mild [1, 2]. In addition, the menopause transition is accompanied of critical biological, psychological, and social factors and comorbid conditions unrelated to the menopause transition that may exacerbate muscle-skeletal symptoms and

F. R. Pérez-López (✉)
Department of Obstetrics and Gynecology, Universidad de Zaragoza Facultad de Medicina, Zaragoza, Spain
e-mail: faustino.perez@unizar.es

P. García-Alfaro · I. Rodríguez
Department of Obstetrics and Gynecology, Hospital Universitario Dexeus, Barcelona, Spain
e-mail: PASGAR@dexeus.com; NACROD@dexeus.com

contribute to changes in body composition [3]. Skeletal muscles are responsible for contracting and producing movements, maintaining posture and body temperature, stabilizing joints, and storing nutrients. In addition, they accumulate proteins, are a source of biochemical products, and react to external temperatures [4]. From the fifth decade of life, there is a reduction of the functional capacity of skeletal muscles (dynapenia) and a gradual reduction of muscle mass (sarcopenia). This process is more evident and prevalent in women, suggesting some relationship with gonadal function decline that is more abrupt in women than in men. A significant number of older people will be at increased risk of sarcopenia with a severe reduction of muscle mass, which is a predictor of all-cause mortality [5]. For sarcopenia and frailty assessment apart from the clinical exam, there are image methods for muscle quantification, although muscle strength assessment can also be useful when appendicular skeletal muscle index is evaluated in patients with sarcopenia and comorbidity [6]. The myopenia concept can be considered when the muscle mass is reduced by at least 5% in 6–12 months or when it is below the fifth centile of healthy 30-year-old subjects [7].

Clark and Manini [8] were the first to postulate the difference between sarcopenia and dynapenia. A significant proportion of peri- and postmenopausal women will display muscle discomfort and reduction of strength as a sarcopenia covariate [9]. Dynapenia is the age-related reduction of muscle strength without an objective cause, increasing the risk of physical incapacity and limited performance. It is frequently associated with changes in muscle composition and function, including sarcopenia, other comorbid conditions, and even increased mortality risk. However, the limit between dynapenia and sarcopenia is not sufficiently clear. The handgrip strength is a simple dynapenia screening test widely reported in the literature, both in otherwise healthy subjects and particular populations with pathology, which provide valid information when muscle mass measurements are not feasible [10, 11]. Other tests to evaluate muscle strength are the 30-second chair-stand test, the timed-up-and-go test, and the walking speed test to assess the lower extremity strength and physical performance and are appropriate to evaluate subjects with arthritis, joint conditions, or among older subjects [12]. The application of some of these tests to young postmenopausal women (< 65 years) is not reliable and has low precision and different cutoffs [13].

For sarcopenia and frailty assessment apart from physical examination, there are specific image methods for muscle quantification although handgrip strength can be a useful complement when appendicular skeletal muscle index is evaluated [6, 14]. Dual-energy X-ray absorptiometry is a more widely available instrument to determine noninvasively muscle quantity (total body lean tissue mass or appendicular skeletal muscle mass). However, results are variable according to different instrument brands and inconsistent for muscle mass assessment.

20.2 Handgrip Strength and Hormones in Postmenopausal Women

Handgrip strength, measured with a dynamometer, is a quick and reproducible test with good correlation with other more complex tools like the chair-stand test or the one-leg stance test. In addition, handgrip strength has a predictive value of brain function, physical capacity, or mortality, being associations stronger between muscular strength and events in women than men. We studied muscle strength in 392 otherwise healthy postmenopausal women living in Spain, aged younger than 65 years (57.30 ± 3.69 years), with normal vitamin D status (≥ 30.0 ng/mL), mean body mass index of 24.9 ± 3.8 kg/m^2, and no physical disabilities [15]. They had a mean handgrip strength in the dominant arm of 24.10 ± 3.88 kg, and they displayed mild significant inverse correlations between handgrip strength and age ($r = -0.131$) and between handgrip strength and early menopause age ($r = -0.033$). Furthermore, early age of menopause was associated with significant higher risk of dynapenia (OR: 2.74, 95% CI: 1.23–6.11). In a posterior analysis of 402 postmenopausal women aged 47 to 83 years, we used a directed acyclic graph to identify causal and confounding factors of dynapenia [16]. We found significant differences for follicle-stimulating hormone (OR: 0.99; 95% CI: 0.98–1.00), cortisol (OR: 1.07, 95% CI: 1.02–1.12), and dehydroepiandrosterone sulfate (OR: 0.99; 95% CI: 0.98–1.00) between postmenopausal women with normal handgrip strength and those with dynapenia. However, there were no significant associations between hormones and handgrip strength after adjustment for confounding variables.

The de Souza Mâcedo et al. [17] meta-analysis of four cross-sectional studies demonstrated that menopause at early age is associated with worse physical function as evaluated by handgrip strength, gait speed, and self-reported functional limitations. However, the heterogeneity of studies does not allow to obtain clear conclusions. Lee et al. [18] reported the influence of reproductive period duration on the handgrip strength in a large cohort of Korean postmenopausal women aged 45–75 years. The authors defined women by the reproductive function duration in tertiles and handgrip strength into four quartiles. It is relevant that the long duration of reproductive function was associated with low risk of absolute handgrip strength (OR: 0.75; 95% CI: 0.56–1.00) for the second tertile and 0.68 (95% CI: 0.51–0.90) for the third tertile reproductive duration period, as compared with the first tertile reproductive period. Therefore, the longer reproductive period was associated with reduced risk of low handgrip strength in postmenopausal women.

20.3 Vitamin D and Muscle Strength

Vitamin D has pleiotropic beneficial effects on different organ and systems, including a positive calcium and mineral balance on muscle metabolism [19–21]. The presence of vitamin D receptor in skeletal muscle suggests a relevant role in the physiology and prevention of muscle weakness during aging. Thus, vitamin D is involved in skeletal muscle function on gait, tone, and balance [22]. Postmenopausal women with low 25-hydroxyvitamin D (25(OH)D) levels are at risk muscle dysfunction and fractures [23], and older adults with plasma 25(OH)D < 25 nmol/L display low handgrip strength [24]. The Fox et al. [25] study described a community cohort of 2576 participants living in Bonn (Germany), reporting handgrip strength according to circulating 25(OH) D levels, being grip strength higher in those with adequate 25 (OH)D levels (≥ 50 to ≤125 nmol/L) than in those with inadequate (30 to <50 nmol/L). In addition, older people showed weaker effects of 25(OH)D levels on grip strength than younger adults. However, some studies from Asia populations did not find associations between vitamin D levels, and handgrip strength is discordant among different countries in older populations [26, 27]. The effects of vitamin D supplementation versus placebo has been investigated in a meta-analysis of randomized placebo-controlled trials [28], concluding that available evidence does not support a beneficial effect of vitamin D supplementation on muscle health [28]. However, the analysis did not include participants with severe vitamin D deficiency (25(OH)D levels ≤20 nmol/L), and this subgroup is of most interest to study.

Mendelian randomization analyses of subjects with probable sarcopenia and sarcopenic obesity were studied for a relation between high 25(OH)D and skeletal muscle traits and grip strength, confirming that genetically higher 25(OH)D had a linear 0.11 kg greater contractile force for 10 units higher 25(OH)D [29]. On the other hand, there are vitamin D receptor mutations which create a complete hormone-resistant status which can manifest in children and in adults affecting bone mineral content, osteoporosis risk, and other complications [30, 31]. García-Vigara et al. [32] have demonstrated that some gene variations of the vitamin D receptor are associated with reduced handgrip strength and the dynapenia risk. This is a new area of research to be developed in the near future to advance on the associations of vitamin D mutations with handgrip strength. Future studies should define genetic factors influencing vitamin D levels and metabolism [33].

20.4 Muscle Strength and Sarcopenia Risk

The European Working Group on Sarcopenia in Older People (EWGSOP) considers that muscle strength is the principal determinant of sarcopenia [34]. Muscle strength, fat mass, and bone metabolism functions are interconnected. Orprayoon et al. [35] studied pre-sarcopenia and sarcopenia prevalence using appendicular muscle mass and associated factors in middle-aged postmenopausal women (45–65 years, mean age 57.8 ± 4.5 years) living in Thailand. They, respectively, reported 11.8%, 2.7%, and 85.6% of pre-sarcopenic, sarcopenic, and nonsarcopenic women. The sarcopenia risk is increased in women with early menopause and ovarian insufficiency. Women with spontaneous premature ovarian insufficiency show low muscle mass compatible with sarcopenia, including appendicular skeletal muscle mass and their quotient with weight, body mass index, total skeletal muscle mass, and weight compared to healthy premenopausal control women [36]. A systematic review and meta-analysis evaluated appendicular skeletal muscle mass and body mass index of women with early menopause (< 45 years) and premature ovary insufficiency (< 40 years), reporting that women with early menopause displayed reduced appendicular muscle mass and no difference in handgrip strength [37], which suggest that ovarian hormones have a positive protective effect on muscle mass preservation.

In a general French population of people aged 18–74 years, including 103 with an acute disease and 200 with a chronic disease, the handgrip values were below the 10 centile in those with chronic diseases and 19.4% of those with acute diseases. Maximum handgrip strength values were at age 41.5 ± 13.6 years for women. In this particular population, the rate of malnourished patients was 20.0% in those with chronic diseases and 23.3% in those with acute diseases [38]. Among Chinese women with the dynapenia definition set at <18 Kg, the prevalence was 25.6% [39]. Therefore, ethnicity, environment, lifestyle, and nutrition should be considered variable factors for muscle strength comparative studies or meta-analyses. Lee et al. [18] studied a large population of postmenopausal women aged 45–75 years using handgrip strength classified in four quartiles. Women with a long reproductive period displayed the lower risk of low absolute muscle grip strength as compared to the first tertile reproductive period, supporting the protective effect of ovarian function duration on muscle strength.

Tessier et al. [40] reported an exhaustive analysis of physical performance in a large community-dwelling Canadian Caucasian older adults (age 65–86 years), evaluating with gait speed, timed up-and-go, chair rise, balance tests, and a weighted-sum score. In addition, handgrip strength and low appendicular lean mass index were considered predictors of low strength. In women, appendicular lean mass index was not an independent predictor, and the prevalence of dynapenia (<20.4 kg) was 24.0%, sarcopenia (< 5.72 kg/m^2) 13.7%, and sarco-dynapenia 5.5%. In addition, low grip strength predicted more precisely low physical performance compared to muscle mass. Also, they were older, less physically active and had lower weight and fat mass.

20.5 Body Composition and Inflammation

Body composition changes along female life due to endocrine and metabolic factors, reproductive history, nutrition, physical activity, skeletal muscle deterioration, and fat accumulation and redistribution. Reproductive factors and menopause transition may contribute with some specific characteristics on body composition and muscle strength and mass. The consequences will be a trend for increased risks of obesity, insulin resistance and metabolic syndrome, reduction of both muscle strength (dynapenia) or muscle mass (sarcopenia), and osteopenia or osteoporosis [3, 9]. Adiposity and intramuscular fat accumulation are linked to mitochondrial damage and increased proinflammatory cytokines inducing muscle dysfunction [37], suggesting that subclinical chronic inflammation may play a role in handgrip strength reduction [38]. Inflammation is associated with increased production of cytokines and acute phase proteins and muscle dysfunction and atrophy. The Tuttle et al. [41] meta-analysis reported higher levels of blood inflammatory cytokines, including C-reactive protein, interleukin-6, and tumor necrosis factor- associated with lower handgrip strength and knee extension strength in people with sarcopenia or low skeletal muscle strength.

The associations between handgrip strength and adiposity was studied in a large cohort of postmenopausal women aged 50–84 years, and for every year in age and for each 1% of adiposity, women were more likely to have dynapenia with odd ratio (OR): 1.09; 95% and confidence interval (CI): 1.04 to 1.14, and OR: 1.06; 95% CI: 1.00 to 1.13, respectively [42]. These results support a link between increased fat mass and low muscle quality. Miranda et al. [43] reported the association between handgrip strength, physical fitness, and body composition studied by bioelectrical impedance in postmenopausal women with the metabolic syndrome. The mechanism of the association may be related to the fact that subjects with less fat mass are less exposed to systemic and regional inflammation [44], preserving muscle function and strength. Future research should analyze nutritional factors to improve handgrip strength and dynapenia risk reduction for postmenopausal women according to nutrient intakes.

20.6 Handgrip Strength, Osteoporosis, and Fracture Risk

Low handgrip strength has been related with osteoporosis and fracture risks. The Lin et al. [45] cross-sectional study of Asian people reported a positive causal relationship between handgrip strength as predictor of osteoporosis in both women and men. In women, a threshold of 21.9 kg handgrip strength had a sensitivity of 59%, specificity of 59%, and area under the curve of 0.75. Therefore, handgrip strength is a simple method to identify women at risk of osteoporosis. In the Knutsor et al. [46] meta-analysis of 19 population-based prospective cohort studies (including 22,577 participants and 9,199 fractures), the adjusted relative fracture risk for incident fracture was 0.70 (95% confidence interval 0.61–0.80) and for hip fracture (9 studies) was 0.61 (95% CI 0.61 (95% CI: 0.54–0.70). The analysis support that high handgrip strength is associated with reduced future fracture risk.

Handgrip strength is a marker of the future evolution of hip fractures in terms of muscle strength in relation to walking ability 4 months after hip fracture treatment [47]. Results demonstrate that improvement in postoperative handgrip strength predicts walking ability 4 months after surgery. Furthermore, Dowling et al. [48] reported the risk of fractures in 16,147 women (60–82 years) with obesity and dynapenia ($\leq$ 21 kg) included in the UK Biobank. Both factors were associated with greater rate of lower extremity fracture risk independently of bone mineral density. Therefore, programs to improve muscle strength are convenient in postmenopausal women to maintain and improve their health.

20.7 Final Remarks

Handgrip strength is (1) a simple and consistent tool to evaluate muscle health, dynapenia, and pre-sarcopenia or sarcopenia risks; and (2) related and confounding factors include body mass index, menopause status, physical activity, bone health, and quality of life in diverse circumstances of young and postmenopausal women.

References

1. Chedraui P, Pérez-López FR, Mendoza M, et al. Severe menopausal symptoms in middle-aged women are associated to female and male factors. Arch Gynecol Obstet. 2010;281(5):879–85. https://doi.org/10.1007/s00404-009-1204-z.

2. Pérez-López FR, Fernández-Alonso AM, Pérez-Roncero G, Chedraui P, Monterrosa-Castro A, Llaneza P. Assessment of menopause-related symptoms in mid-aged women with the 10-item Cervantes scale. Maturitas. 2013;76(2):151–4. https://doi.org/10.1016/j.maturitas.2013.07.002.
3. Mitchell WK, Williams J, Atherton P, Larvin M, Lund J, Narici M. Sarcopenia, dynapenia, and the impact of advancing age on human skeletal muscle size and strength; a quantitative review. Front Physiol. 2012;3:260. Published 2012 Jul 11. https://doi.org/10.3389/fphys.2012.00260.
4. McCuller C, Jessu R, Callahan AL. Physiology, skeletal muscle. In: StatPearls. https://www.ncbi.nlm.nih.gov/books/NBK537139/.
5. Liu P, Hao Q, Hai S, Wang H, Cao L, Dong B. Sarcopenia as a predictor of all-cause mortality among community-dwelling older people: a systematic review and meta-analysis. Maturitas. 2017;103:16–22. https://doi.org/10.1016/j.maturitas.2017.04.007.
6. Vaishya R, Misra A, Vaish A, Ursino N, D'Ambrosi R. Hand grip strength as a proposed new vital sign of health: a narrative review of evidences. J Health Popul Nutr. 2024;43(1):7. https://doi.org/10.1186/s41043-024-00500-y.
7. Fearon K, Evans WJ, Anker SD. Myopenia-a new universal term for muscle wasting. J Cachexia Sarcopenia Muscle. 2011;2(1):1–3. https://doi.org/10.1007/s13539-011-0025-7.
8. Clark BC, Manini TM. Sarcopenia =/= dynapenia. J Gerontol A Biol Sci Med Sci. 2008;63:829–34.
9. Pérez-López FR. Dynapenia and sarcopenia. In: Cano A, editor. Chapter 20: menopause: a comprehensive approach. Berlin: Springer; 2017. p. 317–31. https://doi.org/10.1007/978-3-319-59318-0_20.
10. Angst F, Drerup S, Werle S, Herren DB, Simmen BR, Goldhahn J. Prediction of grip and key pinch strength in 978 healthy subjects. BMC Muscoskel Disord. 2010;11:94.
11. López-Bueno R, Andersen LL, Koyanagi A, Nunez-Cortes R, Calatayud J, Casana J, et al. Thresholds of handgrip strength for all-cause, cancer, and cardiovascular mortality: a systematic review with dose-response metaanalysis. Ageing Res Rev. 2022;82:101778.
12. Manning KM, Hall KS, Sloane R, et al. Longitudinal analysis of physical function in older adults: the effects of physical inactivity and exercise training. Aging Cell. 2024;23(1):e13987. https://doi.org/10.1111/acel.13987.
13. Assis Silva SH, Orsatti FL, de Lima ML, et al. Assessing the robustness of muscle strength and physical performance measures in women older than 40 years: a test-retest reliability study. Menopause. 2024;31(1):33–8. https://doi.org/10.1097/GME.0000000000002294.
14. Ruiz-Margáin A, Macías-Rodríguez RU, Flores-García NC, Román Calleja BM, Fierro-Angulo OM, González-Regueiro JA. Assessing nutrition status, sarcopenia, and frailty in adult transplant recipients. Nutr Clin Pract. 2024;39(1):14–26. https://doi.org/10.1002/ncp.11107.
15. Garcia-Alfaro P, Garcia S, Rodríguez I, Tresserra F, Pérez-López FR. Factors related to muscle strength in postmenopausal women aged younger than 65 years with normal vitamin D status. Climacteric. 2019;22(4):390–4. https://doi.org/10.1080/13697137.2018.1554645.
16. García-Alfaro P, García S, Rodriguez I, Bergamaschi L, Pérez-López FR. Relationship between handgrip strength and endogenous hormones in postmenopausal women. Menopause. 2023;30(1):11–7. https://doi.org/10.1097/GME.0000000000002093.
17. De Souza Mâcedo PR, Rocha TN, Gomes Fernandes SG, Apolinário Vieira MC, Jerez-Roig J, Aires da Câmara SM. Possible association of early menopause with worse physical function: a systematic review. Menopause. 2021;28(4):467–75. https://doi.org/10.1097/GME.0000000000001712.
18. Lee SR, Cho YH, Park EJ, et al. The association between reproductive period and handgrip strength in postmenopausal women: a nationwide cross-sectional study. Menopause. 2024;31(1):26–32. https://doi.org/10.1097/GME.0000000000002283.
19. Pérez-López FR, Ara I. Fragility fracture risk and skeletal muscle function. Climacteric. 2016;19(1):37–41. https://doi.org/10.3109/13697137.2015.1115261.
20. Pérez-López FR, Pilz S, Chedraui P. Vitamin D supplementation during pregnancy: an overview. Curr Opin Obstet Gynecol. 2020;32(5):316–21. https://doi.org/10.1097/GCO.0000000000000641.

21. López-Baena MT, Pérez-Roncero GR, Pérez-López FR, Mezones-Holguín E, Chedraui P. Vitamin D, menopause, and aging: *quo vadis*? Climacteric. 2020;23(2):123–9. https://doi.org/10.1080/13697137.2019.1682543.
22. Beaudart C, Buckinx F, Rabenda V, et al. The effects of vitamin D on skeletal muscle strength, muscle mass and muscle power; a systematic review and meta-analysis of randomized controlled trials. J Clin Endocrinol Metab. 2014;99:4336–45. https://doi.org/10.1210/jc.2014-1742.
23. Halfon M, Phan O, Teta D. Vitamin D: a review on its effects on muscle strength, the risk of fall, and frailty. Biomed Res Int. 2015;2015:953241.
24. Ranathunga RMTK, Hill TR, Mathers JC, et al. No effect of monthly supplementation with 12000 IU, 24000 IU or 48000 IU vitamin D3 for one year on muscle function: the vitamin D in older people study. J Steroid Biochem Mol Biol. 2019;190:256–62. https://doi.org/10.1016/j.jsbmb.2018.12.008.
25. Fox FAU, Koch L, Breteler MMB, Ahmad AN. 25-hydroxyvitamin D level is associated with greater grip strength across adult life span: a population-based cohort study. Endocr Connect. 2023;12(4):e220501. https://doi.org/10.1530/EC-22-0501.
26. Kim BJ, Kwak MK, Lee SH, Koh JM. Lack of association between vitamin D and hand grip strength in Asians: a Nationwide population-based study. Calcif Tissue Int. 2019;104(2):152–9. https://doi.org/10.1007/s00223-018-0480-7.
27. Kitsu T, Kabasawa K, Ito Y, et al. Low serum 25-hydroxyvitamin D is associated with low grip strength in an older Japanese population. J Bone Miner Metab. 2020;38(2):198–204. https://doi.org/10.1007/s00774-019-01040-w.
28. Bislev LS, Grove-Laugesen D, Rejnmark L. Vitamin D and muscle health: a systematic review and meta-analysis of randomized placebo-controlled trials. J Bone Miner Res. 2021;36(9):1651–60. https://doi.org/10.1002/jbmr.4412.
29. Sutherland JP, Zhou A, Hyppönen E. Muscle traits, sarcopenia, and Sarcopenic obesity: a vitamin D Mendelian randomization study. Nutrients. 2023;15(12):2703. Published 2023 Jun 9. https://doi.org/10.3390/nu15122703.
30. Geusens P, Vandevyver C, Vanhoof J, Cassiman JJ, Boonen S, Raus J. Quadriceps and grip strength are related to vitamin D receptor genotype in elderly nonobese women. J Bone Miner Res. 1997;12(12):2082–8. https://doi.org/10.1359/jbmr.1997.12.12.2082.
31. Casado-Díaz A, Cuenca-Acevedo R, Navarro-Valverde C, et al. Vitamin D status and the Cdx-2 polymorphism of the vitamin D receptor gene are determining factors of bone mineral density in young healthy postmenopausal women. J Steroid Biochem Mol Biol. 2013;136:187–9. https://doi.org/10.1016/j.jsbmb.2012.09.026.
32. García-Vigara A, Monllor-Tormos A, García-Pérez MÁ, Tarín JJ, Cano A. Genetic variants of the vitamin D receptor are related to dynapenia in postmenopausal women. Maturitas. 2023;171:40–4. https://doi.org/10.1016/j.maturitas.2023.03.002.
33. Shah V, Zia H, Lo DF. Investigating seasonal association between vitamin D concentration, muscle mass and strength in postmenopausal women: a critical analysis. J Nutr Sci. 2023;12(e74):1–2. https://doi.org/10.1017/jns.2023.33.
34. Cruz-Jentoft AJ, Bahat G, Bauer J, et al. Sarcopenia: revised European consensus on definition and diagnosis [published correction appears in Age Ageing. 2019 Jul 1;48(4):601]. Age Ageing. 2019;48(1):16–31. https://doi.org/10.1093/ageing/afy169. *Erratum: Age Ageing*. 2019;48(4):601. doi:10.1093/ageing/afz046.
35. Orprayoon N, Wainipitapong P, Champaiboon J, Wattanachanya L, Jaisamrarn U, Chaikittisilpa S. Prevalence of pre-sarcopenia among postmenopausal women younger than 65 years. Menopause. 2021;28(12):1351–7. https://doi.org/10.1097/GME.0000000000001866.
36. Li S, Ma L, Huang H, et al. Loss of muscle mass in women with premature ovarian insufficiency as compared with healthy controls. Menopause. 2023;30(2):122–7. https://doi.org/10.1097/GME.0000000000002120.
37. Divaris E, Anagnostis P, Gkekas NK, Kouidi E, Goulis DG. Early menopause and premature ovarian insufficiency may increase the risk of sarcopenia: a systematic review and meta-analysis. Maturitas. 2023;175:107782. https://doi.org/10.1016/j.maturitas.2023.05.006.

38. Treuil M, Mahmutovic M, Di Patrizio P, Nguyen-Thi PL, Quilliot D. Assessment of dynapenia and undernutrition in primary care, a systematic screening study in community medicine. Clin Nutr ESPEN. 2023;57:561–8. https://doi.org/10.1016/j.clnesp.2023.08.003.
39. Wang X, Chen L, Lyu M, Wei N. The optimal cut-off values of screening tools for dynapenia: a cross-sectional study. Disabil Rehabil. 2024;46:4540. https://doi.org/10.1080/09638288.2023.2274884.
40. Tessier AJ, Wing SS, Rahme E, Morais JA, Chevalier S. Physical function-derived cut-points for the diagnosis of sarcopenia and dynapenia from the Canadian longitudinal study on aging. J Cachexia Sarcopenia Muscle. 2019;10(5):985–99. https://doi.org/10.1002/jcsm.12462. *Corrigendum* in J Cachexia Sarcopenia Muscle. 2021;12(6):2262-2267.
41. Tuttle CSL, Thang LAN, Maier AB. Markers of inflammation and their association with muscle strength and mass: a systematic review and meta-analysis. Ageing Res Rev. 2020;64:101185. https://doi.org/10.1016/j.arr.2020.101185.
42. García-Alfaro P, Rodriguez I, Pérez-López FR. Plasma homocysteine levels and handgrip strength in postmenopausal women. Climacteric. 2022;25(5):504–9. https://doi.org/10.1080/13697137.2022.2068409.
43. Miranda H, Bentes C, Resende M, et al. Association between handgrip strength and body composition, physical fitness, and biomarkers in postmenopausal women with metabolic syndrome. Rev Assoc Med Bras (1992). 2022;68(3):323–8. https://doi.org/10.1590/1806-9282.20210673.
44. Lim JP, Chong MS, Tay L, et al. Inter-muscular adipose tissue is associated with adipose tissue inflammation and poorer functional performance in central adiposity. Arch Gerontol Geriatr. 2018;13:1–7. https://doi.org/10.1016/j.archger.2018.11.006.
45. Lin YH, Chen HC, Hsu NW, Chou P, Teng MMH. Hand grip strength in predicting the risk of osteoporosis in Asian adults. J Bone Miner Metab. 2021;39(2):289–94. https://doi.org/10.1007/s00774-020-01150-w.
46. Kunutsor SK, Seidu S, Voutilainen A, Blom AW, Laukkanen JA. Handgrip strength-a risk indicator for future fractures in the general population: findings from a prospective study and meta-analysis of 19 prospective cohort studies. Geroscience. 2021;43(2):869–80. https://doi.org/10.1007/s11357-020-00251-8.
47. Probert N, Andersson ÅG. Functional outcome in patients with hip fracture from 2008 to 2018, and the significance of hand-grip strength—a cross-sectional comparative study. BMC Geriatr. 2023;23(1):686. https://doi.org/10.1186/s12877-023-04398-9.
48. Dowling L, Cuthbertson DJ, Walsh JS. Reduced muscle strength (dynapenia) in women with obesity confers a greater risk of falls and fractures in the UK biobank. Obesity (Silver Spring). 2023;31(2):496–505. https://doi.org/10.1002/oby.23609.

21. Empowerment of Women and Lifestyle: The Help of Digital Technologies

Amparo Carrasco-Catena, Gema Ibáñez-Sánchez, Vicente Traver, and Antonio Cano

Abstract

The Stages of Reproductive Aging Workshop (STRAW) + 10 extend from menarche till the end of the lifespan. Much attention has been traditionally given to issues related with the reproductive period, including obstetrical care, contraception, or fertility, while the years around menopause have concentrated attention on the menopausal transition and the early postmenopause. Clinical symptoms and the associated risk to noncommunicable diseases have supported this interest. When considering a more encompassing scope, which extends not only to biological but also to psychological and social changes, the consideration of an age interval, which extends between 40 and 60 years, integrates a broader group of domains. This more comprehensive view has been demanded by the own women, who also request a more participative role. Consequently, the empowerment of women is becoming a new character in the scenario, with a growing share.

A. Carrasco-Catena
Clinical Area Women's Health, Hospital Universitario y Politécnico La Fe, Valencia, Spain
e-mail: Carrasco_ampcat@gva.es

G. Ibáñez-Sánchez
University Institute of Information and Communication Technologies (ITACA), Valencia, Spain
e-mail: geibsan@itaca.upv.es

V. Traver
University Institute of Information and Communication Technologies (ITACA), Valencia, Spain

Joint Unit for Healthcare Processes Reengineering (eRPSS)—Health Research Institute University and Polytechnic Hospital La Fe, Valencia, Spain
e-mail: vtraver@itaca.upv.es

A. Cano (✉)
Full Professor of Obstetrics and Gynecology, Salus Vitae Women's Health Clinical Center, Valencia, Spain
e-mail: Antonio.cano@uv.es

One important measure to keep and promote health is lifestyle. Empowerment is crucial for lifestyle, since the commitment of the individual is required. Adherence is the most important barrier to maintain healthy lifestyle in the long run. Digital technology, with an easy access to Internet, has been proposed as a very cost-effective enabler with a global reach. Modern smartphones represent easy-to-use devices with a high potential, although experience is still short.

21.1 Introduction

The Stages of Reproductive Aging Workshop (STRAW) + 10 criteria are based on the different stages of ovarian aging established by the evolution of the menstrual pattern and parallel hormonal changes [1]. This approach drew attention to the concept of reproductive life as a continuum, which begins with menarche and also includes the late postmenopausal years.

The menopausal transition and the postmenopause, which define the two postreproductive phases in STRAW +10, extend up to the rest of the lifespan. Far from being a uniform period, they include different stages with specific traits. Among them, menopause emerges as a strong event together with adaptation to other important scenarios, like the definitive loss of fertility.

21.1.1 The 40+ Stage

Biological changes occurring along the menopausal transition and early postmenopause are concomitant with others that involve the sexual and couple relationships, adaptation of family roles with the concurrence of those of mother and daughter, a more senior role at work, etc. This group of challenges is relevant and offers evolving profiles in the years that follow the evident deterioration of fertility, which may be set at around 40 years. This defines a 40+ scenario, which would embrace the array of changes experienced by women in areas exceeding the pure biological changes but with an impact in their lives. This broader concept adds a new perspective in which, in line with the World Health Organization's (WHO) notion of global health [2], it is necessary to include other accompanying variables, primarily psychosocial ones. The psychosocial perspective, consequently, is crucial to address some issues of special interest to women's health, such as contraception, sexuality, or fertility [3–5]. In this way, a more comprehensive approach is achieved, in which the biological stages are integrated into a broader vision.

Menopause, in that context, is one more challenge with a highly varied profile, which may pass undetected in some women while be a source of bothersome symptoms in others. Quality of life will consequently be an issue, together with the required attention to noncommunicable diseases (NCD) that in most cases start developing their subclinical progression during those years. Important threats like those affecting the central nervous system, the cardiovascular tree, musculoskeletal disorders, etc. emerge and require attention [6].

21.2 Empowerment of Women

The end-users of the health systems, traditionally referred to as patients, increasingly play a more active role in the management of their health issues, so from certain perspectives, the term "patient" is becoming less and less appropriate. This is not only so because the massive access to information, though not always correct, is mainly provided by Internet as the most at-hand source but also because there is a growing view that one is, and has to be, concerned in the management of the own health. The "user-led-self management" was proposed as a new approach to NCDs [7]. It was hypothesized that the skills and insights from users of the health system might lead to improvement of services. The participation as key decision-makers was another step that, finally, is strongly reflected in the concept of users' empowerment. This worldwide spread current is coexistent with figures like the "expert patient," which have been supported by governmental agencies, like the UK Department of Health [7].

The WHO soon adopted the term, which appears in its Health Promotion Glossary in 1998. Empowerment was defined as a "process through which people gain greater control over decisions and actions affecting their health" [8].

21.2.1 Knowledge to Boost Empowerment

Empowerment requires some knowledge of the health topic in question. This condition has been understood by users themselves and by institutions at all levels. In this regard, scientific societies, government agencies, and also groups of health professionals are increasingly using new tools, such as, for example, sections for end users in their Internet portals [9]. Concomitant end-user initiatives have emerged in the form of associations, which strengthen the potential of users, further increase their knowledge, create complicity, facilitate mutual support, and progressively become essential actors in any health initiative of institutions and scientific societies. This is already a reality, extended to all dimensions, from the local to the global. Change, also sociological, increases engagement and, possibly, the improvement in users' reported outcomes [10]. Furthermore, sustainability, a major challenge for public and private health systems, can be improved by promoting various facilitators, such as engagement, self-care, or adherence to management plans [11]. So far, a new paradigm described as participatory medicine is being consolidated [12].

In the case of women's health, the first steps were represented by actions in the field of women's activism in the fight for equality [13]. But over the years, the progression towards a more specific health profile of the term has also been extended. Consequently, everything that has the potential to be included under the umbrella of the concept of women's health has been incorporating the conditions implied by the modern understanding of empowerment.

21.2.2 Empowerment of Women in the 40+ Years

Most initiatives related to the empowerment of women over 40 have focused around menopause, which is widely perceived as a significant milestone in that period of life [14]. One important reason is the universality of the phenomenon, which is experienced by all women if they live long enough. Another important point is defined by the holistic impact of menopause, with (1) a strong biological component, which conditions a frequent appearance of disturbing symptoms with potential impact on quality of life and a greater susceptibility to some NCDs; (2) a social effect, often influenced by accompanying symptoms, among other factors; and (3) a psychological reset affecting areas such as mood, sexuality, and others.

Despite advances at all levels, more and better knowledge is required especially to face the challenges in this new scenario, to undertake the appropriate strategy and implement a shared decision-making policy. The pursuit of high standards of health throughout the years that extend into post-reproductive life, or 40+, in women involves strategies with influence across the different domains involved. An important message from the chapters in this book is that such strategies must be individualized. A tailored approach is required to design a response specific to the needs of each woman. Sometimes counseling and psychological support may be all that is required. In other women, pharmacological treatment will be necessary, and hormone therapy, anti-osteoporotic drugs, or ad hoc compounds for vasomotor symptoms are good examples. For other women, a variety of alternative measures may be offered, such as cognitive behavioral therapy, hypnosis, or intake of any of the other evidence-based complementary and alternative therapies [15].

In addition to this list of options, it is important to note that lifestyle defines a first resource for support in most women. The help of lifestyle will extend, more or less directly, to all three domains: biological, psychological, and social. This general benefit is not exclusive to menopause, but is especially appropriate during these years, when the variety of stressors mentioned above tend to accumulate [16–19].

21.3 Technology to Empower Women

The technological advances in the recent years have open a new field that can offer options to enhance the empowerment of women. A major technological breakthrough has been provided by portable devices, such as tablets, smartphones, watches, and other wearables. The case of smartphones is unique, as the number of handsets is increasing exponentially worldwide, with an estimated 6.3 billion smartphone subscriptions globally and a global population of 7.4 billion users by 2022 [20].

The explosion of technological tools has facilitated access to rapidly growing software designed to improve women's education, interpersonal communication, and health promotion. Aware of the potential of technology, official bodies, scientific societies, and groups of health professionals are creating increasingly sophisticated tools in parallel with the rapid development of information and communication technology (ICT) support. Institutional Internet portals are a consolidated example where areas for improving patient education occupy defined spaces. New applications with specific designs are also continually emerging. The DAISY application for women with premature ovarian failure (POI) [21] is a good example. A further step in women's empowerment has materialized through the participation of women themselves in the design of digital resources to provide the specific information of their greatest interest, as in a recent experience in Australia [22]. The resulting app [23] is now available on the web. There is a list of other initiatives that can be found by a quick search on a widely accessible search engine such as Google or others. Websites can also be useful to directly facilitate in-person interaction for women, such as menopause cafes in the UK [24].

Finally, another advantage of ICTs is their efficiency, as they are widely accessible to large numbers of the population and can be very cost-effective, with a relatively low investment in terms of time and resources compared to face-to-face interventions.

21.4 Lifestyle and Empowerment

Lifestyle defines the most suitable setting for implementing empowerment, as it requires the specific commitment of the person concerned. It is necessary to implement an action plan that includes avoiding toxins such as tobacco or excessive alcohol and maintaining a normal weight, regular physical activity (PA), and a healthy diet. This often requires behavioral changes that can entail considerable difficulty [25].

21.4.1 Physical Activity

The health benefits of regular PA practice in menopausal women have been well established [26]. The cardiovascular tree, bone metabolism, or cognition is just some of the systems favorably affected by PA in menopausal and older women [27]. In addition, physical and mental well-being are also improved through the release of endorphins and other modulators of the central nervous system [28, 29].

Despite these multiple benefits, sedentary lifestyle is a global phenomenon that affects both developed and underdeveloped countries [30]. In fact, the WHO highlights the strong relationship between increased time spent in sedentary behaviors and increased mortality from all causes, cardiovascular mortality, incidence of cardiovascular diseases, and type 2 diabetes. The high prevalence of sedentary lifestyle requires a global strategy. Scientific societies, policymakers, and global health organizations have created guidelines and programs to promote the long-term practice of PA [31, 32].

21.4.2 Nutrition

A healthy diet is another key variable to maintain good health [33]. Analysis of 2017 data from 195 countries concluded that 11 million deaths and 255 million DALYs were attributable to poor dietary conditions [34]. Dietary risk factors often determine overweight or obesity, which is reaching pandemic levels worldwide. Data from 32 OECD countries show that 54% of the population was overweight or obese and 18% was obese in 2021 [35].

Menopause is accompanied by an increase in the proportion of fat, which shows a preferential distribution in visceral territories [36]. This central accumulation of fat, measured by a method as simple as waist circumference, is an additional factor to the body mass index (BMI) for predicting morbidity and mortality [37]. A healthy diet is therefore a particularly urgent need in the post-reproductive period of women.

21.5 Adherence to Healthy Lifestyle

One main problem with the long-term implementation of healthy lifestyle is the requirement for the change of habits that are deeply embedded in daily routine. The purpose to change is not enough in the case of many individuals, who face how the renounce to the gratification provided by the unhealthy behavior, like smoking, unlimited eating, or inactivity, drastically undermines the daily efforts to set aside habits that are profoundly implanted in their lives for years. Quitting smoking is a good example [25, 38] in which the challenge is further complicated by the involvement of different neurobiological circuits creating dependence [39]. A real addition is therefore the problem, which makes the task a difficult one. Therefore, a strategy to accomplish effective interventions targeting behavioral change is required.

A first step to achieve success is sufficient motivation, which operates at individual level. An analysis of the barriers and facilitators is then required. There is a wealth of factors, which change at both the individual and the environmental levels, but the global analysis of the published evidence shows that, with minor differences, some big motifs emerge [40, 41]. Social support is a common environmental facilitator. Reinforcement, as for example, the finding that physical changes are identified in response to the intervention, strengthens adherence to the implemented behavioral change. Work schedules, inappropriate resources to implement the intervention, and family life are frequent factors acting as barriers at individual level [40].

The literature on PA adherence rates is sparse and varies from one setting to another or across different types of programs. A representative example is the Exercise Referral Schemes in the UK or the community groups so popular in other public health systems [42]. A review on PA programs lasting ≥ 6 months found an average adherence rate of 69.1% [43]. Another more recent experience based on a community group achieved an adherence of 56.4%, defined as participants attending 75% of the sessions [44].

As with PA, adherence to the diet remains an unresolved issue with unsatisfactory rates [40, 45]. Among the wide range of options available, the Mediterranean diet (MedDiet) has been a fairly well-researched option [46]. The flexibility of implementation, which stems from the general recommendations of the dietary pyramid [47], has been considered as a strength that favors adherence. Consequently, the MedDiet has been proposed as an optimal option for menopausal health in a guideline of the European Menopause and Andropause Society [48]. Despite this easy fit, adherence to the MedDiet is low or moderate, even in countries of the Mediterranean basin where there is a long tradition in favor of its implementation [49, 50].

21.5.1 Adherence to Lifestyle and ICT

Information and communication technologies have been investigated as an enabler to engage people in healthy lifestyles. In parallel to technological support, a number of software modalities are being developed with capabilities to engage the user and promote motivation. Among the most frequently selected actions, gamification facilitates adherence by providing virtual competitions and rewards for achievements [51, 52]. Furthermore, easy access to social media has paved the way for providing contact and interaction and building supportive social networks [53, 54]. Interest in the role of social networks as a digital tool has spread to different areas such as research [55, 56], education [57, 58], or prevention [59]. Furthermore, social media offers avenues for social prescribing, which, among other benefits, encourages people to take responsibility for their health [60].

Social intervention has also been shown to promote behavior change [61], which is a useful option to encourage adherence to a healthy lifestyle. However, further studies on this topic are still needed [62] particularly to overcome the misinformation potential, a weakness of this technological resource [63].

21.5.1.1 Physical Activity

Technological developments enable smartphones to offer functionalities specifically designed to increase engagement with PA. These include the ability to monitor PA along with other functions, such as the assessment of related parameters, energy expenditure, and number of steps per day, among others. Biological functions such as heart rate, sleep hours, etc. can also be monitored. Recent experiences have confirmed the what and how of an intervention in which the fluid use of WhatsApp among groups of women gathered in a public health scheme has been shown to be useful in supporting a positive behavior change to promote adherence to PA. The intervention achieved an acceptable long-term adherence rate, 56.4% at 1 year [44].

21.5.1.2 Nutrition

Insufficient data creates a large gap in knowledge on how technology can help improve adherence to healthier nutrition. Barriers to adherence may present specific characteristics. For example, socioeconomic status may have an impact influenced by the price of fresh food, but also by access to better cooking skills or a better understanding of nutritional guidelines [64].

Data from smartphone and app use have opened avenues to key determinants of adherence, such as access to theoretical background, ability to tailor the intervention, coaching option, and reward provided for milestone achievement to meet the need for tangible outcomes [65].

A systematic review including literature published up to April 2020 found that digital interventions, including 10 online and 5 delivered by smartphone, improved adherence to MedDiet in different settings and populations [66]. The diversity of countries analyzed supports the idea that the intervention can be successful even in non-Mediterranean countries, which is interesting given the urgent need to implement the so-called Great Food Transformation, as called by the EAT Commission, a manifesto of experts that advocates the global implementation of diets compatible with the United Nations Sustainable Development Goals and the Paris Agreement [46].

21.6 Conclusion

The post-reproductive years span a broad time period, starting with the drastic reduction in fertility around age 40 until the end of life. The notion of the 40+ period helps to include the psychological and social domains in addition to the biological domain. While they may seem relatively independent, there are strong connections between them.

Menopause represents a milestone in that interval, with its own impact and specific circumstances. The extension of the concept of individual empowerment has gained momentum in the field of women's health, such that an increasing number of women demand their direct involvement in managing their needs. This should strengthen commitment to achieving health and quality of life goals. Lifestyle is a background strategy that supports every health initiative at any time in life, also in this period. However, a strong limiting factor in all lifestyle plans is adherence. Modern digital technology is uniquely positioned as a tool to potentially provide large-scale, cost-effective adherence support. The experience is still short, but rapid technological advances are creating new opportunities that generate many expectations.

References

1. Harlow SD, Gass M, Hall JE, Lobo R, Maki P, Rebar RW, et al. STRAW + 10 collaborative group. Executive summary of the stages of reproductive aging workshop + 10: addressing the unfinished agenda of staging reproductive aging. Fertil Steril. 2012;97:843–51. https://doi.org/10.1016/j.fertnstert.2012.01.128.
2. World Health Organization. 1948. Summary Reports on Proceedings Minutes and Final Acts of the International Health Conference held in New York from 19 June to 22 July 1946. World Health Organization. https://apps.who.int/iris/handle/10665/85573. Accessed 1 Aug 2024.
3. Boivin J, Appleton TC, Baetens P, Baron J, Bitzer J, Corrigan E, et al. European Society of Human Reproduction and Embryology. Guidelines for counselling in infertility: outline version. Hum Reprod. 2001;16:1301–4. https://doi.org/10.1093/humrep/16.6.1301.
4. Bitzer J, Giraldi A, Pfaus J. A standardized diagnostic interview for hypoactive sexual desire disorder in women: standard operating procedure (SOP part 2). J Sex Med. 2013;10:50–7. https://doi.org/10.1111/j.1743-6109.2012.02817.x.

5. Bitzer J. Overview of perimenopausal contraception. Climacteric. 2019;22:44–50. https://doi.org/10.1080/13697137.2018.1540566.
6. Vos T, Flaxman AD, Naghavi M, Lozano R, Michaud C, Ezzati M, et al. Years lived with disability (YLDs) for 1160 sequelae of 289 diseases and injuries 1990-2010: a systematic analysis for the global burden of disease study 2010. Lancet. 2012;380:2163–96. https://doi.org/10.1016/S0140-6736(12)61729-2.
7. Tattersall RL. The expert patient: a new approach to chronic disease management for the twenty-first century. Clin Med (Lond). 2002;2:227–9. https://doi.org/10.7861/clinmedicine.2-3-227.
8. World Health Organization. Promotion glossary. https://www.who.int/publications/i/item/WHO-HPR-HEP-98.1. Accessed 1 Aug 2024.
9. Lee PS, Tsao LI, Lee CL, Liu CY. The effect of the electronic platform of menopausal health screen system and counseling intervention on the empowerment of menopausal women: a quasi-experimental study. Health Care Women Int. 2021;42:127–42. https://doi.org/10.1080/07399332.2020.1811283.
10. Löfgren S, Hedström M, Ekström W, Lindberg L, Flodin L, Ryd L. Power to the patient: care tracks and empowerment a recipe for improving rehabilitation for hip fracture patients. Scand J Caring Sci. 2015;29:462–9. https://doi.org/10.1111/scs.12157.
11. Doubova SV, Infante-Castañeda C, Martinez-Vega I, Pérez-Cuevas R. Toward healthy aging through empowering self-care during the climacteric stage. Climacteric. 2012;15:563–72. https://doi.org/10.3109/13697137.2011.635824.
12. deBronkart D. The patient's voice in the emerging era of participatory medicine. Int J Psychiatry Med. 2018;53:350–60. https://doi.org/10.1177/0091217418791461.
13. Grabe S. An empirical examination of women's empowerment and transformative change in the context of international development. Am J Community Psychol. 2012;49:233–45. https://doi.org/10.1007/s10464-011-9453-y.
14. Hickey M, LaCroix AZ, Doust J, Mishra GD, Sivakami M, Garlick D, et al. An empowerment model for managing menopause. Lancet. 2024;403:947–57. https://doi.org/10.1016/S0140-6736(23)02799-X.
15. The 2023 Nonhormone Therapy Position Statement of The North American Menopause Society Advisory Panel. The 2023 Nonhormone therapy position statement of the North American Menopause Society. Menopause. 2023;30:573–90. https://doi.org/10.1097/GME.0000000000002200.
16. Stampfer MJ, Hu FB, Manson JE, Rimm EB, Willett WC. Primary prevention of coronary heart disease in women through diet and lifestyle. N Engl J Med. 2000;343:16–22.
17. Ruiz-Cabello P, Coll-Risco I, Acosta-Manzano P, Borges-Cosic M, Gallo-Vallejo FJ, Aranda P, et al. Influence of the degree of adherence to the Mediterranean diet on the cardiometabolic risk in peri and menopausal women. The flamenco project. Nutr Metab Cardiovasc Dis. 2016;27:217–24. https://doi.org/10.1016/j.numecd.2016.10.008.
18. Chomistek AK, Chiuve SE, Eliassen AH, Mukamal KJ, Willett WC, Rimm EB. Healthy lifestyle in the primordial prevention of cardiovascular disease among young women. J Am Coll Cardiol. 2015;65:43–51.
19. Khera AV, Emdin CA, Drake I, Natarajan P, Bick AG, Cook NR, et al. Genetic risk, adherence to a healthy lifestyle, and coronary disease. N Engl J Med. 2016;375:2349–58.
20. Statista. Global smartphone penetration rate as share of population from 2016 to 2023. https://www.statista.com/statistics/203734/global-smartphone-penetration-per-capita-since-2005/. Accessed 1 Aug 2024.
21. Daisy Network. https://www.daisynetwork.org/. Accessed 1 Aug 2024.
22. Yeganeh L, Boyle JA, Johnston-Ataata K, Flore J, Hickey M, Kokanović R, et al. Positive impact of a co-designed digital resource for women with early menopause. Menopause. 2022;29:671–9. https://doi.org/10.1097/GME.0000000000001972.
23. AskEM. https://www.askearlymenopause.org/. Accessed 1 Aug 2024.
24. Menopause Cafe. https://www.menopausecafe.net/our-history/. Accessed 1 Aug 2024.
25. Hatsukami DK, Stead LF, Gupta PC. Tobacco addiction. Lancet. 2008;371:2027–38.

26. Mendoza N, De Teresa C, Cano A, Godoy D, Hita-Contreras F, Lapotka M, et al. Benefits of physical exercise in postmenopausal women. Maturitas. 2016;93:83–8.
27. Woodward MJ, Lu CW, Levandowski R, Kostis J, Bachmann G. The exercise prescription for enhancing overall health of midlife and older women. Maturitas. 2015;82:65–71.
28. Pedersen BK, Febbraio MA. Muscles, exercise and obesity: skeletal muscle as a secretory organ. Nat Rev Endocrinol. 2012;8:457–65.
29. Borer KT, De Sousa MJ, Nindl BC, Stanford KI, Pedersen BK. Integrative exercise endocrinology. Front Endocrinol (Lausanne). 2024;14:1350462. https://doi.org/10.3389/fendo.2023.1350462.
30. Hallal PC, Andersen LB, Bull FC, Guthold R, Haskell W, Ekelund U. Global physical activity levels: surveillance progress, pitfalls, and prospects. Lancet. 2012;380:247–57.
31. World Health Organization. Global action plan on physical activity 2018–2030: more active people for a healthier world. https://www.who.int/publications/i/item/9789241514187. Accessed 1 Aug 2024.
32. World Health Organization. WHO Guidelines on physical activity and sedentary behavior. https://www.who.int/publications/i/item/9789240015128. Accessed 1 Aug 2024.
33. Downer S, Berkowitz SA, Harlan TS, Olstad DL, Mozaffarian D. Food is medicine: actions to integrate food and nutrition into healthcare. BMJ. 2020;369:m2482. https://doi.org/10.1136/bmj.m2482.
34. GBD 2017 Diet Collaborators. Health effects of dietary risks in 195 countries, 1990–2017: a systematic analysis for the Global Burden of Disease Study 2017. Lancet. 2019;393:1958–72. https://doi.org/10.1016/S0140-6736(19)30041-8.
35. OECD. Obesity, diet and physical activity. https://www.oecd.org/en/topics/obesity-diet-and-physical-activity.html. Accessed 1 Aug 2024.
36. Abildgaard J, Ploug T, Al-Saoudi E, Wagner T, Thomsen C, Ewertsen C, et al. Changes in abdominal subcutaneous adipose tissue phenotype following menopause is associated with increased visceral fat mass. Sci Rep. 2021;11:14750. https://doi.org/10.1038/s41598-021-94189-2.
37. Ross R, Neeland IJ, Yamashita S, Shai I, Seidell J, Magni P, et al. Waist circumference as a vital sign in clinical practice: a consensus statement from the IAS and ICCR working group on visceral obesity. Nat Rev Endocrinol. 2020;16:177–89. https://doi.org/10.1038/s41574-019-0310-7.
38. Warren GW, Sobus S, Gritz ER. The biological and clinical effects of smoking by patients with cancer and strategies to implement evidence-based tobacco cessation support. Lancet Oncol. 2014;15:e568–80.
39. Molas S, DeGroot SR, Zhao-Shea R, Tapper AR. Anxiety and nicotine dependence: emerging role of the Habenulo-Interpeduncular Axis. Trends Pharmacol Sci. 2017;38:169–80.
40. Deslippe AL, Soanes A, Bouchaud CC, Beckenstein H, Slim M, Plourde H, et al. Barriers and facilitators to diet, physical activity and lifestyle behavior intervention adherence: a qualitative systematic review of the literature. Int J Behav Nutr Phys Act. 2023;20:14. https://doi.org/10.1186/s12966-023-01424-2.
41. Spiteri K, Broom D, Bekhet AH, de Caro JX, Laventure B, Grafton K. Barriers and motivators of physical activity participation in middle-aged and older-adults—a systematic review. J Aging Phys Act. 2019;27:929–44. https://doi.org/10.1123/japa.2018-0343.
42. Pavey T, Taylor A, Hillsdon M, Fox K, Campbell J, Foster C, et al. Levels and predictors of exercise referral scheme uptake and adherence: a systematic review. J Epidemiol Community Health. 2012;66:737–44. https://doi.org/10.1136/jech-2011-200354.
43. Farrance C, Tsofliou F, Clark C. Adherence to community based group exercise interventions for older people: a mixed-methods systematic review. Prev Med. 2016;87:155–66. https://doi.org/10.1016/j.ypmed.2016.02.037.
44. García-Vigara A, Fernandez-Garrido J, Carbonell-Asíns JA, Sánchez-Sánchez ML, Monllor-Tormos A, García-Pérez MÁ, et al. Physical activity to reduce the burden of frailty after menopause: effectiveness and adherence rate of a resource saving exercise plan. Menopause. 2024;31:634–40. https://doi.org/10.1097/GME.0000000000002372.

45. Jefcoate PW, Robertson MD, Ogden J, Johnston JD. Exploring rates of adherence and barriers to time-restricted eating. Nutrients. 2023;15:2336. https://doi.org/10.3390/nu15102336.
46. Willett W, Rockström J, Loken B, Springmann M, Lang T, Vermeulen S, et al. Food in the Anthropocene: the EAT-lancet commission on healthy diets from sustainable food systems. Lancet. 2019;393:447–92. https://doi.org/10.1016/S0140-6736(18)31788-4.
47. Hidalgo-Mora JJ, García-Vigara A, Sánchez-Sánchez ML, García-Pérez MÁ, Tarín J, Cano A. The Mediterranean diet: a historical perspective on food for health. Maturitas. 2020;132:65–9. https://doi.org/10.1016/j.maturitas.2019.12.002.
48. Cano A, Marshall S, Zolfaroli I, Bitzer J, Ceausu I, Chedraui P, et al. The Mediterranean diet and menopausal health: an EMAS position statement. Maturitas. 2020;139:90–7. https://doi.org/10.1016/j.maturitas.2020.07.001.
49. Obeid CA, Gubbels JS, Jaalouk D, Kremers SPJ, Oenema A. Adherence to the Mediterranean diet among adults in Mediterranean countries: a systematic literature review. Eur J Nutr. 2022;61:3327–44. https://doi.org/10.1007/s00394-022-02885-0.
50. Damigou E, Faka A, Kouvari M, Anastasiou C, Kosti RI, Chalkias C, et al. Adherence to a Mediterranean type of diet in the world: a geographical analysis based on a systematic review of 57 studies with 1,125,560 participants. Int J Food Sci Nutr. 2023;74:799–813. https://doi.org/10.1080/09637486.2023.2262781.
51. Godfrey A, Stuart S, Tenaerts P. Tech world and medicine come together to harness digital medicine. Maturitas. 2019;127:95–6. https://doi.org/10.1016/j.maturitas.2019.05.004.
52. Rivera-Romero O, Gabarron E, Ropero J, Denecke K. Designing personalised mHealth solutions: an overview. J Biomed Inform. 2023;146:104500. https://doi.org/10.1016/j.jbi.2023.104500.
53. Chen J, Wang Y. Social media use for health purposes: systematic review. J Med Internet Res. 2021;23:e17917. https://doi.org/10.2196/17917.
54. King-Mullins E, McElroy IE. Social media for patient engagement. Surgery. 2023;174:1092–3. https://doi.org/10.1016/j.surg.2023.07.005.
55. Guthrie KA, Caan B, Diem S, Ensrud KE, Greaves SR, Larson JC, et al. Facebook advertising for recruitment of midlife women with bothersome vaginal symptoms: a pilot study. Clin Trials. 2019;16:476–80. https://doi.org/10.1177/1740774519846862.
56. Sedrak MS, Sun CL, Hershman DL, Unger JM, Liu J, Dale W, et al. Use of social Media for Recruitment of patients for cancer clinical trials. JAMA Netw Open. 2020;3:e2031202. https://doi.org/10.1001/jamanetworkopen.2020.31202.
57. Harrell KN, Vervoort D, Luc JGY, Tracy BM, Daniel SJ. Social media in surgery. Am Surg. 2021;87:1021–4. https://doi.org/10.1177/0003134820972979.
58. Chirumamilla S, Gulati M. Patient education and engagement through social media. Curr Cardiol Rev. 2021;17:137–43. https://doi.org/10.2174/1573403X15666191120115107.
59. Prochaska JJ, Coughlin SS, Lyons EJ. Social media and mobile technology for cancer prevention and treatment. Am Soc Clin Oncol Educ Book. 2017;37:128–37. https://doi.org/10.1200/EDBK_173841.
60. Roland M, Everington S, Marshall M. Social prescribing—transforming the relationship between physicians and their patients. N Engl J Med. 2020;383:97–9. https://doi.org/10.1056/NEJMp1917060.
61. Laranjo L, Arguel A, Neves AL, Gallagher AM, Kaplan R, Mortimer N, et al. The influence of social networking sites on health behavior change: a systematic review and meta-analysis. J Am Med Inform Assoc. 2015;22:243–56. https://doi.org/10.1136/amiajnl-2014-002841.
62. Petkovic J, Duench S, Trawin J, Dewidar O, Pardo Pardo J, Simeon R, et al. Interventions delivered through interactive social media for health behaviour change, health outcomes, and health equity in the adult population. Cochrane Database Syst Rev. 2021;5:CD012932. https://doi.org/10.1002/14651858.CD012932.pub2.
63. Weiss R. Menopause and social media: pros and cons for the general public. Maturitas. 2023;174:67–8. https://doi.org/10.1016/j.maturitas.2023.02.006.

64. Schoufour JD, de Jonge EAL, Kiefte-de Jong JC, van Lenthe FJ, Hofman A, Nunn SPT, et al. Socio-economic indicators and diet quality in an older population. Maturitas. 2018;107:71–7. https://doi.org/10.1016/j.maturitas.2017.10.010.
65. McAleese D, Linardakis M, Papadaki A. Quality and presence of behaviour change techniques in Mobile apps for the Mediterranean diet: a content analysis of android Google play and apple app store apps. Nutrients. 2022;14:1290. https://doi.org/10.3390/nu14061290.
66. Benajiba N, Dodge E, Khaled MB, Chavarria EA, Sammartino CJ, Aboul-Enein BH. Technology-based nutrition interventions using the Mediterranean diet: a systematic review. Nutr Rev. 2022;80:1419–33. https://doi.org/10.1093/nutrit/nuab076.